Activation to Acquisition

Activation to Acquisition

Functional Aspects of the Basal Forebrain Cholinergic System

Russell T. Richardson
Editor

Birkhäuser
Boston • Basel • Berlin

Russell T. Richardson
Department of Neurology
School of Medicine
Johns Hopkins University
Baltimore, MD 21205

Library of Congress Cataloging-in-Publication Data
Activation to acquisition: functional aspects of the basal forebrain cholinergic system / edited by Russell T. Richardson; [contributors, John H. Ashe . . . [et al.]].
p. cm.
Includes bibliographical references and index.
ISBN 0-8176-3467-3 (hardcover : alk. paper). -- ISBN 3-7643-3467-3 (alk. paper).
1. Prosencephalon. 2. Cholinergic mechanisms. I. Richardson, Russell T., 1954- . II. Ashe, John H.
[DNLM: 1. Basal Ganglia--physiology. 2. Cholinergic Fibers--physiology. WL 307 A 188]
OP382.F7A37 1991
612.8 ' 25--dc20
DLC 91-11515
for Library of Congress CIP

Printed on acid-free paper.

Typeset by ARK Publications, Newton Centre, MA using TeX.
Printed and bound by Edwards Brothers, Inc., Ann Arbor, Michigan.
Printed in the U.S.A.

9 8 7 6 5 4 3 2 1

ISBN 0-8176-3467-3
ISBN 3-7643-3467-3

CONTENTS

Contributors

John H. Ashe, Ph.D Center for the Neurobiology of Learning and Memory, University of California, Irvine, CA 92717, and Department of Psychology, University of California, Riverside, CA 92521, USA

Mark F. Bear, Ph.D Center for Neural Science, Brown University, Providence, RI 02912, USA

Larry L. Butcher, M.D. Department of Psychology, University of California, Los Angeles, CA 90024, USA

György Buzsáki, M.D., Ph.D Center for Molecular and Behavioral Neuroscience, Rutgers University, 195 University Avenue, Newark, NJ 07102, USA

Kenneth M. Carnes, Ph.D Department of Anatomy and Neurobiology, Washington University School of Medicine, 600 S. Euclid Avenue, St. Louis, MO 63110, USA

Mahlon R. DeLong, M.D. Departments of Neurology and Neuroscience, The Johns Hopkins University School of Medicine, Meyer 5-185, 600 North Wolfe Street, Baltimore, MD 21205, USA

Robert W. Dykes, Ph.D Department of Physiology, Faculty of Medicine, University of Montreal, Montreal, Quebec, Canada H 3C 357

Fred H. Gage, Ph.D Department of Neuroscience, University of California at San Diego, La Jolla, CA 92093, USA

Linda K. Gorman, Ph.D Mental Retardation Research Center, Brain Research Institute, Departments of Anatomy and Psychiatry, UCLA Medical Center, Los Angeles, CA 90024, USA

Kazuyuki Imamura, Ph.D Department of Neuroscience, Osaka Bioscience Institute, Furue-dai, Suita-shi, Osaka, 565 Japan

Debra L. Johnson, Ph.D Department of Psychology, University of Utah, Salt Lake City, UT 84112, USA

Takuji Kasamatsu, M.D. Smith-Kettlewell Eye Research Institute, 2232 Webster Street, San Francisco, CA 94115, USA

Raymond P. Kesner, Ph.D Department of Psychology, University of Utah, Salt Lake City, UT 84112, USA

Vassilis E. Koliatsos, M.D. Departments of Neurology and Pathology, The Johns Hopkins University School of Medicine, Meyer 5-185, 600 North Wolfe Street, Baltimore, MD 21205, USA

Alicja M. Markowska, Ph.D Department of Psychology, The Johns Hopkins University, Baltimore, MD 21218, USA

M.-Marsel Mesulam, M.D. Neurology Unit, Beth Israel Hospital, 330 Brookline Avenue, Boston, MA 02215, USA

David S. Olton, Ph.D Department of Psychology, The Johns Hopkins University, Baltimore, MD 21218, USA

Donald L. Price, M.D. Departments of Neurology and Pathology, The Johns Hopkins University School of Medicine, Meyer 5-185, 600 North Wolfe Street, Baltimore, MD 21205, USA

Joseph L. Price, M.D. Department of Anatomy and Neurobiology, Washington University School of Medicine, 660 S. Euclid Avenue, St. Louis, MO 63110, USA

Russell T. Richardson, Ph.D Department of Neurology, The Johns Hopkins University School of Medicine, Meyer 5-185, 600 North Wolfe Street, Baltimore, MD 21205, USA

Nicole Tremblay, Ph.D Department of Dental Medicine, Faculty of Dentistry, University of Montreal, Montreal, Quebec, Canada H3C 357

Richard A. Warren, Ph.D Department of Neurology and Neurosurgery, Faculty of Medicine, McGill University, Montreal, Quebec, Canada

Norman M. Weinberger, M.D. Center for the Neurobiology of Learning and Memory, University of California, Irvine, CA 92717, and Department of Psychobiology, University of California, Irvine, CA 92717, USA

Gary L. Wenk, Ph.D Department of Psychology, The Johns Hopkins University, Baltimore, MD 21218, USA

Charles D. Woody, M.D. Mental Retardation Research Center, Brain Research Institute, Departments of Anatomy and Psychiatry, UCLA Medical Center, Los Angeles, CA 90024, USA

Nancy J. Woolf, M.D. Department of Psychology, University of California, Los Angeles, CA 90024, USA

Current Status of the Basal Forebrain Cholinergic System: A Preview and Commentary

Russell T. Richardson

Too seldom are scientists provided a format to discuss theoretical issues openly. Investigators might outline hypotheses in the introduction or discussion sections of their written works, but such hypotheses, if presented at all, often remain within the limited scope of the data presented in the article. New experiments are often performed without a clear theoretical framework and without an expressed objective of supporting or refuting a specific hypothesis. As John Platt states in his classic 1964 article, "Strong Inference,"

> "Biology... is a 'high information' field, where years and decades can easily be wasted on the usual type of 'low information' observations or experiments if one does not think carefully in advance about what the most important and conclusive experiments would be."

Platt argues that strong inference is the most effective method for making progress in science. It is the process in which investigators (1) formulate multiple, testable hypotheses to explain a set of observations, (2) perform experiments that could disprove one or more of the hypotheses, and (3) based on the results of the experiments, reject some hypotheses, formulate new ones, and repeat the process again. This procedure provides a steady progression towards a fuller understanding of a scientific problem and is therefore preferable to collecting loosely related bits of information in hopes that someday they will fall into a coherent picture.

The ultimate goal of this book is to facilitate the path towards a better understanding of the basal forebrain cholinergic system (BFCS); to learn what it does and how it does it. More rapid and efficient progress toward this goal may be attained if the methods of strong inference are applied to studies of the BFCS. Since the first step in the process is to formulate testable hypotheses, the focus of this book is on current views of the functions of the BFCS.

Naturally, hypotheses must be based on observations, and only a few years ago, data pertaining to the BFCS were scarce. Although components of the BFCS were described as early as 1872, (see the chapter by Koliatsos and Price), it has become a major focus of interest only in the past 10 to 15 years. Formulating more than rudimentary hypotheses is difficult without sufficient information, but researchers have been steadily uncovering new facts about the BFCS, from electron microscopic studies of its ultrastructure to clinical studies of its role in dementia. There is now a sufficient understanding of the basic neurobiological properties of the BFCS to warrant detailed hypotheses of what its functions are and the mechanisms by which those functions are achieved. The study of the BFCS has grown out of its infancy to the point where the methods of strong inference can be applied to accelerate our understanding of it.

Some of the leading investigators of the BFCS have contributed chapters to this book. Each one was requested to address the following question: "Based on your critical evaluation of relevant studies, what is the most likely function of the basal forebrain cholinergic system?" Thus, this book attempts to accomplish the initial step in the strong inference process by bringing together multiple, testable hypotheses regarding the functions of the BFCS. This consolidation of views should help to guide future investigations of the BFCS and provide them the goal of disproving one or more of the hypotheses expressed in this book. Future studies may likewise attempt to provide support for a given hypothesis, but the main strength of supporting evidence is its ability to disprove alternative hypotheses. The more confidently we can state what the BFCS does not do, the more precisely we can define what it does do.

The contributors to this book, in addition to presenting their views of the functions of the BFCS, have also provided a thorough review of what is currently known about the BFCS. The initial chapter (by Koliatsos and Price) provides a historical perspective of the BFCS from its earliest descriptions to its most recent relations to dementia. That chapter and the following two (by Mesulam; Price and Carnes) also focus on the anatomical organization of the BFCS and its implications for the function of the system. The next four chapters (by Buzsáki and Gage; Richardson and DeLong; Gorman and Woody; Ashe and Weinberger) are based primarily on physiological studies of the neuromodulatory effects of ACh on cortical neurons, the activity of BFCS neurons, and the potential role of the cholinergic system in cortical activation, learning, and memory. The BFCS role in learning and memory is also the focus of the two subsequent chapters (by Olton, Wenk, and Markowska; Kesner and Johnson), but from more of a behavioral viewpoint in which the relations of the BFCS to other brain structures and their functions are scrutinized. The next two chapters (by Kasamatsu and Imamura; Dykes, Tremblay, Warren, and Bear) present different views of the role of the BFCS and ACh in developmental processes, specifically in ocular dominance plasticity in striate cortex. Dykes et al. also examine the role of the BFCS in ongoing dynamic processes that may continually shape the functional properties of cortical neurons. This theme is expanded in the final chapter (by Woolf and Butcher) in which the BFCS is viewed as being involved in cognition by altering the anatomical connections among different groups of neurons representing specific bits of information. Thus, the body of information regarding the BFCS in this book is both broad and deep. The hypotheses put forth by the contributors are supported by substantial reviews of relevant data, thereby making this volume the most complete account to date of the BFCS.

A considerable range of hypotheses are presented here. At one end of the spectrum, the BFCS is viewed as merely ensuring that its target structures operate efficiently. At the other extreme, the BFCS is seen as having a direct causal effect in various forms of plasticity. Some authors have developed specific models of how the BFCS may function. Such models are advantageous because they lead to specific predictions that can be tested experimentally. Regardless of the correctness of the models, the process of testing them can provide an efficient means of learning more about the BFCS and understanding it better. Finally, some authors have raised serious doubts whether the BFCS is directly involved in some processes, such as cortical development and certain forms of learning. Such questions are beneficial because they help to stimulate and focus research efforts to clearly delineate what the BFCS does and does not do.

The BFCS has been suggested to be involved in the following processes:

Cortical Activation

The release of ACh from BFCS neurons is hypothesized to play a major role in cortical activation by altering specific ion conductances in cortical neurons (see chapters by Price and Carnes; Buzsáki and Gage; Richardson and DeLong). This hypothesis ties together several classic observations, such as the effects of cholinergic drugs on EEG and the function of the ventral branch of brainstem ascending pathways. The BFCS may also indirectly affect cortical activation through its influence on the reticular thalamic nucleus. On a shorter time scale, the cholinergic system may produce brief changes in ion currents in target neurons similar to those occurring with cortical activation.

Learning and Memory

Views of the BFCS role in learning and memory vary considerably. The BFCS is generally not considered to be the site of the neuronal changes essential for learning, but areas to which it projects, specifically neocortex, hippocampus, and amygdala, are believed to be critically involved in learning and memory (see Olton et al.; Kesner and Johnson). Hence, the role of the BFCS in learning and memory may only be related to its ability to maintain normal neuronal activity in its target structures. Alternatively, the BFCS may produce changes in neuronal activity in target areas and thereby contribute more directly to learning and memory. Two models are proposed for how the BFCS may induce learning related changes in cortical neurons, either by transmitting an "arousal" type signal (see Richardson and DeLong) or by amplifying a "conditioning" signal generated in specific thalamic nuclei (see Ashe and Weinberger). In either case, learning is contingent on long-lasting changes in the response properties of cortical neurons. ACh may directly produce long-lasting increases in excitability (see Gorman and Woody), or it may create only a transient increase in excitability, thereby enabling more permanent forms of enhancement to be expressed, such as long-term potentiation via NMDA receptors (see Ashe and Weinberger; Dykes et al.).

Cortical Reorganization

Changes in the responses of cortical neurons induced by the BFCS may be related not only to learning and memory, but also to more extensive modifications of the functional organization of cortex (see Dykes et al.; Woolf and Butcher). Such changes in cortical organization may occur following marked decreases (from lesions) or increases (from extensive use) in sensory input or as a normal, ongoing process. The resulting cortical reorganization may be due to changes in synaptic strengths or actual structural changes, both of which are hypothesized to be influenced by the BFCS. Such changes may alter the receptive field properties of cortical neurons (see Ashe and Weinberger; Dykes et al.) or the interconnections among cortical and BFCS neurons (see Woolf and Butcher).

Development

Recent evidence suggests that the BFCS may play an important role in development, specifically in ocular dominance plasticity in monocularly deprived kittens (see Kasamatsu and Imamura; Dykes et al.). ACh may work synergistically with norepinephrine (NE) to promote normal development, but the relative effectiveness and importance of ACh compared to NE is debatable. The role of the BFCS in ocular dominance plasticity may provide a useful model for its role in development and possibly other forms of plasticity.

Attention

A potential role of the BFCS in attention is considered by several authors. The BFCS may be related to an animal's ability to attend to several channels of input simultaneously (divided attention) (see Ashe and Weinberger; Olton et al.) or to focus on a single channel while excluding others (selective attention) (see Price and Carnes; Richardson and DeLong). The BFCS has been hypothesized to control the flow of sensory information along multi-synaptic pathways through cortical areas to the hippocampus and amygdala (see Mesulam), and this gating function may constitute a form of attention. Moreover, the role of the BFCS in development may be related to attentional processes since ocular dominance plasticity appears to depend on the animal attending to altered visual input (see Kasamatsu and Imamura; Dykes et al.).

Obviously, a wide range of functions may be influenced by the BFCS. Most of the hypotheses presented here are not mutually exclusive, and many of them suggest similar mechanisms of BFCS function. In almost every hypothesis, ACh is considered to be a *neuromodulator*, and, hence, the BFCS is seen as a system that modifies the response properties of target neurons. Such neuronal changes may be critically involved in all of the processes mentioned above, namely, cortical activation, learning and memory, cortical reorganization, development, and attention.

In all of these processes, the cholinergic system is viewed as altering the functional properties of other brain structures over time. The main difference between the role of the BFCS in these processes may be the *time course* or permanence of the changes, from a time span of minutes to an entire lifetime. For example, enhanced neuronal response properties during cortical activation do not persist into periods of slow wave sleep, whereas learning related changes can be relatively permanent. The normal development of the telencephalon may depend on input from the cholinergic system and is fairly permanent. However, recent studies have demonstrated considerable plasticity in the organization of the adult cerebral cortex (Merzenich et al., 1983), and cortical reorganization may also involve the BFCS.

The aforementioned processes may also differ in the *spatial domain* of the changes induced by the BFCS. The unique anatomical organization of the BFCS gives it the potential to affect both large and small areas of the forebrain (see Price and Carnes). The BFCS as a whole projects to the entire neocortical mantle as well as to the hippocampal formation and amygdaloid complex. However, single BFCS neurons appear to project to small, restricted areas and may therefore have more localized effects. It is not yet clear whether all BFCS neurons work in concert to influence all target neurons equally or whether they act more independently to have differential effects on separate groups of neurons. The changes induced by the BFCS that are related to cortical activation and early development may encompass most of the forebrain, whereas changes related to learning or cortical reorganization may be restricted to selected groups of neurons.

If the BFCS actually does play a role in the several processes mentioned above, it could be viewed as a multidimensional modulatory system, as shown in Fig. 1. Its modulatory effects may vary across both time (i.e., the permanence of the effect) and space (i.e., the size and selectivity of the affected target neurons), depending on the nature of the process. For example, in cortical activation, the entire neocortex is affected (large spatial domain) and the modulation is transient (short temporal domain). In cortical reorganization or in learning, only selected neurons are affected (small spatial domain) and the modulation is persistent (long temporal domain). Likewise, the BFCS role in development may entail a large spatial domain and a long temporal domain, and its role in attention may entail a small spatial domain and a short temporal domain. The BFCS may therefore have the capacity to modulate neuronal activity across both spatial and temporal dimensions, and the resulting changes may contribute to a number of different processes.

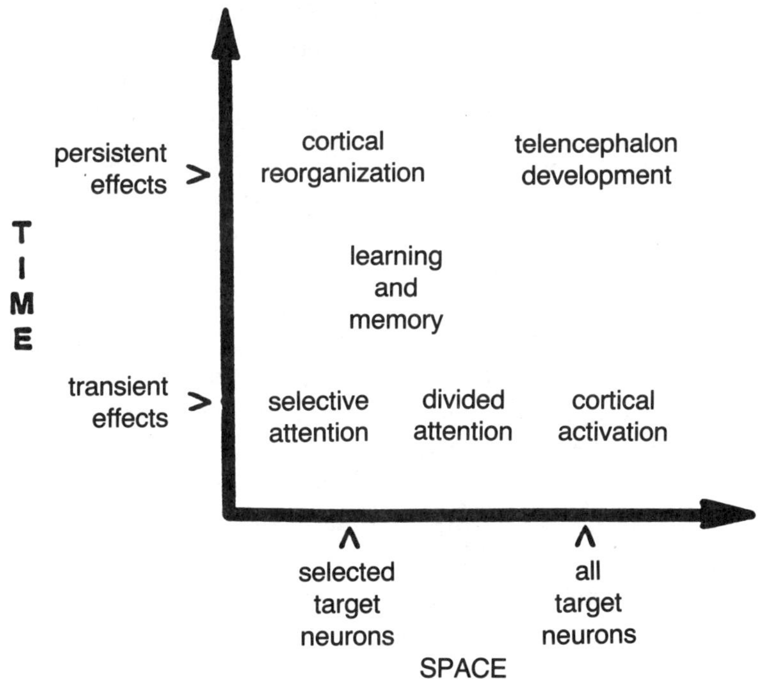

Figure 1. Schematic diagram of the BFCS as a multidimensional modulatory system. Many of the processes that may involve the BFCS can be organized along spatial and temporal dimensions.

Finally, a discussion of the BFCS would not be complete without commenting on its role in Alzheimer's disease (AD). Much of the interest in the BFCS can be attributed to its possible role in AD, and at one time the cholinergic hypothesis of AD was probably the primary focus of AD research. However, one of the main outcomes of that research has been the finding that the BFCS is clearly not the only area affected in AD, nor could the loss of BFCS neurons easily account for the vast number of neurochemical, pathological, and behavioral manifestations of AD. The focus of research efforts has shifted to include other aspects of AD such as abnormalities in other brain regions, cytoarchitectonic changes, the origins of amyloid and neurofibrillary tangles, and the genetic basis of AD (Deary and Whalley, 1988; Glenner, 1989; Price et al., 1989).

Nevertheless, despite the broadening of the focus of AD research, experimental treatment of AD continues to consist primarily of attempts to compensate for damage to the cholinergic system. Numerous clinical studies have evaluated the effects of administering various cholinergic agonists to AD patients, and, as a whole, such studies have been remarkably unsuccessful in achieving consistent or marked improvements. However, some encouraging (although sometimes controversial) results have come from long-term administration of physostigmine (Thal et al., 1986; Stern et al., 1988) or a combination of tetrahydroaminoacridine (THA) and lecithin (Summers et al., 1986). Consequently, many planned experimental treatments for AD will also focus on the cholinergic system. Some of these treatments will use cholinergic agonists that act on specific subtypes of muscarinic or nicotinic receptors (Roberts and Lazareno, 1990) or a combination of cholinergic and noradrenergic agonists (Ashford et al., 1989). Another proposal is to use nerve growth factor (NGF) to promote survival of BFCS neurons in AD patients (see Koliatsos and Price). Thus, the role of the BFCS in the treatment of AD continues to be a critically important area of research.

An improved understanding of the normal functions of the BFCS may help to improve treatment designs for AD, to indicate why some approaches are ineffective, and to suggest new strategies for treatment. Hence, a better understanding of the BFCS is clearly needed, and the issues discussed in this book should facilitate progress in this area of research. Given the rapidly expanding body of information regarding the BFCS, future works may soon be able to provide a much clearer view of what the BFCS does, how it does it, and what practical uses can be derived from this new knowledge.

REFERENCES

Ashford, J.W., Sherman, K.A., and Kumar, V. (1989): Advances in Alzheimer therapy: cholinesterase inhibitors. *Neurobiol. Aging* 10:99-105

Deary, I.J. and Whalley L.J. (1988): Recent research on the causes of Alzheimer's disease. *Brit. Med. J.* 297:807-810

Glenner, G.G. (1989): The pathobiology of Alzheimer's disease. *Ann. Rev. Med.* 40:45-51

Merzenich, M.M., Kaas, J.H., Wall, J.T., Nelson, R.J., Sur, M. and Felleman, D.J. (1983): Topographic reorganization of somatosensory cortical areas 3b and 1 in adult monkeys following restricted deafferentation. *Neurosci.* 8:33-55

Platt, J.R. (1964): Strong inference. *Science* 146:347-353

Price, D.L., Koo, E.H. and Unterbeck, A. (1989): Cellular and molecular biology of Alzheimer's disease. *BioEssays* 10:69-74

Roberts, F. and Lazareno, S. (1990): Cholinergic treatments for Alzheimer's disease. *Biochem. Soc. Trans.* 17:76-79

Stern, Y., Sano, M. and Mayeux, R. (1988): Long-term administration of oral physostigmine in Alzheimer's disease. *Neurol.* 38:1837-1841

Summers, W.K., Majovski, L.V., Marsh, G.M., Tachiki, K. and Kling, A. (1986): Oral tetrahydroaminoacridine in long-term treatment of senile dementia, Alzheimer type. *N. Engl. J. Med.* 315:1241-1245

Thal, L.J., Masur, D.M., Sharpless, N., Fuld, P. and Davies, P. (1986): Acute and chronic effect of oral physostigmine and lecithin in Alzheimer's disease. *Prog. Neuropsychopharmacol. Biol. Psych.* 10:627-636

The Basal Forebrain Cholinergic System: An Evolving Concept in the Neurobiology of the Forebrain

Vassilis E. Koliatsos and Donald L. Price

THE BASAL FOREBRAIN CHOLINERGIC SYSTEM AND THE BASAL FOREBRAIN MAGNOCELLULAR COMPLEX

The basal forebrain cholinergic system (BFCS) is the cholinergic component of a broader population of conspicuous neurons in the basal forebrain, recently retermed the basal forebrain magnocellular complex (BFMC) (Hedreen et al., 1984; Koliatsos et al., in press, a). These neurons, which are large (15-18 × 20-30 μm in the rat; *ca.* 40 × 50 μm in the human), isodendritic, and intensely basophilic, are located in the medial septum, diagonal band of Broca (DBB), substantia innominata, and substriatal gray substance (Kimura et al., 1981; Hedreen et al., 1983; Mesulam et al., 1983b, 1984; Arendt et al., 1986; Dinopoulos et al., 1986; Mesulam and Geula, 1988). Individual cells of the BFMC project to restricted zones within cortex (Table I) (iso- and mesocortex) and limbic structures (hippocampus, piriform cortex, basolateral amygdala) and to the olfactory bulb. In various telencephalic targets of the system, terminal fields of these cells are organized differently, both in terms of cholinergic fiber densities and the extent of terminal domains of individual neurons (Koliatsos et al., in press, a). Inputs to BFMC neurons arise mainly from a limited number of limbic and paralimbic peripiriform regions that reciprocate their innervation by the BFMC and from a multitude of diencephalic and brainstem regions characterized by long ascending projections to telencephalon such as midline thalamus and hypothalamus, ventral tegmental area, raphe, and locus coeruleus (Záborszky, 1989).

Table 1. Distribution and Nomenclature of BFMC Cell Groups in Three Mammalian Orders.

Anatomical Location	BFMC Groups	BFCS Groups	Rodents	Carnivores	Primates (incl. humans)
Medial septum	Medial septal nucleus	Ch1*	+	+	+
Vertical limb of the DBB	Nucleus of vertical limb of the DBB	Ch2	+	+	+
Horizontal limb of the DBB	Nucleus of horizontal limb of the DBB	Ch3	+	+	Not clearly delineated
Medial forebrain bundle	Nucleus of horizontal limb of the DBB or magno-cellular preoptic nucleus	Ch4	+	+	+
Substantia innominata	NBM	Ch4	+	+	+
Globus pallidus	"	"	+	+	Only in medullary laminae
Ventral pallidum	"	"	+	+	±
Substriatal gray	"	"	+	+	+
Ansa lenticularis	"	"	+	+	+
Entopeduncular nucleus	"	"	+	+	Some cells in supraoptic commissure of Meynert

Although a large number of cells in the BFMC use acetylcholine as their transmitter, other cells of the complex contain γ-aminobutyric acid (GABA). Relative proportions of cholinergic and GABAergic neurons differ characteristically in various subdivisions of the BFMC, and these patterns are maintained across mammalian evolution (Köhler and Chan-Palay, 1983; Brashear et al., 1986; Walker et al., 1989b; Koliatsos et al., in press, a). The peptide galanin has been colocalized in cholinergic cells of the BFMC (Melander et al., 1985; Melander and Staines, 1986; Walker et al., 1989a,c). Other putative transmitters have not been localized definitively within these cells. Intermingled with magnocellular neurons in certain subdivisions of the BFMC are cells containing neurotensin, somatostatin, leucine-encephalin, neuropeptide Y, or tyrosine hydroxylase (Walker et al., 1989a; V.E. Koliatsos, personal observations). In general, the latter classes of neurons differ in size and morphology from typical BFMC cells and may belong to adjacent basal forebrain systems (Koliatsos et al., in press, a).

The BFMC, thought to play a key role in such functions as learning and memory (as reviewed by Bartus et al., 1986, and Olton and Wenk, 1987), degenerates in certain types of dementia, including Alzheimer's disease (AD), Down's syndrome, progressive supranuclear palsy, and in some cases of Parkinson's disease (Price et al., 1985). In AD, degeneration of neurons of the BFMC appears to be an early and consistent abnormality (Francis et al., 1985). The significance of these cells for cognitive processes and their involvement in neurological disease have stimulated research aimed at a better understanding of the role of this forebrain system in normal brain function and in the clinical manifestations of dementia. Recent research activity on the BFMC is at variance with earlier periods in neuroscience when this forebrain system received little attention. However, the relatively few works of early neuroanatomists and experimental neurologists outlined areas of interest that still represent exciting topics of investigation. The present review discusses: the development of our understanding of the BFMC/BFCS

Table 1 [Note]. * Mesulam nomenclature. Since the choice of terms for the different neuronal populations within the BFMC varies among investigators, the classification proposed in this table reflects the authors' views primarily. In the construction of the table, the major factors considered are usage and practicality. True anatomical criteria for parcellation can apply only to a limited degree, since BFMC and BFCS represent anatomical continua. A recent review has addressed major issues associated with subparcellation and nomenclature of the BFMC (Butcher and Semba, 1989).

during the last 120 years; major issues of current research; and finally, some future directions of study. Since the present volume focuses on the cholinergic cells of the BFMC, the term BFCS will be primarily used in the remainder of this review, although in most cases, issues under discussion involve the whole BFMC. It must be emphasized that the term BFCS has only limited value and that the role of cholinergic cells of the basal forebrain cannot be understood outside the context of the BFMC, which also includes a large number of noncholinergic neurons.

BFCS: AN HISTORICAL PERSPECTIVE (1872 TO LATE 1980s)

Early Descriptive Neuroanatomy: From Meynert (1872) *to Brockhaus* (1942)

The first description of the major component—in higher mammals—of the BFCS, presently known as the nucleus basalis of Meynert (NBM), was made by Theodor Meynert (1872) in a chapter on the anatomy of the brain in Stricker's *Manual of Histology* and did not exceed ten printed lines (Fig. 1A). In the pre-Meynert era, Johann C. Reil (1809) had described fairly extensively the subcommissural area where the majority of BFMC cells is located, but in the absence of any clues about its actual organization and anatomical affiliations, he called it "ungenannte Marksubstanz" (unnamed substance). Karl Reichert (1861) recognized the same area as a separate anatomical entity in his famous atlas of the human brain (Fig. 1B), but he did not give this structure a specific name. The failure to assign a term to this brain structure by these authorities prompted neuroanatomists in Meynert's time to refer to the NBM area as the "substantia innominata of Reil" (e.g., von Kölliker, 1896). Despite its somewhat negative connotation, the term substantia innominata is still useful in topographic descriptions of the extremely complicated region of the subcommissural gray in which several systems of the basal forebrain come together (Paxinos and Watson, 1986). However, some contemporary authors consider the term obsolete and even confusing (Heimer et al., 1989). Meynert termed the NBM as the "nucleus of the ansa peduncularis" ("Ganglion der Hirnschenkelschlinge") to emphasize its association with the transverse bundle in which fibers of the inferior thalamic peduncle converge with axons of the ventral amygdalofugal pathway caudal to the decussation of the anterior commissure. Meynert's report was based on gross dissections, fresh brain slices, and material fixed with potassium dichromate and stained with gold chloride or carmine. Due in part to the nature of these preparations, Meynert noted a close association of the NBM with ascending longitudinal fiber bundles. The "posterior longitudinal fasciculus" (an older neuroanatomical term for the medial longitudinal fasciculus), which Meynert thought might bear a major affiliation with the NBM (Fig. 1A), is now known to be part of the vestibular system and to terminate in medial thalamus, having no functional or anatomical relationship to the NBM. However, the concept of an extensive innervation of the NBM by brainstem afferents recently has been brought back into focus, primarily as a result of the wide application of tract-tracing techniques, and may be of major functional significance.

Von Kölliker (1896), who revisited the human basal forebrain in the sixth edition of his *Handbuch der Gewebelehre des Menschen* using Weigert stains, is credited with the first complete description of the topography of the NBM. He used, for the first time, the term "basal ganglion" to include the whole BFCS from the septal plane rostrally to the mammilary bodies caudally; his observations hold valid today. A complete English translation of this description was provided in the classical comparative paper of Gorry (1963).

A detailed morphological description of the NBM, made possible with the advent in the 1870s of silver impregnation methods (Golgi, 1873, 1885) was done by Beccari (1911), who studied the cytology of the human anterior perforated substance employing Nissl, Golgi/Golgi-Cox, and Weigert stains. Beccari described the cells of the NBM as having large multipolar somata and long dendrites that display little branching. He also described populations of smaller stellate neurons closely associated with large cells of the BFCS in the most superficial layers of the basal forebrain. These components of the BFCS are very complex and possibly represent an interface between the BFCS and other basal forebrain systems; some of Beccari's stellate cells may correspond to small neurotensin-, somatostatin-, and neuropeptide Y-containing neurons, identified recently with immunocytochemistry in this area of the brain (Walker et al., 1989a).

Aniline dyes (Nissl), available since 1894 (Nissl, 1894, 1895), appeared in studies of the BFCS primarily with a short report by Ramón y Cajal (1955) in his *Textura del Sistema Nervioso del Hombre y de los Vertebrados* (translated in French as *Histologie du Système Nerveux*). Ramón y Cajal was impressed with the intense basophilia and large size of BFCS cells and went so far as to compare them with motor neurons, based on size, Nissl substance, and amounts of lipofuscin. Cajal, misled by the dispersed topography of BFCS cells, did not include them in a single system, and like

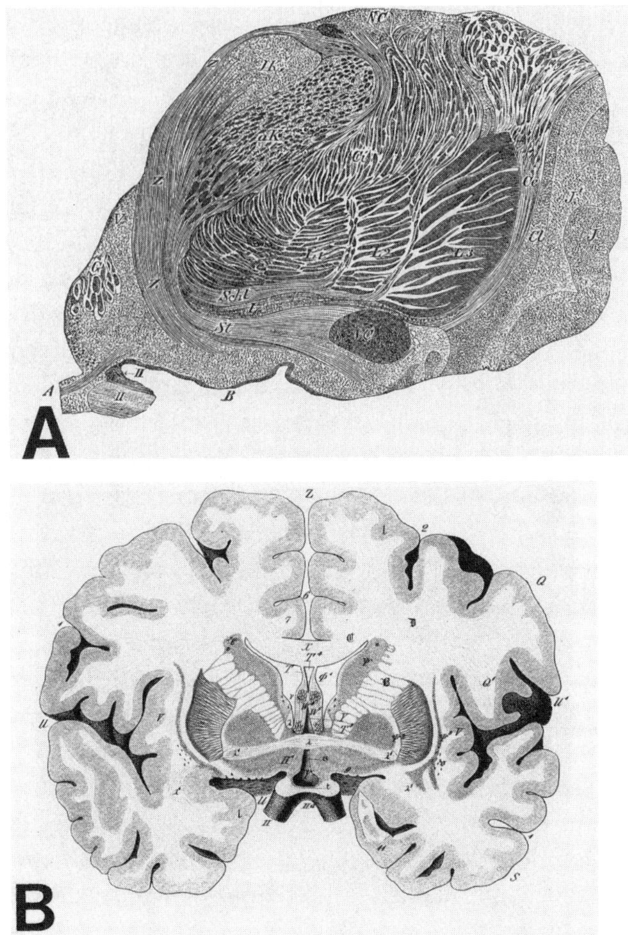

Figure 1. The classical era in investigations of the BFCS commences with Meynert's first description of the homonymous nucleus which he called "nucleus of ansa peduncularis." **A.** As reproduced from Meynert's chapter in Stricker's handbook of histology (Meynert, 1872), the position of the NBM is denoted in the second layer (L) of the substantia innominata (the four layers of which, in this transverse section of human forebrain, are labeled as SchL, L, St, and Z). It is noteworthy that the position of the NBM is demarcated by the presence of abundant fibers that belong, according to Meynert, to the medial longitudinal fasciculus; the nature of this preparation—transparent, unfixed section of the brain—facilitates the visualization of fiber tracts. **B.** The area occupied by NBM is left unlabeled in the classical atlas of the human brain edited by Reichert (1861). The explanation given for number 9, used to label the substantia innominata in Reichert's drawing, actually deals with the striate arteries that vertically penetrate this area of the brain and give its surface anatomy a "perforated" picture.

Becarri, he considered them as the deep layer of the anterior perforated substance (or olfactory tubercle in nonprimate species). Ayala (1915) is responsible for the first major description of the BFCS based on Nissl methods. He focused on the variable morphology of magnocellular, basophilic cells in the substantia innominata and substriatal gray and separated these nerve cells in a lateral-posterior sector (which he named "nucleus subputaminalis") and a rostral-medial sector, which he thought of as the NBM proper ("nucleus of the ansa lenticularis").

Foix and Nicolesco (Foix and Nicolesco, 1925; Nicolesco and Nicolesco, 1929), using Nissl stains, redescribed the cytology of BFCS cells, which they classified by virtue of topography, structure and connections, and histopathology, together with a number of hypothalamic nuclei (e.g., supraoptic and periventricular nucleus) in the telencephalo-diencephalic component of the "vegetative" (autonomic) centers of the base of the brain. In a period when patterns of basophilia were the major determinants of neuronal phenotype, cells of this "system" were thought of as intensely basophilic, with a peripheral distribution of Nissl bodies.

Until the early 1940s, except for von Kölliker's inclusive description, neuroanatomists tended to view the BFCS as a succession of separate cell groups or nuclei that they usually ascribed to other major neighboring structures or "systems." It is characteristic that in the 1942 edition of Mettler's influential *Neuroanatomy* (Mettler, 1942), the intermediate sector of the NBM is divided into the nucleus of ansa lenticularis (corresponding mostly to the intermediodorsal NBM), which Mettler considered part of the entopeduncular nucleus, and nucleus of the ansa peduncularis (intermedioventral NBM). Similar trends are obvious in other major publications of that time (Papez and Aronson, 1934; Riley, 1943).

The BFCS was seen again as a single system by Brockhaus (1942) in a Nissl study focusing on the topography of magnocellular groups in the basal forebrain and comparable in thoroughness with the earlier description of von Kölliker with Weigert stain. Brockhaus examined the basal forebrain in several primate species (from lemurs to humans) and paid much attention to magnocellular populations in the basal forebrain beyond the NBM, such as the "nucleus of the tuberculum olfactorium" (corresponding to the current notion of the nucleus of the horizontal limb of the DBB) and the "nucleus of the diagonal band of Broca" (corresponding to the current definition of the nucleus of the vertical limb of the DBB) (Fig. 2A). He included the NBM with these other populations of cells in what he collectively termed "basal nucleus complex" ("Basalkernkomplex"). This concept, solidified in the

1970s and 1980s by the common histochemical and connectional features of these collections of neurons, is identical to the present topographic definition of the BFCS.

Early Experimental Neurology:
Kodama (1926-28) *and Akert-Pilleri* (*Late* 1950s)

S. Kodama studied extensively the developmental, comparative, and connectional aspects of basal ganglia and their accessory structures, including the BFCS, in a series of papers published in the *Swiss Archives of Neurology and Psychiatry* (Kodama, 1926a,b, 1927, 1928a,b). This excellent but rarely cited work represents the most thorough investigation of the BFCS until the 1960s. Kodama's ideas about the connectivity of basal ganglia were based on studies of anterograde and retrograde degeneration, the only tracing method available at that time. He used autopsy cases with a variety of focal lesions in telencephalon and brainstem as well as experimental animal cases (dogs, cats, and rabbits) in which he reproduced some of the lesions found in human cases. Kodama carefully categorized his material into cases with telencephalic lesions, which he used to study possible associations of basal ganglia with cortex (Kodama, 1927), and cases with diencephalic/mesencephalic lesions, which were used for studies of the subcortical connections of the basal ganglia (Kodama, 1928a). Among the first group of cases were: a 31-year-old man with a traumatic hemorrhagic cyst of the temporal lobe that had induced antero- and retrograde degeneration of the BFCS; and a 9 1/2-year-old girl with a meningeal tumor that destroyed wide areas of the temporal lobe in which Kodama observed complete cell loss in the posterior NBM. Kodama reproduced these patterns of degeneration in newborn dogs and cats by removing the temporal lobe or by extensive hemispheric ablations. Among the second group of cases, he reported on a man with a midline tumor of the pontine tegmentum, who showed partial degeneration of the NBM; Kodama then induced atrophy of the NBM in rabbits with collicular/thalamic lesions. These latter observations may indicate an anterograde degeneration of the BFCS after removal of its widespread brainstem afferents. The above observations and Kodama's earlier work on the NBM were summarized in a final drawing of the possible connections of the BFCS, including reciprocal connectivity with the temporal lobe (see Fig. 89 in Kodama, 1928b). Nearly 50 years ahead of their time, these observations predicted innervation of the NBM by anterior temporal/temporopolar areas; these areas are among the few cortical regions that project to the NBM, as has been shown recently with more modern anatomical methods (Mesulam and Mufson, 1984).

Twenty years later Pilleri and Akert repeated Kodama's ablation experiments on rhesus monkeys. They removed the temporal lobe up to the rhinal sulcus without damaging the hippocampus and found loss of nerve cells in the posterior NBM, especially in the external medullary lamina (Pilleri, 1962) (for a more thorough review of these experiments, see Gorry, 1963). Deviating slightly from Kodama's conclusions, these investigators interpreted these changes in the NBM as signs of anterograde—as opposed to combined anterograde/retrograde (according to Kodama)—degeneration. It is noteworthy that Pilleri and Akert found no effects on the NBM of frontal or parietal cortical ablations, an observation in keeping with recent studies that showed persistence of NBM neurons after extensive neocortical ablations in the rat (Sofroniew et al., 1983). Pilleri extended his transneuronal degeneration strategies to observations in human autopsy cases, including individuals with stroke (Pilleri, 1966), and cases with Pick's disease and AD (Pilleri, 1966b). In the latter study, he reported severe cell loss in the NBM of one individual with AD, a finding he contrasted with the apparently healthy NBM in Pick's disease. A present explanation of the profound effects of temporal ablations on the BFCS may be that, besides the reciprocal innervation resulting in both antero- and retrograde degeneration, these lesions lie fairly proximal to the NBM and may remove all existing proximal collaterals of BFCS axons, therefore inflicting severe damage to parent cell bodies (Sofroniew and Isacson, 1988; Koliatsos et al., 1989a).

Gorry (1963) *and the Comparative Neuroanatomy of the BFCS*

The comparative anatomist J. Gorry characterized the NBM as an "obscure texture" when he approached its functional role from a developmental-comparative vantage point (Gorry, 1963). Based on observations on 35 brains belonging to 11 orders of mammals, Gorry found that the size and differentiation of the NBM increase with increasing cerebralization (the latter defined by brain weight and the ratio length of hypothalamus to length of cerebrum) and that cell size in the NBM corresponds to animal size. This positive correlation was shown to exist between different species as well as between different orders of animals. Stephan and Andy reached similar conclusions after extensive studies of the comparative neuroanatomy of the septal area (Andy and Stephan, 1959, 1961, 1966, 1968; Stephan and Andy, 1962, 1964). These investigators found that the septum, including septal components of the BFCS, increase in size and complexity in the ascending

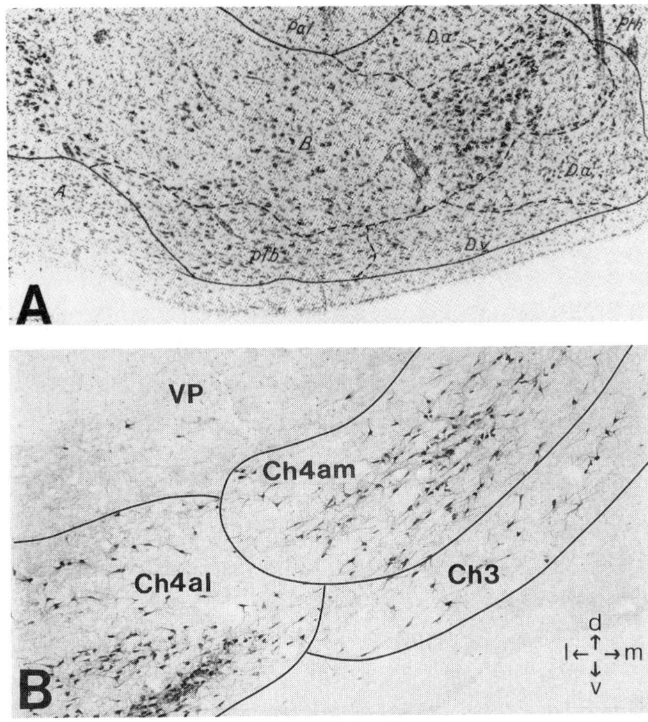

Figure 2. An old (A) and a recent (B) attempt for a topographical parcellation of the BFCS. Illustration A is based on Nissl and is taken from Brockhaus's classical study of the anatomical organization of the basal forebrain (Brockhaus, 1942). Illustration B is a recent ChAT-immunostained preparation labeled according to Mesulam's "Ch" nomenclature schema (Mesulam et al., 1983a). Both preparations represent a coronal plane through the monkey basal forebrain caudal to the commissural decussation. Although such topographic approaches do justice to the efferent organization of the system, which follows topographical rules as well (see text), some peripheral intermingling among individual projection groups renders the anatomical organization of the BFCS much more complex (see also Fig. 3). Partial abbreviations in A: A, amygdala; B, nucleus basalis; D.a, nucleus of the DBB, pars angularis[1]; D.v, nucleus of the DBB, pars ventralis[2]; Pal, globus pallidus; pTb, nucleus paratubercularis[3]. Abbreviations in B: Ch3, cholinergic cells in the nucleus of the horizontal limb of the DBB; Ch4al, cholinergic cells in the NBM, anterolateral portion; Ch4am, cholinergic cells in the NBM, anteromedial portion; VP, ventral pallidum. Orientation is the same in A and B: d, dorsal; l, lateral; m, medial; v, ventral.

[1] Corresponding to the nucleus of the vertical limb of the DBB according to the nomenclature used in this chapter

[2] Corresponding to the nucleus of the horizontal limb of the DBB

[3] Corresponding to the lateral parts of the nucleus of the horizontal limb

primate scale. Some interesting comparative notes on the NBM had also been contributed by Kodama (1926a) and Pilleri (1962, 1966c). Kodama (1926b) insisted on the incomplete differentiation of the NBM from globus pallidus and on its close association with the latter. Feremutsch (1961) followed up on Kodama's point on the incomplete differentiation of the NBM from globus pallidus in a monograph, based on Nissl methods, that dealt with the primate basal ganglia. Although Feremutsch focused on the cytoarchitectonic organization and comparative anatomy of the neostriatum and globus pallidus, his need to differentiate these structures from the NBM led him to undertake a fairly extensive comparative study of this nucleus as well. Feremutsch postulated that the NBM essentially replaces the caudal part of the external segment of the globus pallidus in lower primates (lemurs) and its differentiation from the globus pallidus increases in the ascending scale of lemurs → prosimians → simians → great apes → man. A quite different statement on the relationships between the globus pallidus and NBM was made by Grünthal (1932, 1933), who assumed that the NBM in lower mammals corresponded to the external segment of the globus pallidus in primates. In the latter, Grünthal thought the NBM to be rudimentary, a view later disproved by Gorry (1963). The lack of precise delineation between the globus pallidus and NBM, as seen with conventional stains, is particularly evident in lower mammals and was the primary reason why Gorry failed to recognize any elements of the NBM in the rat. Although the inclusion of the NBM with the globus pallidus is an oversimplification due to inadequate labeling methods, it is congruent with the constant affiliation of the two structures throughout phylogeny (Parent et al., 1979) and also with current ideas for a possible common anlage between the NBM and globus pallidus (Bayer, 1985; S. Bayer, personal communication).

The BFCS and the Isodendritic Core of the Brain (1960s)

In the late 1960s, Ramon-Moliner and Nauta (1966) used the Golgi-Cox method to classify neurons of the BFCS, together with cells in the brainstem, into a common morphological unit they termed "isodendritic core of the brain." This core generally corresponded to regions regarded as the reticular formation. Criteria for inclusion of a cell group or nucleus in this system were multipolar and polymorphic somata; "generalized" dendrites (long and rectilinear, with sparse branching and without directional preference); a considerable degree of dendritic overlap among individual neurons; and free intermingling of dendrites and passing fiber bundles. According to these authors, the apposition of groups of isodendritic cells with the above features to one another from the lower medulla to the basal diencephalon generates a continuum of overlapping dendritic fields capable of processing afferent signals of very heterogeneous origin. Similar observations were made by Leontovitch and Zhukova (1963). Das and Kreutzberg (Das and Kreutzberg, 1968; Das, 1971) used Ramón y Cajal's term "interstitial" to describe the same groups of cells and found a coincidence between isodendritic morphology and intense AChE staining; they clearly considered the BFCS as the most rostral part of the reticular formation. At approximately the same time, Shute and Lewis (1967) associated the above groups of cells with ascending "cholinergic" projections, and physiological evidence suggested that reticular-activating influences on cortex might be associated with acetylcholine release, mediated, at least in part, by cortically projecting neurons of the BFCS (Miller et al., 1940; Kanai and Szerb, 1965; Celesia and Jasper, 1966; Szerb, 1967; Jasper and Tessier, 1971).

Ideas for a close association of the BFCS with the reticular formation have been revived recently in a variety of ways. In the early 1980s, when neuropathological studies revealed that a variety of brainstem groups with "isodendritic" neurons degenerate together with the NBM in several neurodegenerative diseases including AD and Parkinson's disease, Rossor (1981) proposed the term "diseases of the isodendritic core." More recently, Saper (1987) included the BFCS in the broader category of subcortical nonthalamic nuclei that provide major input to the cerebral cortex and presumably do not directly drive cortical cells but rather modulate responses of the latter to their more specific inputs. Saper predicted that all these groups scattered throughout the base of the brain should be intensely interconnected. Although such hypotheses can only be verified with multiple retrograde tracing strategies that involve injections of retrograde tracers in fiber-rich subcortical areas and bear the risk of labeling irrelevent pathways, there is some evidence that such interconnectivity exists, at least in the ascending fashion (Záborszky, 1989). Tracing-immunohistochemical experiments have shown a substantial projection from the BFCS to the reticular nucleus of thalamus (Hallanger et al., 1987; Levey et al., 1987; Steriade et al., 1987), an area that influences specific thalamic nuclei in their modulation of cortical activity. These findings provide additional arguments for considering the BFCS as the most rostral component of the reticular activating system. Finally, physiological studies on the role of NBM cells in cortical activation still attract substantial interest (Stewart et al., 1984; Detári and Vanderwolf, 1987; Buzsáki et al., 1988).

The BFCS as a Source of Widespread Cholinergic Innervation of the Telencephalon (*Late* 1960s *and* 1970s; *Early* 1980s)

The process of specification of projections and transmitter identity of the BFCS began with the pioneering work of Shute and Lewis (Lewis and Shute, 1967; Shute and Lewis, 1967), who described the distribution of major cholinergic pathways of the brain, using a combination of stereotaxic lesions with the thiocholine method for the histochemical detection of cholinesterases (Koelle and Friedenwald, 1949). Shute and Lewis worked on the assumption that central cholinergic neurons, like those of the peripheral nervous system, should contain acetylcholinesterase (AChE)—the enzyme that hydrolyzes acetylcholine—not only in cell bodies but also in the axon and nerve terminals. Their work predicted the origin and termination of cholinergic pathways in the telencephalon with some notable exceptions, such as the anterior thalamic "cholinergic" projection to cortex or the olfactory tubercle "cholinergic" projection to the olfactory bulb. A number of accurate descriptions were also made by Shute and Lewis (1967) for thalamic/brainstem cholinergic pathways, including the pontine cholinergic projection to thalamus and the habenulo-interpeduncular tract (Shute and Lewis, 1967). In the early to mid 1970s, the advent of horseradish peroxidase (HRP) and its various conjugates as axonal tracers made possible the discovery that the BFCS is a source of diffuse projections to cortex (including hippocampus), olfactory bulb, and basolateral amygdala (Das, 1971; Divac, 1975; Kievit and Kuypers, 1975; Ottersen, 1980). At about the same time, Mesulam and Van Hoesen (1976) were able to colocalize AChE histochemical product in NBM cells retrogradely labeled from HRP injections into motor/premotor cortex. A strong perikaryal histochemical reaction for AChE was then still considered a marker of cholinergic neurotransmission (Jacobowitz and Palkovits, 1974; Mesulam and Van Hoesen, 1976; Parent et al., 1979). The pharmacohistochemical procedure for AChE histochemistry introduced by Butcher et al. (1975) was an additional step in the precise characterization of central cholinergic pathways, including those originating in the BFCS. This protocol called for treatment of animals with the irreversible AChE inhibitor diisopropylfluorophosphate (DFP) 4-6 hours prior to sacrifice (Parent et al., 1977, 1981; Bigl et al., 1982; Woolf and Butcher, 1982; Mesulam et al., 1983a; Smith and Parent, 1984; Woolf et al., 1984). This technique proved to be a more reliable method for cholinergic neurons than AChE histochemistry alone, provided that the DFP-sacrifice interval was shortened to 2-3 hours (Butcher et al., 1975; Butcher and Woolf, 1984). However, the cholinergic nature of telencephalic projections of the BFCS was confirmed in the 1980s, with the advent and use of polyclonal (Peng et al., 1981) and, in particular, monoclonal (Crawford et al., 1982; Eckenstein and Thoenen, 1983; Levey et al., 1983) antibodies against choline acetyltransferase (ChAT) (Fig. 2B) and with basal forebrain lesions combined with biochemical determinations of cortical ChAT levels. In the first setting, ChAT immunohistochemistry was used to localize neurons of the BFCS (Kimura et al., 1981; Hedreen et al., 1982; Mesulam et al., 1983b, 1984) or was combined with retrograde tracing (HRP, fluorescent dyes) from neocortex, amygdala, and olfactory bulb to show that numerous cells located in various sectors of the BFCS were double labeled (Rye et al., 1984; Woolf et al., 1984; Mesulam et al., 1986; Koliatsos et al., 1988; Koliatsos and Price, submitted for publication). In the second setting, excitotoxic (Johnston et al., 1979, 1981; Lehmann et al., 1980; Wenk et al., 1984; Struble et al., 1986) or electrolytic (Wenk et al., 1980) lesions of the NBM were associated with reductions in cortical ChAT. Since those first reports, the idea of the BFCS as the principal source of cholinergic innervation of cortex, olfactory bulb, and amygdala has been amply confirmed by several groups using a variety of methods, including, more recently, induction of acetylcholine release in cortex following electric stimulation of the NBM (Casamenti et al., 1986; Kurosawa et al., 1989).

The BFCS and Mechanisms of Reward (1971)

The first attempt at a physiological characterization of BFCS neurons was made in the early 1970s, in the course of a study focused on the activity of pallidal neurons (DeLong, 1971). This study showed that neurons of the NBM discharge continuously, but exhibit phasic changes in discharge rate when a water reward is delivered. These findings were extended a few years later by Rolls and associates (Burton et al., 1976; Mora et al., 1976), who showed that NBM neurons respond to visual stimuli linked with food or juice rewards and that these responses are reduced as animals became satiated, or when the presentation of the stimulus is not followed by reward. The above observations have been confirmed repeatedly in subsequent studies (Richardson and DeLong, 1986; Richardson et al., 1988), all of which indicate that reinforcement is associated with clear changes in the activity of NBM cells and hence acetylcholine release in cortex. Such changes in acetylcholine release lead to either a transient (Krnjević and Ropert, 1982; Cole and Nicoll, 1984) or a more prolonged increase in the responsiveness of hippocampal and cortical neurons (Woody et al., 1978; Sillito and Kemp, 1983; Metherate et al., 1987). A transient increase in cortical responsiveness may be associated with an arousal response (Sillito and Kemp, 1983), whereas more persistent changes in the responsiveness of cortical neurons may contribute to learning (Richardson et al., 1988).

The BFCS and Alzheimer's Disease (1982)

A cholinergic cortical deficit was suspected as a hallmark of AD as early as the mid 1960s, when Pope and coworkers (1964) reported on reduced AChE in the cortex of AD patients. However, the so-called "cholinergic hypothesis" of AD did not evolve until the demonstration in the mid 1970s that ChAT activity was also reduced in cortices of affected individuals (Bowen et al., 1976; Perry et al., 1977; Davies, 1979). These reductions were shown to correlate with the severity of intellectual impairment and regional densities of senile plaques (Blessed et al., 1968; Perry et al., 1978). The discovery in the late 1970s that the BFCS is the major source of cortical cholinergic innervation directed investigators to reexamine the BFCS in light of the cholinergic hypothesis of AD. The index case of a major loss of neurons in the NBM was a 72-year-old man with a 14-year history of dementia and brain abnormalities typical of AD (Whitehouse et al., 1981, 1982). Marked degeneration of NBM neurons in individuals with AD has since been confirmed in numerous laboratories (Perry et al., 1982; Arendt et al., 1983; Candy et al., 1983; Pearson et al., 1983b; Tagliavini and Pilleri, 1983; McGeer et al., 1984c; Mann et al., 1984; Rogers et al., 1985; Rinne et al., 1987; Allen et al., 1988), although in some of the above studies (Candy et al., 1983; Pearson et al., 1983b; Perry et al., 1982; Rinne et al., 1987; Allen et al., 1988), emphasis is placed on cell shrinkage and dysfunction rather than on cell loss. The BFCS is also affected in disorders other than AD, including Down's syndrome in older individuals (Casanova et al., 1985), Parkinson's disease with dementia (Arendt et al., 1983; Whitehouse et al., 1983), and progressive supranuclear palsy (Tagliavini et al., 1984; Rogers et al., 1985; Agid et al., 1986). The major pathological changes in neurons of the NBM in AD and other dementias include: reductions in cell size and transmitter markers; cytoskeletal abnormalities; appearance of abnormal proteins in cells; participation of axons/terminals of these cells in neurite formation; and cell degeneration (Koo and Price, in press).

The cholinergic hypothesis of AD has also received support from basic animal research showing that acetylcholine plays a major role in normal memory (Deutsch, 1971) as well as from clinical studies in human subjects showing that cholinergic synapse blockers produce amnesia in normal individuals (Drachman and Leavitt, 1974). In addition, more recent work suggested that cholinesterase inhibitors provide some therapeutic benefit in patients with AD (Thal et al., 1983). The involvement of cholinergic transmission in central processes associated with memory and learning becomes more significant considering the modest and less-specific role of other neurotransmitters, such as catecholamines (Ashton, 1987). However, in most studies involving pharmacological manipulations of the central cholinergic transmission, anatomical specificity is not possible. Cholinomimetic as well as anticholinergic effects of drugs affect nonselectively the central cholinergic synapses, involving, in addition to the BFCS cells, other cholinergic systems (e.g., the caudal cholinergic chain including the pedunculopontine and lateral dorsal tegmental nucleus, the habenulo-interpeduncular tract, and neostriatal cholinergic neurons). The implication of the BFCS in the effects of these drugs on complex behavior is only a matter of course, since cholinergic pathways of the diencephalon and brainstem are not intimately associated with major sites of memory processing, such as the hippocampus and limbic system.

CURRENT UNDERSTANDING OF THE ANATOMICAL ORGANIZATION OF THE BFCS

Local Circuitry

Very few studies have addressed, directly or indirectly, issues of intrinsic organization of the BFMC/BFCS, and the available information is insufficient to allow for the construction of a local synaptic model, as in the case of the cerebral cortex, cerebellum, thalamus, or spinal cord. Undoubtedly, the two major contributors to local circuitry of the BFMC are the cholinergic and GABAergic projection neurons, cells that are morphologically identical (Brashear et al., 1986). Using a variety of methods, smaller neurons have been found to mingle with larger projection cells (Beccari, 1911; Walker et al., 1989a); some of these small cells contain galanin (Chan-Palay, 1988b; Walker et al., 1989c; Kordower and Mufson, in press). Although many of these neurons may represent admixtures of other neighboring basal forebrain systems, particularly in the problematic area of the substantia innominata (Koliatsos et al., in press, a), some galanin-containing neurons are local-circuit neurons (Chan-Palay, 1988b). Cholinergic and GABAergic BFMC neurons have been shown to form synaptic contacts with each other: GABAergic boutons with synaptic specializations appose cholinergic dendrites and somata in ventral pallidum (Záborszky et al., 1986b; Ingham et al., 1988) and may represent terminals from local collaterals of corticopetal axons (Semba et al., 1988b). In addition, cholinergic terminals have been shown to synapse on GABAergic cells of the ventral pallidum (Záborszky et al., 1986b) and upon GABAergic neurons of the medial septal-DBB nuclei (Léránth and Frotscher, 1989). Cholinergic-cholinergic interactions have not been found in the ventral pallidum and NBM (Záborszky et al., 1986b; Martínez-Murillo et al., 1988), although a few such interactions have been observed in the medial septal nucleus and the nucleus of the DBB (Bialowas and Frotscher, 1987). A special role has been recently proposed for local galanin-containing terminals in the human NBM that originate primarily from smaller galaninergic neurons interspersed among projection cells of the BFMC: these putative inhibitory terminals are thought to hypertrophy and hyperinnervate remaining cholinergic neurons in the brains of individuals with AD, further suppressing their function (Chan-Palay, 1988a). On a larger scale, different components of the BFCS appear to be intensely interconnected (Conrad and Pfaff, 1976; Swanson, 1976; Swanson and Cowan, 1979; V. E. Koliatsos, personal observations). It appears, thus, that depolarization in a given group of BFMC cells (e.g., after a stimulation by a common afferent bundle of fibers) leads to changes within a broader area of the complex. Furthermore, every time a signal is transmitted to a distal target of the system, GABAergic projection neurons inhibit the activity of cholinergic projection neurons and the latter influence the activity of GABAergic neurons with an as yet unknown polarity. The outcome of this local modulation will depend on whether interconnections between the two projection neurons are also affected by local-circuit neurons and whether various excitatory and inhibitory afferents to the BFMC preferentially address GABAergic or cholinergic neurons (see below, *Afferent Organization*). Wider application of intracellular recording/tracing in conjuction with studies of inputs to the BFMC (see below) will help to resolve these issues and to illuminate the significance of the complex intrinsic organization of the BFMC/BFCS.

Efferent Organization

Although the BFCS belongs to a group of subcortical systems that diffusely projects to telencephalon, it has a unique efferent organization that distinguishes it from the other systems, i.e., the ascending noradrenergic system originating in locus coeruleus, serotoninergic pathways originating in the raphe complex, and dopaminergic axons from the ventral tegmental area. First, the BFCS has undergone a remarkable expansion and differentiation with increasing cerebralization, whereas the other diffuse ascending systems have remained relatively stable (Gorry, 1963; Parent et al., 1984). Second, BFCS axons innervate relatively restricted zones within telencephalic targets of the BFCS, which, in neocortex, do not exceed an idealized circular area with a diameter of 1.5 mm; the extent of these terminal fields may be greater in allocortex, where some BFCS axons appear to cover fields with a diameter >3 mm (Price and Stern, 1983; Saper, 1984; Woolf et al., 1984; Carlsen et al., 1985; Walker et al., 1985; Koliatsos et al., 1988; Koliatsos and Price, submitted for publication). In contrast, axons from other ascending pathways, e.g., the noradrenergic or serotoninergic system, branch profusely and widely so that a single axon can innervate not only large areas within a confined telencephalic structure but also targets widely apart and located in different telencephalic/diencephalic structures (van der Kooy and Hattori, 1980; Nagai et al., 1981; Fallon and Loughlin, 1982; de Olmos and Heimer, 1980). Third, there is a considerable degree of topographic organization in efferents of the BFCS: rostrally located components of the system tend to innervate rostral targets in the telencephalon; and similar associations exist along the ventralateral-dorsomedial plane (Luiten et al., 1987). This pattern in the efferent organization of the BFCS has prompted some investigators to consider cyto- and chemoarchitectonic parcellations of the BFCS to be also useful as projection maps of the system (Mesulam et al., 1983a,b, 1986) (Fig. 2B). However, there is a significant peripheral intermingling among individual projection groups of the BFCS and, in some cases, such as the nucleus of the horizontal limb of the DBB, the efferent organization is quite complex (Divac, 1981; Koliatsos and Price, submitted for publication) (Fig. 3). Fourth, the cellular organization of the BFCS may be influenced by organization and functional patterns in its telencephalic target fields. For example, in the rat, interconnected cortical/subcortical targets of the BFCS tend to be innervated by single BFCS cells in rates that exceed, by far, the incidence of BFCS neurons branching to innervate two randomly selected cortical/subcortical sites (V. E. Koliatsos, personal observations). Fifth, there is a remarkable, species-consistent variability in the ratio of cholinergic/noncholinergic BFMC neurons that innervate each telencephalic target of the complex. Projections to allocortical hippocampus originate from at least as many noncholinergic (mostly GABAergic) as cholinergic BFMC neurons, whereas cholinergic BFMC neurons innervating any isocortical field are eight- to ninefold more than noncholinergic BFMC cells that project to the same field; mesocortical regions represent an intermediate case (Köhler et al., 1984; Rye et al., 1984; Amaral and Kurz,

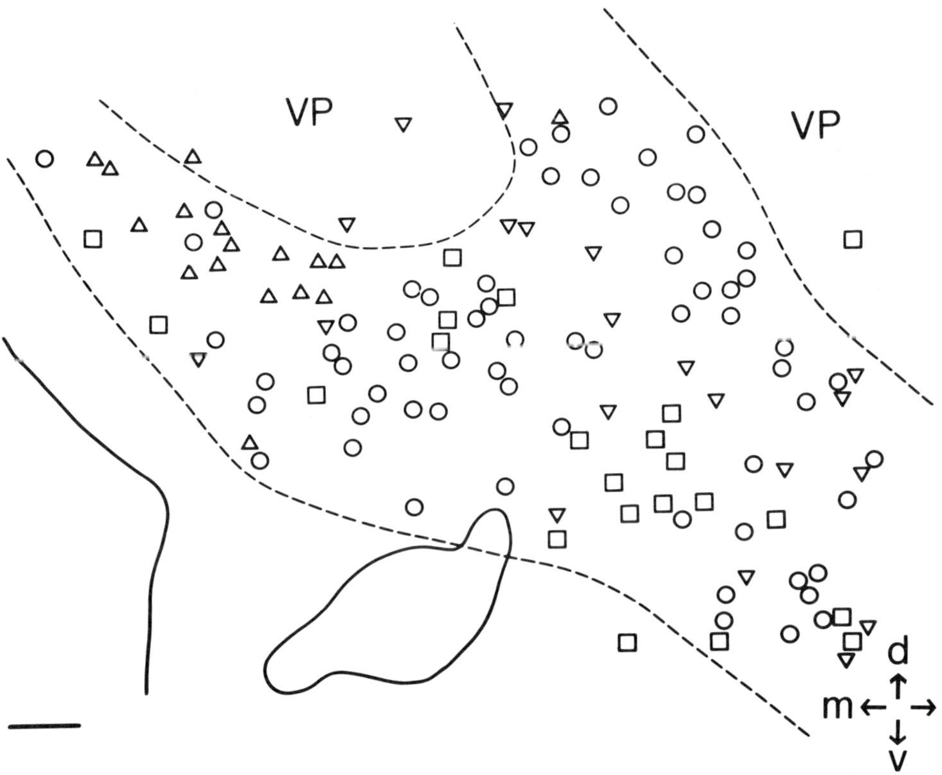

Figure 3. Despite their topographical organization, axons of the BFCS directed at specific telencephalic targets originate in BFCS populations of neurons that overlap each other, especially in BFCS sectors such as the nucleus of the horizontal limb of the DBB (depicted in this figure). In the case illustrated here, different fluorescent retrograde tracers were used to label different projection groups in the BFCS: True Blue (triangles pointing up) was injected into septal hippocampus; Fluoro-Gold (triangles pointing down) was injected into temporal hippocampus/entorhinal cortex; Evans Blue (circles) was injected into olfactory bulb; and Diamidino Yellow (squares) was injected into basolateral amygdala. Although there is a fair degree of topography (e.g., cells projecting to septal hippocampus are located more medially and dorsally than cells projecting to basolateral amygdala or temporal hippocampus), significant intermingling exists among the individual projection groups. Scale bar: 60 μm.

1985; Koliatsos et al., 1988; Koliatsos and Price, submitted for publication). Finally, the peptide galanin is colocalized in cholinergic cells throughout the BFCS in monkeys (Melander and Staines, 1986; Walker et al., 1989a,c; but only in medial septal-DBB neurons in rats (Melander et al., 1985), which project primarily to hippocampal allocortex (Fig. 4). The vast majority of magnocellular BFCS neurons in humans do not contain galanin (Walker et al., 1989c; Kordower and Mufson, in press).

The above points illustrate the remarkable way in which the organization of the telencephalic targets of the BFCS—including their phylo- and ontogenetic qualities—is reflected in the cyto- and chemoarchitecture of the BFMC/BFCS. This high level of organization is further maintained within the microcircuitry of the innervated telencephalic area. In hippocampus, cholinergic BFMC axons (although not exclusively) contact pyramidal neurons in Ammon's horn and granule cells within the dentate gyrus (both types of cells using excitatory amino acids as transmitters), whereas GABAergic axons selectively innervate GABAergic interneurons in a basket-like arrangement (Frotscher and Léránth, 1985, 1986; Freund and Antal, 1988). This GABAergic-GABAergic interaction introduces to the physiology of the hippocampus a GABA-mediated disinhibitory circuit that can assist in eliciting N-methyl-D-aspartate (NMDA)-receptor-mediated responses, including long-term potentiation (Collingridge et al., 1988). Recent studies have shown that the latter is preferentially induced under conditions of maximal excitation (Larson et al., 1986; Pavlides et al., 1988). It is conceivable that both the GABAergic disinhibitory septohippocampal axon and the presumably excitatory cholinergic BFCS terminal at the hippocampal projection neuron (Bird and Aghajanian, 1976; Benardo and Prince, 1982; Krnjević and Ropert, 1982) could contribute to this state of increased excitation.

Another complicating factor in BFCS efferents originates in preliminary observations that different components of the system innervate different layers within the same cortical area (e.g., entorhinal cortex) (Luiten et al., 1987). Further investigations need to address whether there is a differential innervation of superficial vs. deep cortical layers by distinct cells of the BFCS or even a more general subdivision of the BFCS into cell groups that project to superficial cortical layers and other groups that innervate deep cortical layers.

The remarkable complexity in the efferent organization of the BFCS demands more research in a variety of frontiers, including further elucidation of transmitters and other phenotypic features of individual projection neurons using multiple tract tracing/immunohistochemical/ *in situ* hybridization techniques; clarification of patterns of proximal and distal branching, course, and termination of individual BFCS fibers, using high-resolution intracellular or intraaxonal labeling methods (Sugiura et al., 1986); and further analysis of the microcircuitry in terminal fields of the BFCS, including

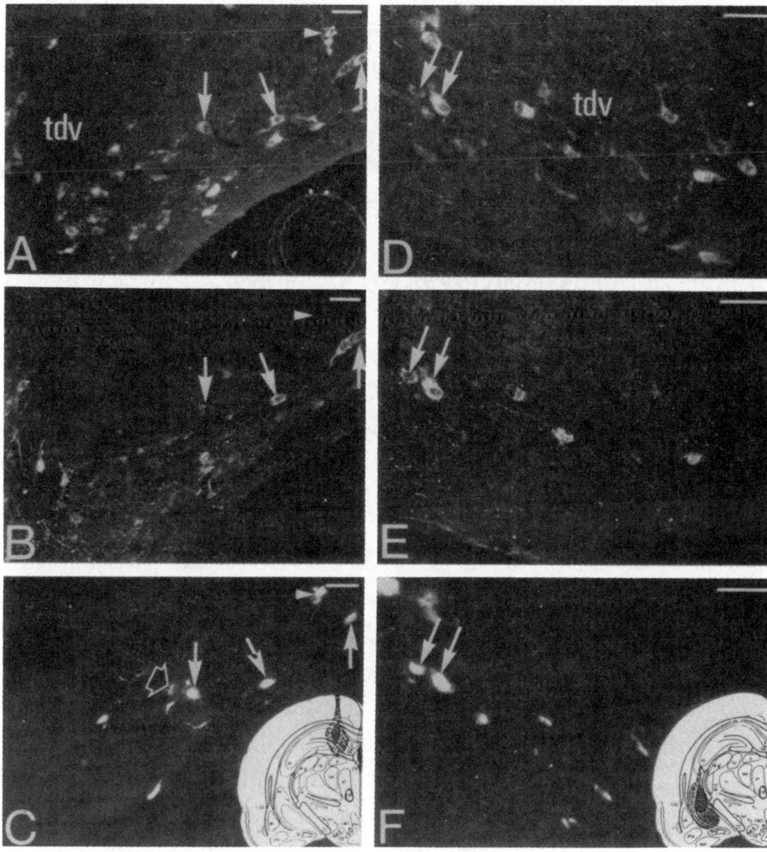

Figure 4. The era of chemical neuroanatomy investigations of the BFCS is best exemplified by combinations of tract-tracing techniques with immunohistochemistry. In this illustration, retrogradely labeled neurons from injections of the fluorescent dye True Blue in septal (C) and temporal (F) hippocampus colocalize ChAT-immunoreactivity visualized with fluorescein (A,D) and galanin immunoreactivity visualized with rhodamine (B,E). Triple-labeled cells are indicated by arrows. Retrogradely labeled cells, which are only cholinergic, are labeled with arrowheads (A,C). A few True Blue-labeled neurons are not immunoreactive for either ChAT or galanin (open arrow in C). Reproduced with permission of Elsevier Science Publishers, Amsterdam from Melander et al. (1985): Galanin-like immunoreactivity in cholinergic neurons of the septum-basal forebrain complex projecting to the hippocampus of the rat, *Brain Res.* 360:133. Abbreviation: tdv, tractus diagonalis, ventral part (corresponding to the horizontal limb of the DBB according to the nomenclature of the present chapter). Scale bar: 50 μm.

neuronal (and nonneuronal) targets of cholinergic and GABAergic BFMC axons, as well as of the anatomical relationships of these axons with cholinergic and other receptors on postsynaptic structures. Although the latter is expected to involve laborious electron microscopic methods, labeling of postsynaptic structures will certainly be facilitated by recent progress in the molecular biology/neurobiology of cholinergic receptors, including the advent of monoclonal antibodies (Lindstrom et al., 1987) to localize various types of neuronal cholinergic receptors (Swanson et al., 1987; Levey et al., 1989), and the availability of cDNA probes for muscarinic (Bonner et al., 1987) and nicotinic (Lindstrom et al., 1987) receptors, which have been already used to localize messenger ribonucleic acid (mRNA) for these receptors in the brain by *in situ* hybridization (Buckley et al., 1988; Wada et al., 1989).

Afferent Organization

Although the efferent organization of the BFCS is extremely specific, the system is thought to receive variable and widespread afferents. This condition is not surprising, in view of the position of the BFCS in the course of major fiber systems of the forebrain, including basal longitudinal forebrain bundles, i.e., the medial forebrain bundle (containing dopaminergic mesencephalic axons, noradrenergic fibers from locus coeruleus, and serotoninergic axons mostly from central superior and dorsal raphe nuclei) and the ansa lenticularis; transverse pathways, including the inferior thalamic peduncle, the ventral amygdalofugal pathway and the fornix; commissural pathways, i.e., the anterior commissure; and the internal capsule. The abundance of fiber bundles in the vicinity of the BFCS, although suggestive of highly diverse and rich inputs, imposes formidable difficulties when tract-tracing methods are employed to determine the precise sources of BFCS afferents. Although injection of retrograde axonal tracers (HRP, fluorescent dyes) in the area of the BFCS is the most practical and representative way to map nuclei that innervate the BFCS, the invariable uptake of these tracers by fibers of passage precludes them from yielding conclusive results. Unfortunately, from the extensive literature that deals with inputs to the BFCS, only a moderate number of studies has used anterograde tracer injections in brain areas considered as possible sources of innervation of the BFCS. These experiments have labeled terminal fibers in the area of the BFCS originating from: a limited number of cortical limbic (i.e., piriform cortex) and paralimbic (i.e., orbitofrontal, insular, entorhinal, or prelimbic) areas (Whitlock and Nauta, 1956; Aggleton et al., 1980; Mesulam and Mufson, 1984; Russchen et al., 1985); amygdala (mostly the basolateral complex) (Krettek and Price, 1978; Price and Amaral, 1981; Kelley et al., 1982; Záborszky et al., 1984; Russchen et al., 1985); lateral septum (Swanson and Cowan, 1979); nucleus accumbens (Groenewegen and Russchen, 1984; Mesulam and Mufson, 1984) and dorsal striatum (Grove et al., 1986); a number of hypothalamic nuclei (Conrad and Pfaff, 1976; Saper et al., 1976; Amaral et al., 1982); the substantia nigra/ventral tegmental area (Simon et al., 1979); the peripeduncular nucleus (Jones et al., 1976); the midbrain/pontine/medullary reticular formation (Edwards and deOlmos, 1976; Vertes and Martin, 1988), pedunculopontine and lateral dorsal tegmental nuclei (Semba et al., 1988a); locus coeruleus (Jones and Moore, 1977); and the raphe complex (Azmitia and Segal, 1978; Semba et al., 1988a; Vertes and Martin, 1988). Only a handful of these anterograde tracing studies has used double-labeling methodology to identify the precise targets of the anterogradely labeled terminals in the basal forebrain. In these cases, it has been found, for instance, that *Phaseolus vulgaris* leucoagglutinin (PHA-L)-labeled striatal (Grove et al., 1986), lateral hypothalamic (Záborszky and Cullinan, 1989), and ventral tegmental, peripeduncular, and raphe axons (Grove, 1988) appose cholinergic somata/dendrites of the BFCS. The previous studies are supplemented by an additional small number of experiments employing double-immunohistochemical labeling with ChAT (for cholinergic BFCS neurons) and another enzyme or transmitter antibody representing a catecholaminergic (Záborszky, 1989), peptidergic (Bolam et al., 1986; Chang et al., 1987; Martínez-Murillo et al., 1988), or GABAergic (Záborszky et al., 1986b; Ingham et al., 1988) input. Finally, exceptionally few of the previous inputs to BFCS neurons have been confirmed with electron microscopy, such as: terminals from the lateral septum (Léránth and Frotscher, 1989); amygdala (Záborszky et al., 1984) and lateral hypothalamus (Záborszky and Cullinan, 1989) (Fig. 5); unspecified, presumably striatal, enkephalinergic (Chang et al., 1987; Martínez-Murillo et al., 1988) or substance P-containing (Bolam et al., 1986) terminals; and neuropeptide Y, somatostatin (Záborszky, 1989), or catecholaminergic (Záborszky, 1989) terminals of unknown origin. In addition, most of the ultrastructural studies employing double-transmitter immunohistochemistry, including our own unpublished data (L.J. Martin and V.E. Koliatsos, personal observations), have shown that immunolabeled peptidergic or catecholaminergic terminals also synapse upon noncholinergic dendrites/somata. It appears likely, therefore, that cholinergic and GABAergic projection neurons of the

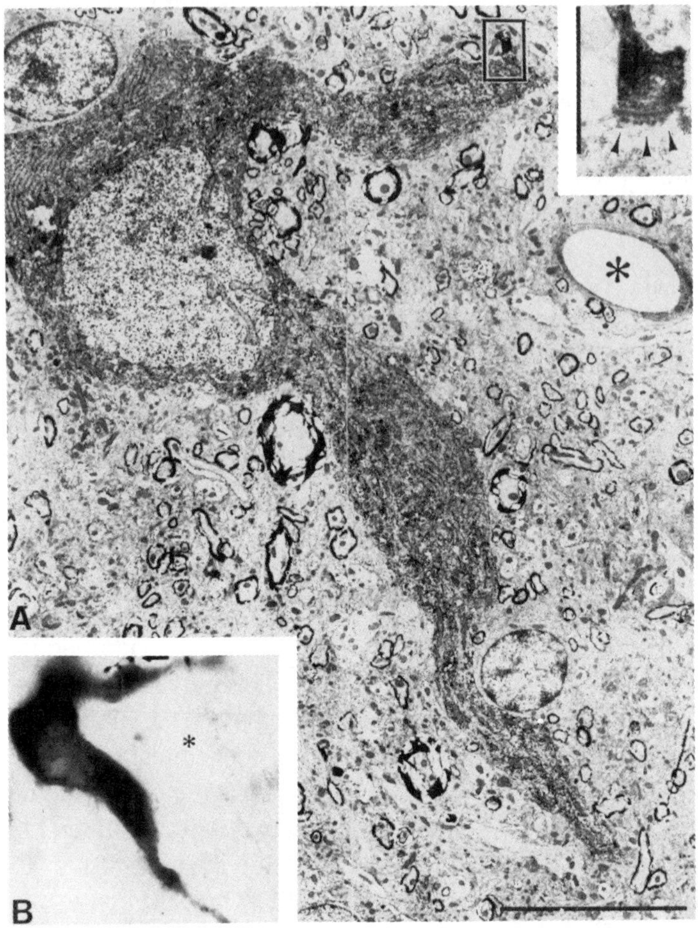

Figure 5. This electron micrograph taken from the intrapallidal sector of the NBM respresents an excellent example of anatomical research aimed at elucidating the transmitter specificity or origins of inputs to individual BFCS neurons. The section was processed with dual-labeling preembedding immunocytochemistry for PHA-L and ChAT. PHA-L had been injected in the lateral hypothalamus and visualized with a nickel ammonium sulfate-intensified diaminobenzidine chromagen reaction. ChAT was visualized with a standard diaminobenzidine procedure. The cell in B represents a light microscope picture of the neuron in A. The arrow indicates a PHA-L terminal synapsing on the cholinergic neuron, which is boxed in A and further magnified in the inset (upper right corner). Arrowheads in inset denote synaptic densities in the BFCS neuron. Scale bars: A = 10 μm; inset = 1 μm. Reproduced with permission of Elsevier Publishers, Amsterdam, from Záborszky and Cullinan (1989): Hypothalamic axons terminate on forebrain cholinergic neurons: an ultrastructural double-labeling study using PHA-L tracing and ChAT immunocytochemistry, *Brain Res.* 479:181.

BFMC are recipients of the same transmitter-specific subcortical inputs to the system (L. Záborszky, personal communication).

Since one cannot predict, at present, the emergence of a new generation of retrograde tracers that will not be taken up by fibers of passage, future studies of afferents to the BFCS will continue to use mostly anterograde tracing strategies from candidate sources of inputs to the BFCS or physiological methods (Semba et al., 1988a). Hopefully, at least some of these studies will continue to determine the precise basal forebrain targets of traced axons with multiple-labeling/ultrastructural approaches.

The BFCS as a Source of Cholinergic Innervation of Cortical Vessels

Several lines of anatomical evidence indicate that cortical microvessels and capillaries may be nonneuronal targets of cholinergic projections arising in the BFCS: cerebral capillaries and endothelial cells bind at equal rates to tritiated quinuclidinyl benzilate (QNB), a ligand for muscarinic sites; in addition, cerebral vessels show moderate levels of ChAT biochemical activity (Estrada et al., 1983). Following PHA-L injections in various components of the BFCS, anterogradely labeled terminals have been shown to appose cortical microvessels by light microscopy (Luiten et al., 1987). At the ultrastructural level, ChAT immunoreactivity has been localized in endothelial cells of brain vessels (Parnavelas et al., 1985). More recent studies measuring cortical blood flow after stimulation of BFCS cells or damage to the BFCS have confirmed the previous evidence and indicated vasodilative effects of the BFCS on cortical vessels. Lesions of the NBM appear to be at least partly responsible for acetylcholine-mediated increases in cortical blood flow as induced by cismethrin (a sodium channel toxin) (Lister and Ray, 1988). Focal electrical stimulation of NBM cells or microinjections of L-glutamate in the NBM increase cerebral blood flow in urethane-anesthetized rats; this response is abolished by muscarinic and nicotinic blockers (Biesold et al., 1989). In a very recent paradigm employing electrical stimulation of the NBM, the primary vasodilative effect was dissociated from a secondary metabolic response with the aid of concomitant measurements of local cerebral blood flow and tissue gas partial pressures; the observed increases in blood flow were potentiated with AChE inhibitors (Lacombe et al., 1989). The previous research has added a new dimension in the possible role of the BFCS in the physiology of the forebrain and may prove to be of some importance in evaluating the role of the BFCS in human disease, including AD.

Functional and Behavioral Implications

Aspects of the anatomical organization of the BFCS have prompted hypotheses about its functional role. For instance, departing from the limbic/paralimbic inputs to the BFCS (conveying, among other things, multisensory information) and the rich innervation of the BFCS by areas such as hypothalamus (containing information associated with motivational states), Mesulam and Mufson (1984) postulated that BFCS neurons are in a unique position to influence the activity of the entire neocortex according to the prevailing motivational state but only when the appropriate stimulus is present. This view is consistent with the physiological experiments of Rolls and associates (Burton et al., 1975, 1976; Mora et al., 1976), who found that BFCS neurons alter their firing rate in relation to the availability of food as well as food preference and state of hunger. The introduction of a multitude of brainstem afferents makes the above picture even more perplexing.

Mishkin and Appenzeller (1987) viewed the BFCS as a major subcortical station for visual recognition memory. According to their schema, the BFCS is one of two relay stations by which visual information, generated in striate/peristriate cortical areas and subsequently forwarded to amygdala/hippocampus via a parietal-inferotemporal-limbic pathway, gains access back to cortex; the other feedback station is the anterior thalamic complex.

We and others have discussed previously that the precise organization of the efferents of the BFCS—in contrast to the organization of other subcortical systems projecting to the cortex, such as locus coeruleus and raphe—suggests that different parts of this system influence information processing in selected and anatomically limited areas of cortex (Koliatsos et al., in press, a). This generalization would predict that the specificity in the efferent organization of the BFCS is accompanied by a similar specificity in the afferents of the system, so that differentially projecting groups of cholinergic basal forebrain cells are influenced by distinct neural systems (Koliatsos and Price, submitted for publication). A potential lateral inhibition within the BFCS, mediated by local collaterals of GABAergic projection neurons, might further enhance the specificity in information flow through the system. The previous notion is supported by physiological studies showing that cortically projecting neurons of the NBM—again, in contrast to cells of locus coeruleus—are markedly heterogeneous in impulse-conduction velocities, spike waveforms, spontaneous activity, and certain sensory-behavioral discharge properties (Aston-Jones et al., 1984, 1985; Grant and Aston-Jones,

1986). Obviously, further anatomical studies employing multiple labeling with antero- and retrograde tracing methods are nessessary to determine the relationship between afferents and efferents in the BFCS. However, the very extensive and variable projection targets of the BFCS make it unlikely that the system will be finally associated with a single function, unless there is considerable local coordination among BFCS cells projecting to different cortical areas.

Some conflicting results generated by behavioral studies may be better understood when viewed from a neuroanatomical perspective. Rhesus monkeys show impairments in visual recognition memory only when the medial septal nucleus-DBB and NBM sectors are concomitantly damaged, suggesting that each of these components of the BFCS is necessary but not sufficient for processing this type of memory (Aigner et al., submitted for publication). In squirrel monkeys, lesions in the NBM are sufficient to produce deficits in the same type of memory (Irle and Markowitsch, 1987). In rats, damage to the NBM produces more severe impairments in a spatial memory task than do lesions of the septal area (Miyamoto et al., 1987). However, in aged rodents, only degeneration in the medial septal nucleus and the nucleus of the DBB correlates at statistically significant levels with impairments in the same spatial memory task (Morris maze) (Fischer et al., 1989). An optimistic interpretation of the above inconsistencies may be that slightly different placements of lesion electrodes in an extremely complex but topographically organized system may entirely alter the implications for different cortical/hippocampal targets, and hence, the behavioral outcomes. Moreover, some of these lesions necessarily impinge upon other interdigitating systems of the basal forebrain with possibly significant roles in complex behavior, such as the ventral pallidum, which projects massively to the mediodorsal thalamic nucleus (Koliatsos et al., in press, a).

MOLECULAR PROCESSES WITHIN THE BFCS

The BFCS Cell as a Cholinergic Neuron

Acetylcholine was the first neurotransmitter to be discovered (Loewi, 1921), and physiological studies of cholinergic transmission on the experimentally accessible neuromuscular junction of vertebrates laid the paradigm for subsequent studies of other neurotransmitters (Fatt and Katz, 1951). Cholinergic neurons are distributed universally in the nervous system of all species of animals, but they differ in their distribution in different species (Mautner, 1977). Following an action potential, a cholinergic neuron releases acetylcholine by exocytosis in the synaptic cleft; acetylcholine then binds to receptors on the postsynaptic membrane, resulting in excitation or inhibition of the postsynaptic cell; this effect is followed by rapid destruction of acetylcholine via enzymatic hydrolysis and the reuptake of choline by its cholinergic terminals. This process involves four highly specific proteins:

- ChAT, which catalyzes the biosynthesis of acetylcholine in a single step by transfering an acetyl group from acetylcoenzyme A to choline;
- Specific cholinergic receptors at the postsynaptic site;
- The hydrolytic enzyme AChE; and
- The choline transport system.

In the following paragraphs, we briefly discuss current issues related to the function and significance of these four proteins.

As discussed previously, the cholinergic phenotype of neurons of the BFCS was determined with certainty through the use of monoclonal antibodies against ChAT in immunohistochemical staining protocols. ChAT was one of the first enzymes in neurobiology to be described (Nachmansohn and Machado, 1943). Although the enzymatic activity of ChAT has been considered one of the rate-limiting steps in the synthesis of acetylcholine (Tuček, 1982), inhibitors of ChAT do not decrease acetylcholine synthesis *in vivo*, an observation that switches the emphasis to the intracellular concentrations of the acetylcholine precursors (see below, end of this passage) (Taylor and Brown, 1989). The substrates for ChAT (choline and acetylCoA) are common cellular components that are being used in other important biochemical pathways as well (e.g., biosynthesis of membrane phospholipids, such as phosphatidylcholine). Their conversion into ACh by ChAT has prompted speculations for increased vulnerability of cholinergic neurons under abnormal metabolic conditions via a process termed "autocannibalism" that employs digestion by the cell of its cell membrane (Wurtman et al., 1990).

The ChAT protein sequence in Drosophila is highly homologous with Torpedo AChE and presents similarities to the binding domain of a neuronal α-type nicotinic receptor from rat (Mori et al., 1987; Salvaterra, 1987). Some of these homologies not only suggest a divergent evolution of cholinergic macromolecules from a common ancestral gene but also point towards domains in the enzyme that may be functionally important. Complementary deoxyribonucleic acid (cDNA) clones encoding the complete sequence of porcine (Berrard et al., 1987), rat (Brice et al., 1989) and *ca.* one-third of the coding region of human (Hersh et al., 1989) ChAT have been isolated.

An interesting issue in the molecular biology of ChAT is the factor(s) that regulates the life-term commitment of a neuron to express ChAT and not another transmitter phenotype. Factors or conditions that can induce, maintain, or alter neurotransmitter phenotype have recently become an intense field of study. Thus far, at least three factors have been isolated that can convert *in vivo* superior cervical ganglion adrenergic neurons to a cholinergic phenotype: an instructive differentiation factor purified from cultured heart cells (cholinergic differentiation factor [CDF]) (Fukada, 1985); ciliary neurotrophic factor (CNTF) from rat sciatic nerve (Saadat et al., 1989), and membrane-associated neurotransmitter induction substance (MANS) from rat spinal cord (Wong and Kessler, 1987). CDF is biochemically different from CNTF and MANS (Rao et al., 1989). It is anticipated that production of larger amounts of these purified factors, used in conjunction with available probes for ChAT mRNA, will elucidate molecular mechanisms of neurotransmitter phenotype expression. Such strategies may also provide an additional, more easy-to-manipulate source of cholinergic neurons for grafts into desirable targets in adult brain (Mahanthappa et al., in press). Another focus of intense current interest is the production of immortal cholinergic cell lines for use either as transplants or for further studies of the biology of the cholinergic neuron (Hammond et al., 1986).

Cholinergic receptors were originally classified as muscarinic and nicotinic on the basis of resemblance of acetylcholine effects to those of naturally occurring alcaloids. Both types of receptors are found in the central nervous system and have been further subclassified with the aid of various synthetic ligands (Taylor, 1985; Hammer et al., 1989). Recently, various cholinergic receptors have been characterized biochemically (Lindstrom et al., 1987; Nathanson, 1987; Haga et al., 1988) and their respective cDNAs have been cloned and sequenced (Boulter et al., 1986; Bonner et al., 1987; Peralta et al., 1988). Currently, there are five known genes coding for muscarinic receptors and seven genes coding for nicotinic receptors. This development opens the transition from the pharmacological to the molecular era of the central cholinergic synapse. Although some relationships between receptor subtypes defined with the two methods of classification have been clarified (e.g., the pharmacologically defined M_2 receptor corresponds to the m_2 muscarinic receptor protein), overall patterns appear to be very complex

(McCormick, 1989).

AChE, concentrated at both pre- and postsynaptic sites of cholinergic transmission, has one of the highest turnover rates of any mammalian enzyme (approximately 80 μsec) (Koelle, 1987). Therefore, following the activation of a postsynaptic receptor by acetylcholine, the transmitter concentration can be reduced to subeffective levels within a fraction of a millisecond. The structure, mechanisms of action, and subcellular distribution of AChE are known in great detail, and excellent reviews are available (e.g., Koelle, 1963, 1987; Massoulié and Bon, 1982). Agents that bind AChE (anticholinesterases) occupy a significant position in cholinergic pharmacology both as toxic compounds (i.e., organophosphates, which irreversibly bind AChE) and therapeutic substances, used in a variety of disorders from bladder dysfunction to myasthenia gravis. The introduction of a new generation of anticholinesterases as enhancers of cholinergic transmission in the targets of the BFCS has elevated hopes for ameliorating some of the memory deficits associated with AD (for review, see Growdon, in press).

The choline transport system, called the sodium-dependent high-affinity choline uptake (SDHACU) system, is located at cholinergic terminals and is an exclusive feature of the cholinergic neuron, whereas a low-affinity choline uptake mechanism is present in all tissues (Taylor and Brown, 1989). The SDHACU system concentrates choline from a low level in the extracellular fluid to a value several magnitudes higher in the axonal cytoplasm and is also linked to acetylcholine release (Taylor and Brown, 1989). Blocking of SDHACU system by hemicholinium-3 greatly decreases acetylcholine synthesis and release (Jope, 1979), an observation suggesting that choline uptake is the major rate-limiting factor in the biosynthesis of acetylcholine.

The BFCS Cell as a Target for a Prototypical Trophic Factor

In the early 1980s, it was discovered (Honneger and Lenoir, 1982; Gnahn et al., 1983) that cultured embryonic BFCS cells increase ChAT production in the presence of a peptide, introduced 30 years earlier as a trophic ("nourishing," "feeding") agent for peripheral sensory and sympathetic embryonic neurons (Levi-Montalcini and Hamburger, 1951, 1953) and subsequently widely hailed as the prototypical trophic factor (Levi-Montalcini, 1987; Snider and Johnson, 1989). This peptide is the nerve growth factor (NGF), a dimer comprised of two identical subunits, each with 118 amino acids and a molecular weight of 13.25 kiloDaltons (Angeletti and Bradshaw, 1971). cells of the BFCS, together with the cholinergic interneurons of the striatum (Mobley et al., 1985) are the main targets of NGF actions in the central nervous system. The discovery of these forebrain cholinergic targets of NGF was serendipitous, since initial investigations had predicted that the central catecholaminergic neurons would be the brain responders to NGF, as are their counterparts in the peripheral nervous system (Schwab et al., 1979).

During the last few years, a considerable body of information has been generated dealing with actions of NGF on BFCS neurons. It is now known that BFCS neurons express NGF receptor mRNA (Schatteman et al., 1988; Higgins and Mufson, 1989; Koh et al., 1989) (Fig. 6) and protein (Hcfti

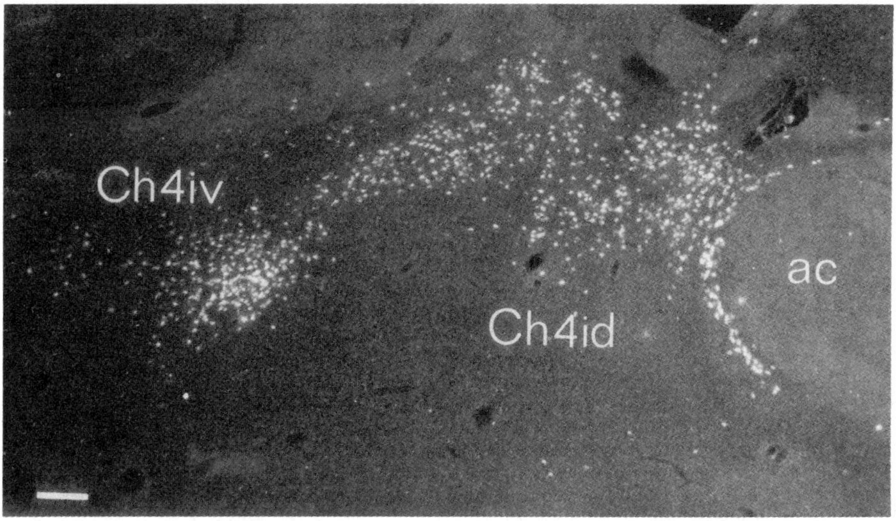

Figure 6. A recent trend in research on the BFCS utilizes molecular biological methods to address issues of normal phenotype and plasticity of BFCS neurons. This *in situ* hybridization preparation from the human brain utilized a [^{35}S]-labeled RNA probe, hydrolyzed to 100-nucleotide fragments, for the localization of NGF receptor transcripts in the NBM. Abbreviations: ac, anterior commissure; Ch4iv, intermedioventral component of cholinergic neurons in the NBM (Mesulam nomenclature); Ch4id, intermediodorsal component of cholinergic neurons in the NBM. Scale bar: 250 μm. Reproduced with permission of Academic Press, Orlando, from Higgins and Mufson (1989): NGF receptor gene expression is decreased in the nucleus basalis in Alzheimer's disease, *Exp. Neurol.* 106:226.

et al., 1986; Kordower et al., 1988; Schatteman et al., 1988; Koh et al., 1989), whereas their target cells in neocortex and hippocampus (e.g., pyramidal cells in Ammon's horn and granule cells in the dentate gyrus) appear to be the main sites of NGF mRNA and protein production in the central nervous system (Korsching et al., 1985; Shelton and Reichardt, 1986; Ayer-LeLievre et al., 1988). NGF is taken up by high-affinity receptors on terminals and transported retrogradely to the cell body (Seiler and Schwab, 1984), where it has a number of actions, including apparent enhancement of cell viability. Injections of NGF into the ventricles of developing rodents cause BFCS neurons to increase ChAT activity (Mobley et al., 1986) and to express several genes, including those coding for the prion protein and amyloid precursor protein (Mobley et al., 1988). Following nerve injury, treatment with NGF (Hefti, 1986; Williams et al., 1986; Kromer, 1987; Gage et al., 1988; Koliatsos et al., in press, b; Koliatsos et al., submitted for publication; Whittemore et al., 1989) or with implanted NGF-engineered cells (Rosenberg et al., 1988; Stromberg et al., 1990) prevents degenerative changes in BFCS neurons. NGF treatment may partially restore innervation of deafferented terminal fields (Haroutunian et al., 1986) and may, at least transiently, ameliorate behavioral deficits associated with these lesions (Will and Hefti, 1985). Moreover, NGF has been reported to have effects on age-associated deficits in behaviors dependent on the septohippocampal circuit (Fischer et al., 1987), perhaps by ameliorating degenerative changes that occur in BFCS neurons. Thus, in both the axotomy and aging paradigms, NGF seems to partially reverse abnormalities associated with alterations in cholinergic neurons. More recently, it has been shown that primate BFCS neurons also respond to NGF (Koliatsos et al., in press, b) (Fig. 7). This finding is consistent with the fact that the amino acid sequence of NGF, including one hydrophilic domain that may have a role in mediating NGF binding to its receptor, is highly conserved (Angeletti and Bradshaw, 1971; Dunbar et al., 1984; Meier et al., 1986). NGF receptors are also highly conserved in evolution (Johnson et al., 1986) and are present on primate BFCS neurons (Hefti et al., 1986; Kordower et al., 1988; Schatteman et al., 1988; Higgins and Mufson, 1989). Although the efficacy of these trophic influences on noncholinergic cells of the BFMC needs to be clarified further, these recent findings are interesting for a number of reasons. First, they indicate that patterns of NGF (and possibly other trophic factor)-mediated influences remain essentially the same, regardless of brain complexity. Second, slight interspecies differences in the NGF molecule or its receptor do

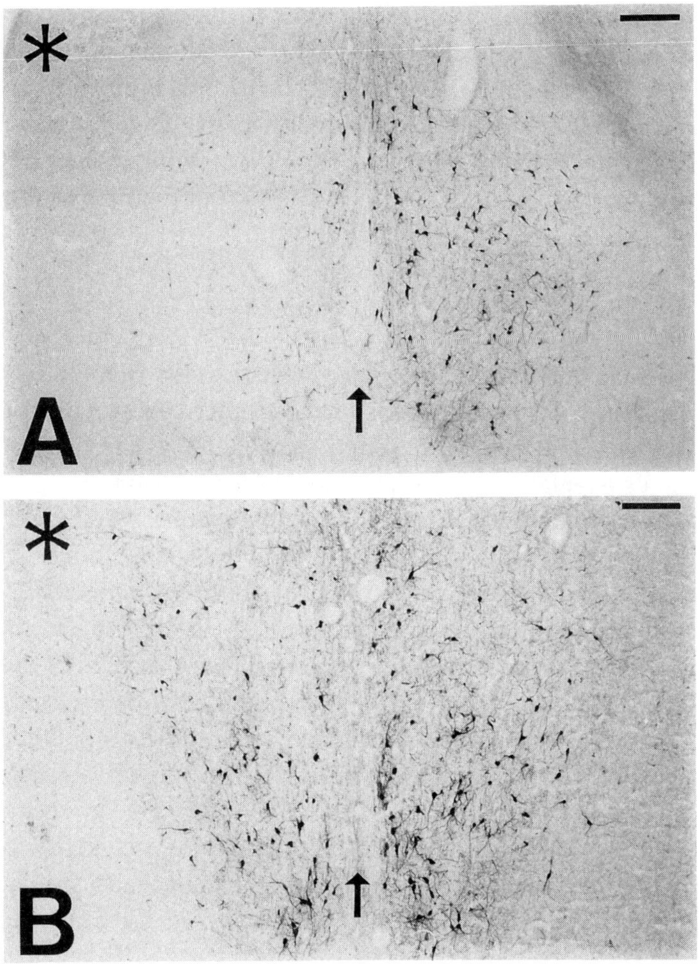

Figure 7. Of potential importance is the possibility of treating experimentally induced or age-associated abnormalities in the BFCS using NGF. In the case illustrated above, macaques were subjected to a unilateral transection of the fornix. This lesion results in a profound down-regulation of ChAT in BFCS neurons located in the medial septal nucleus (A), an abnormality almost entirely restored by intraventricular treatment of these animals with mouse NGF (B). This axotomy-induced pathology has similarities with the neuropathology of AD and is summarized in alterations in transmitter phenotype and morphology in otherwise surviving neurons (Candy et al., 1983). These primate experiments set the stage for future applications of trophic factors in naturally occurring animal or human diseases associated with dysfunction of transmitter-specific populations of neurons. Asterisk indicates lesioned side. Arrow indicates midline. Scale bars: 200 μm.

not influence the responsiveness of neurons to NGF. Third, NGF therapy may have benefits for aged, behaviorally impaired nonhuman primates (Price et al., in press). Finally, if NGF proves effective and nontoxic when chronically administered in monkeys, all the conditions will have been met (Phelps et al., 1989) for considering a trial for NGF therapy in patients with AD, a subject group that shows consistent degeneration of neurons in the BFCS.

CONCLUDING REMARKS

The lengthy—and continuing—effort to understand the BFCS has, in a way, followed the course of investigations of most other cell groups in the brain and other organs. The parallel description of the BFCS from both a topographic and a systematic vantage point represents a good example; the topographic approach dominated in the initial phases of research on the BFCS and its more recent immunocytochemical ramifications (exemplified by the "Ch" nomenclature of Mesulam and colleagues (Mesulam et al., 1983a,b; Mesulam and Geula, 1988) are commonly used in current descriptions of the system. Such approaches are not only useful for purposes of description but may also have functional significance, especially in a system that, at least with respect to its efferents, maintains a fairly strict topographic organization; in most cases, location in the BFCS also implies a specific target in cortex or amygdala. On the other hand, as discussed in the section on the anatomical organization of the BFCS, projections of the system cover the whole cortical mantle and a few subcortical telencephalic structures, and it is quite unlikely that all these projections are associated with a single function. The situation may be analogous to striatum or thalamus structures which, as a whole, are not associated with any particular function. Instead, individual components of both brain areas derive functional specificity from the different cortico-subcortical circuits relayed in these components (e.g., neostriatum; Alexander et al., 1986). Naturally, such structural-functional correlations can hold in systems that maintain a high degree of topographic organization in their afferent-efferent circuitry. In the case of the BFCS, the only part of the subcortico-cortical circuits relayed in the system that is known with certainty to be specific is the projection of BFCS to cortex. Information on the afferents of the system is not sufficient to indicate the degree of specificity in the origins of these inputs or the selectivity in target cells of the BFCS. Also, investigations of the local circuits operating within the BFMC have not yielded definitive answers on the degree or patterns of integration among different types of cells or different cell groups within the BFMC/BFCS. A comparison between afferent and efferent organization and the local circuitry of the BFMC/BFCS will help to clarify whether the BFCS is a telencephalic version of a diffuse ascending system that modulates the state of information processing in the telencephalon (such as midline thalamic nuclei) (Mesulam, 1985; Saper, 1987) or whether it affects the very content of information processing by relaying specific signals through appropriate channels (such as specific thalamic nuclei) (Fig. 8).

The contributions of the neurotransmitter era in neurobiology in the late 1970s, which gave a new thrust to investigations of the BFCS, also relate to the questions discussed above. The discovery of the cholinergic nature

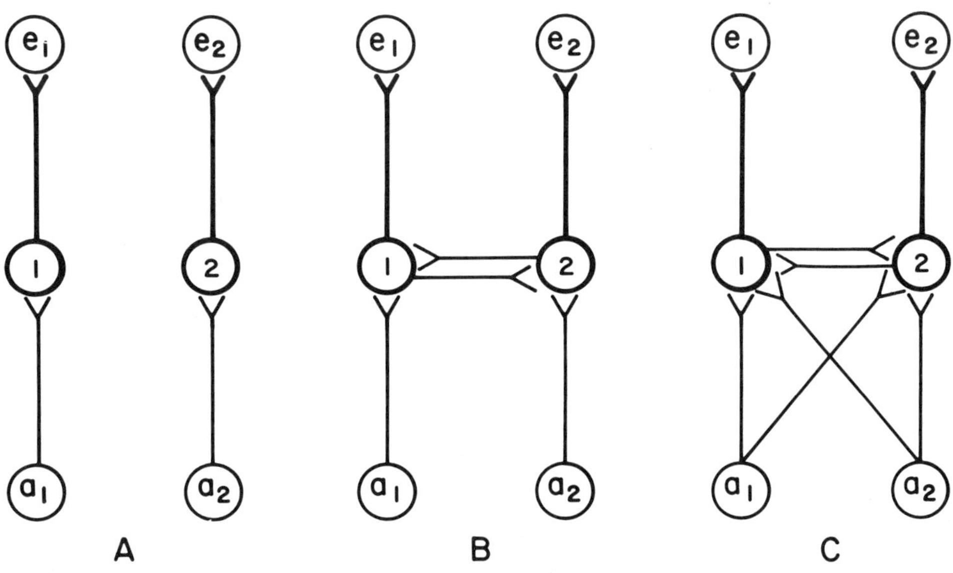

Figure 8. A better understanding of the relationship between afferents/efferents and local circuitry within the BFCS will assist in a fuller functional characterization of the system. This schematic diagram depicts three hypothetical scenarios (A,B,C) of the relationships of two representative BFCS sectors (1 and 2) with their afferent (a) and efferent (e) connections, as well as between themselves. The variable factor is the degree of crosstalking between the two lines of information flow mediated via BFCS sectors 1 and 2. Based on existing data, the organization depicted in scenario A is rather unlikely, and there is little support for scenario C. Most of the anatomical/physiological evidence is consistent with the circuitry depicted in scenario B.

of the BFCS and the prominent role of cholinergic transmission in limbic/paralimbic brain areas explained, among other things, the effects of anticholinergic drugs on complex behavior (i.e., memory) and suggested a pharmacological method to manipulate the physiology of the BFCS. However, it is not clear whether the importance of cholinergic neurotransmission for memory derives from the "memory"-relevant information conveyed by the BFCS (Mishkin and Appenzeller, 1987). An alternative explanation could be that hippocampus and paralimbic cortex, structures very important for memory, are more dependent upon their cholinergic inputs, which are particularly dense, than, for example, the occipital cortex, which receives sparse cholinergic innervation. In more general terms, transmitter-defined systems in the brain do not necessarily coincide with functionally defined systems (for example, refer to the multifunctional roles attributed to the noradrenergic projections originating from locus coeruleus (Amaral and Sinnamon, 1977)). Moreover, there is no reason to believe that there should be any underlying relationship between a functional system and the set of neurotransmitters it employs (Björklund et al., 1989). Attempts to establish one-to-one correlations between neurobiological processes at different levels of complexity (behavior, function, pathways/circuits, cells, molecules) have been rewarded mainly in simple vertebrate systems (Hawkins et al., 1987). Mammalian central nervous systems are much more complex. However, this complexity should not discourage further efforts to understand the functional role(s) of the BFCS. For example, in the area of neuroanatomy, more work is needed before a model circuit is constructed to encompass the major inputs and outputs of the BFCS as well as local cell interactions. Since it is likely that the BFCS will be found to participate in a variety of diverse functions in the brain, a more profound understanding of its anatomical organization might further illuminate its functional roles (as has been the case, for example, with thalamus and basal ganglia). At the same time, integration should be attempted between disciplines in neuroscience that directly complement each other, such as physiology and anatomy or anatomy and cellular/molecular biology. An example of an integrated view of the BFCS utilizing data from its circuitry as well as its cellular and molecular biology is shown in Fig. 9. The strength of multiple complementary approaches to the study of complex systems, such as the BFCS, lies not only in that these strategies result in its fuller characterization but also in that they permit more specific correlations to be made between individual features of the

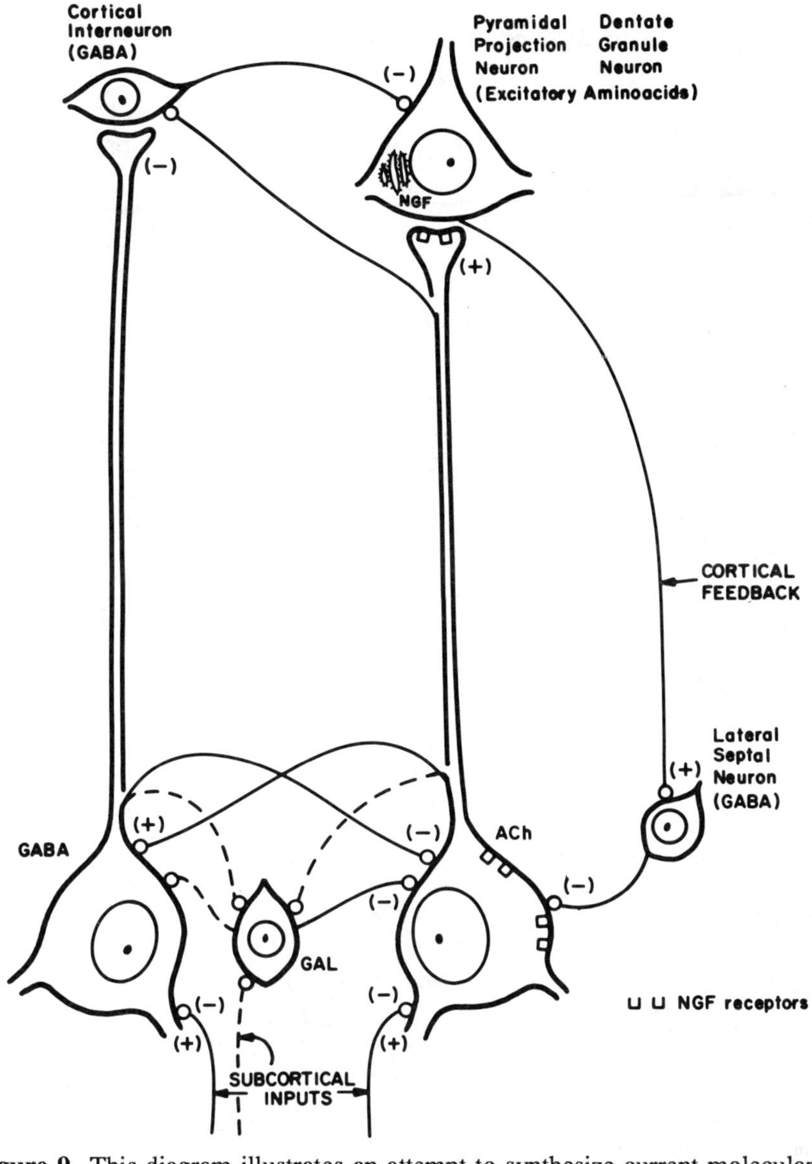

Figure 9. This diagram illustrates an attempt to synthesize current molecular, anatomical, and physiological information into a circuit diagram of the BFMC/BFCS. Key cells in this diagram are the cholinergic and GABAergic projection neurons and their putative targets in cortex (including hippocampus). Signs indicate physiological polarities (excitation or inhibition), and dashed lines suggest likely, but as yet unproven, connections. For the GABAergic neuron, a target-derived neurotrophic factor has not yet been identified.

BFCS as disclosed with different methodologies. For instance, there may be a very specific association between cholinergic phenotype in the BFCS and responsiveness to NGF (Koliatsos et al., in press, b). This and other potential associations may reveal underlying rules of neurobiological organization, hopefully leading to a more fundamental understanding of the BFCS in the not-so-distant future.

ACKNOWLEDGMENTS

The authors thank Doctors Lary C. Walker and Russell T. Richardson for their inputs on the manuscript and Dr. Gunnar Gouras for his assistance in the extensive reviews of the German literature.

This work was supported by grants from the U.S. Public Health Service (NIH NS 20471, AG 04146, AG 03359, and NS 07179). D.L. Price is the recipient of a Javits Neuroscience Investigator Award (NIH NS 10580) and a Leadership and Excellence in Alzheimer's Disease (LEAD) award (NIA AG 07914). This work is also supported by The Robert L. & Clara G. Patterson Trust, The Metropolitan Life Foundation, and the American Health Assistance Foundation.

REFERENCES

Aggleton, J.P., Burton, M.J. and Passingham, R.E. (1980): Cortical and subcortical afferents to the amygdala of the rhesus monkey (*Macaca mulatta*). *Brain Res.* 190:347-368

Agid, Y., Javoy-Agid, F., Ruberg, M., Pillon, B., Dubois, B., Duyckaerts, C., Hauw, J.-J., Baron, J.-C, and Scatton, B. (1986): Progressive supranuclear palsy: anatomo-clinical and biochemical considerations. In: *Parkinson's Disease: Advances in Neurology, Vol. 45*. Yahr, M.D., Bergmann, K.J., eds. New York: Raven Press

Aigner, T.G., Mitchell, S.J., Aggleton, J.P., DeLong, M.R., Struble, R.G., Price, D.L., Wenk, G.L., Pettigrew, K.D. and Mishkin, M. (submitted for publication): Transient impairment of recognition memory following ibotenic-acid lesions of the basal forebrain in macaques

Alexander, G.E., DeLong, M.R. and Strick, P.L. (1986): Parallel organization of functionally segregated circuits linking basal ganglia and cortex. *Ann. Rev. Neurosci.* 9:357-381

Alheid, G.F. and Heimer, L. (1988): New perspectives in basal forebrain organization of special relevance for neuropsychiatric disorders: the striatopallidal, amygdaloid, and corticopetal components of substantia innominata. *Neurosci.* 27:1-39

Allen, S.J., Dawbarn, D. and Wilcock, G.K. (1988): Morphometric immunochemical analysis of neurons in the nucleus basalis of Meynert in Alzheimer's disease. *Brain Res.* 454:275-281

Amaral, D.G. and Kurz, J. (1985): An analysis of the origins of the cholinergic and noncholinergic septal projections to the hippocampal formation of the rat. *J. Comp. Neurol.* 240:37-59

Amaral, D.G. and Sinnamon, H.M. (1977): The locus coeruleus: neurobiology of a central noradrenergic nucleus. *Prog. Neuropathol.* 9:147-196

Amaral, D.G., Veazey, R.B. and Cowan, W.M. (1982): Some observations on hypothalamo-amygdaloid connections in the monkey. *Brain Res.* 252:13-27

Andy, O.J. and Stephan, H. (1959): The nuclear configuration of the septum of Galago demidovii. *J. Comp. Neurol.* 111:503-546

Andy, O.J. and Stephan, H. (1961): Septal nuclei in the Soricidae (insectivores): cytoarchitectonic study. *J. Comp. Neurol.* 117:251-274

Andy, O.J. and Stephan, H. (1966): Septal nuclei in primate phylogeny: a quantitative investigation. *J. Comp. Neurol.* 126:157-170

Andy, O.J. and Stephan, H. (1968): The septum in the human brain. *J. Comp. Neurol.* 133:383-410

Angeletti, R.H. and Bradshaw, R.A. (1971): Nerve growth factor from mouse submaxillary gland: amino acid sequence. *Proc. Natl. Acad. Sci. USA* 68:2417-2420

Arenberg, D. (1990): Longitudinal changes in cognitive performance. In: *Alzheimer's Disease: Advances in Neurology, Vol. 51.* Wurtman, R. J., Corkin, S., Growdon, J. H., Ritter-Walker, E., eds. New York: Raven Press

Arendt, T., Bigl, V., Arendt, A. and Tennstedt, A. (1983): Loss of neurons in the nucleus basalis of Meynert in Alzheimer's disease, paralysis agitans, and Korsakoff's disease. *Acta Neuropathol.* (Berl.) 61:101-108

Arendt, T., Zvegintseva, H.G. and Leontovich, T.A. (1986): Dendritic changes in the basal nucleus of Meynert and in the diagonal band nucleus in Alzheimer's disease a quantitative Golgi investigation. *Neurosci.* 19:1265-1278

Ashton, H. (1987): *Brain Systems, Disorders, and Psychotropic Drugs.* Oxford: Oxford University Press

Aston-Jones, G., Rogers, J., Grant, S., Ennis, M., Shaver, R. and Bartus, R. (1984): Physiology of cortically projecting neurons in monkey nucleus basalis of Meynert. *Soc. Neurosci. Abstr.* 10:808

Aston-Jones, G., Shaver, R. and Dinan, T.G. (1985): Nucleus basalis neurons exhibit axonal branching with decreased impulse conduction velocity in rat cerebrocortex. *Brain Res.* 325:271-285

Ayer-LeLievre, C., Olson, L., Ebendal, T., Seiger, A. and Persson, H. (1988): Expression of the β-nerve growth factor gene in hippocampal neurons. *Science* 240:1339-1341

Ayala, G. (1915): A hitherto undifferentiated nucleus in the forebrain (nucleus subputaminalis). *Brain* 37:433-448

Azmitia, E.C. and Segal, M. (1978): An autoradiographic analysis of the differential ascending projections of the dorsal and median raphe nuclei in the rat. *J. Comp. Neurol.* 179: 641-668

Bartus, R.T., Dean, R.L. and Fisher, S.K. (1986): Cholinergic treatment for age-related memory disturbances. In: *Treatment Development Strategies for Alzheimer's Disease.* Crook, T., Bartus, R. T., Ferris, S., Gershon, S., eds. Madison, Connecticut: Mark Powley Associates

Bayer, S.A. (1985): Neurogenesis of the magnocellular basal telencephalic nuclei in the rat. *Int. Dev. Neurosci.* 3:229-243

Beccari, N. (1911): La sostanza perforata anteriore e i suoi rapporti col rinencefalo mel cervello dell'uomo. *Arch. Ital. Anat. Embriol.* 10:261-328

Benardo, L.S. and Prince, D.A. (1982): Cholinergic excitation of mammalian hippocampal pyramidal cells. *Brain Res.* 249:315-331

Berrard, S., Brice, A., Lottspeich, F., Braun, A., Barde, Y.-A. and Mallet, J. (1987): cDNA cloning and complete sequence of porcine choline acetyltransferase: *in vitro* translation of the corresponding RNA yields an active protein. *Proc. Natl. Acad. Sci. USA* 84:9280-9284

Bialowas, J. and Frotscher, M. (1987): Choline acetyltransferase-immunoreactive neurons and terminals in the rat septal complex: a combined light and electron microscopic study. *J. Comp. Neurol.* 259:298-307

Biesold, D., Inanami, O., Sato, A. and Sato, Y. (1989): Stimulation of the nucleus basalis of Meynert increases cerebral cortical blood flow in rats. *Neurosci. Lett.* 98:39-44

Bigl, V., Woolf, N.J. and Butcher, L.L. (1982): Cholinergic projections from the basal forebrain to frontal, parietal, temporal, occipital, and cingulate cortices: a combined fluorescent tracer and acetylcholinesterase analysis. *Brain Res. Bull.* 8:727-749

Bird, S.J .and Aghajanian, G.K. (1976): The cholinergic pharmacology of hippocampal pyramidal cells: a microiontophoretic study. *Neuropharmacol.* 15: 273-282

Björklund, A., Hökfelt, T. and Swanson, L.W. (1987): Preface. In: *Integrated Systems of the CNS, Part I, Hypothalamus, Hippocampus, Amygala, Retina; Handbook of Chemical Neuroanatomy, Vol 5.* Björklund, A., Hökfelt, T. and Swanson, L.W., eds. Amsterdam: Elsevier

Blessed, G., Tomlinson, B.E. and Roth, M. (1968): The association between quantitative measures of dementia and of senile change in the cerebral grey matter of elderly subjects. *Br. J. Psych.* 114:797-811

Bolam, J.P., Ingham, C.A., Izzo, P.N., Levey, A.I., Rye, D.B., Smith, A.D. and Wainer, B.H. (1986): Substance P-containing terminals in synaptic contact with cholinergic neurons in the neostriatum and basal forebrain: a double immunocytochemical study in the rat. *Brain Res.* 397:279-289

Bonner, T.I., Buckley, N.J., Young, A.C. and Brann, M.R. (1987): Identification of a family of muscarinic acetylcholine receptor genes. *Science* 237:527-532

Boulter, J., Evans, K., Goldman, D., Martin, G., Treco, D., Heinemann, S. and Patrick, J. (1986): Isolation of a cDNA clone coding for a possible neural nicotinic acetylcholine receptor subunit. *Nature* 319:368-374

Bowen, D.M., Smith, C.B., White, P. and Davison, A.N. (1976): Neurotransmitter-related enzymes and indices of hypoxia in senile dementia and other abiotrophies. *Brain* 99:459-496

Brashear, H. R., Záborszky, L. and Heimer, L. (1986): Distribution of GABAergic and cholinergic neurons in the rat diagonal band. *Neurosci.* 17:439-451

Brice, A., Berrard, S., Raynaud, B., Ansieau, S., Coppola, T., Weber, M.J. and Mallet, J. (1989): Complete sequence of a cDNA encoding an active rat choline acetyltransferase: a tool to investigate the plasticity of cholinergic phenotype expression. *J. Neurosci. Res.* 23:266-273

Brockhaus, H. (1942): Vergleichend-anatomische Untersuchungen über den Basalkerncomplex. *J. Psychol. Neurol.* 51:57-95

Buckley, N.J., Bonner, T.I. and Brann, M.R. (1988): Localization of a family of muscarinic receptor mRNAs in rat brain. *J. Neurosci.* 8:4646-4652

Burton, M.J., Mora, F. and Rolls, E.T. (1975): Visual and taste neurones in the lateral hypothalamus and substantia innominata: modulation of responsiveness by hunger. *Exp. J. Physiol.* (Lond.) 252:50P-51P

Burton, M.J., Rolls, E.T., and Mora, F. (1976): Effects of hunger on the responses of neurons in the lateral hypothalamus to the sight and taste of food. *Exp. Neurol.* 51:668-677

Butcher, L.L. and Semba, K. (1989): Reassessing the cholinergic basal forebrain: nomenclature schemata and concepts. *Trends Neurosci.* 12:483-485

Butcher, L.L. and Talbot, K. (1978): Acetylcholinesterase in rat nigro-neostriatal neurons: experimental verification and evidence for cholinergic-dopaminergic interactions in the substantia nigra and caudate-putamen complex. In: *Cholinergic-Monoaminergic Interactions in the Brain.* Butcher, L.L., ed. New York: Academic Press

Butcher, L. and Woolf, N.J. (1984): Histochemical distribution of acetylcholinesterase in the central nervous system: clues to the localization of cholinergic neurons. In: *Classical Transmitters in the CNS, Part II. Handbook of Chemical Neuroanatomy, Vol. 3.* Björklund, A., Hökfelt, T. and Kuhar, M.J., eds. Amsterdam: Elsevier

Butcher, L. L., Talbot, K. and Bilezikjian, L. (1975): Acetylcholinesterase neurons in dopamine-containing regions of the brain. *J. Neurol. Transm.* 37:127-153

Buzsáki, G., Bickford, R.G., Ponomareff, G., Thal, L.J., Mandel, R. and Gage, F.H. (1988): Nucleus basalis and thalamic control of neocortical activity in the freely moving rat. *J. Neurosci.* 8:4007-4026

Candy, J.M., Perry, R.H., Perry, E.K., Irving, D., Blessed, G., Fairbairn, A.F. and Tomlinson, B.E. (1983): Pathological changes in the nucleus of Meynert in Alzheimer's and Parkinson's diseases. *J. Neurol. Sci.* 59:277-289

Carlsen, J., Záborszky, L. and Heimer, L. (1985): Cholinergic projections from the basal forebrain to the basolateral amygdaloid complex: a combined retrograde fluorescent and immunohistochemical study. *J. Comp. Neurol.* 234: 155-167

Casamenti, F., Deffenu, G., Abbamondi, A.L. and Pepeu, G. (1986): Changes in cortical acetylcholine output induced by modulation of the nucleus basalis. *Brain Res. Bull.* 16:689-695

Casanova, M.F., Walker, L.C., Whitehouse, P.J. and Price, D.L. (1985): Abnormalities of the nucleus basalis in Down's syndrome. *Ann. Neurol.* 18:310-313

Celesia, G.G. and Jasper, H.H. (1966): Acetylcholine released from cerebral cortex in relation to state of activation. *Neurol.* 16:1053-1070

Chan-Palay, V. (1988a): Galanin hyperinnervates surviving neurons of the human basal nucleus of Meynert in dementias of Alzheimer's and Parkinson's disease: a hypothesis for the role of galanin in accentuating cholinergic dysfunction in dementia. *J. Comp. Neurol.* 273:543-557

Chan-Palay, V. (1988b): Neurons with galanin innervate cholinergic cells in the human basal forebrain and galanin and acetylcholine coexist. *Brain Res. Bull.* 21:465-472

Chang, H.T., Penny, G.R. and Kitai, S.T. (1987): Enkephalinergic-cholinergic interaction in the rat globus pallidus: a pre-embedding double-labeling immunocytochemistry study. *Brain Res.* 426:197-203

Cole, A.E. and Nicoll, R.A. (1984): Characterization of a slow cholinergic postsynaptic potential recorded *in vitro* from rat hippocampal pyramidal cells. *J. Physiol.* 352:173-188

Collingridge, G.L., Herron, C.E. and Lester, R.A.J. (1988): Synaptic activation of N-methyl-D-aspartate receptors in the Schaffer collateral-commissural pathway of rat hippocampus. *J. Physiol.* 399:283-300

Conrad, L.C.A. and Pfaff, D.W. (1976): Efferents from medial basal forebrain and hypothalamus in the rat. I. An autoradiographic study of the medial preoptic area. *J. Comp. Neurol.* 169:185-220

Crawford, G.D., Correa, L. and Salvaterra, P.M. (1982): Interaction of monoclonal antibodies with mammalian choline acetyltransferase. *Proc. Natl. Acad. Sci. USA* 79:7031-7040

Das, G.D. (1971): Projections of the interstitial nerve cells surrounding the globus pallidus: a study of retrograde changes following cortical ablations in rabbits. *Z. Anat. Entwick-Gesch.* 41:135-160

Das, G.D. and Kreutzberg, G.W. (1968): Evaluation of interstitial nerve cells in the central nervous system: a correlative study using acetylcholinesterase and Golgi techniques. *Ergebu. Anat. EntwGesch.* 41:1-58

Davies, P. (1979): Neurotransmitter-related enzymes in senile dementia of the

Alzheimer type. *Brain Res.* 171:319-327

DeLong, M.R. (1971): Activity of pallidal neurons during movement. *J. Neurophysiol.* 34:414-427

de Olmos, J. and Heimer, L. (1980): Double and triple labeling of neurons with fluorescent substances: the study of collateral pathways in the ascending raphe system. *Neurosci. Lett.* 19:7-12

Detárí, L. and Vanderwolf, C.H. (1987): Activity of identified cortically projecting and other basal forebrain neurones during large slow waves and cortical activation in anaesthetized rats. *Brain Res.* 437:1-8

Deutsch, J. A. (1971): The cholinergic synapse and the site of memory. *Science* 174:788-794

Dinopoulos, A., Parnavelas, J.G. and Eckenstein, F. (1986): Morphological characterization of cholinergic neurons in the horizontal limb of the diagonal band of Broca in the basal forebrain of the rat. *J. Neurocytol.* 15:619-628

Divac, I. (1981): Cortical projections of the magnocellular nuclei of the basal forebrain: a reinvestigation. *Neurosci.* 6:983-984

Divac, I. (1975): Magnocellular nuclei of the basal forebrain project to neocortex, brain stem, and olfactory bulb. Review of some functional correlates. *Brain Res.* 93:385-398

Drachman, D.A. and Leavitt, J.L. (1974): Human memory and the cholinergic system. A relationship to aging? *Arch. Neurol.* 30:113-121

Dunbar, J.C., Tregear, G.W. and Bradshaw, R.A. (1984): Histidine residue modification inhibits binding of murine nerve growth factor to its receptor. *J. Protein. Chem.* 3:349-356

Eckenstein, F. and Thoenen, H. (1983): Cholinergic neurons in the rat cerebral cortex demonstrated by immunohistochemical localization of choline acetyltransferase. *Neurosci. Lett.* 36:211-215

Edwards, S.B. and de Olmos, J.S. (1976): Autoradiographic studies of the projections of the midbrain reticular formation: ascending projections of nucleus cuneiformis. *J. Comp. Neurol.* 165:417-432

Estrada, C., Hamel, E. and Krause, D.N. (1983): Biochemical evidence for cholinergic innervation of intracerebral blood vessels. *Brain Res.* 266:261-270

Fallon, J.H. and Loughlin, S.E. (1982): Monoamine innervation of the forebrain: collateralization. *Brain Res. Bull.* 9:295-307

Fatt, P. and Katz, B. (1951): An analysis of the end-plate potential recorded with an intra-cellular electrode. *J. Physiol.* 115:320-370

Feremutsch, K. (1961): Basalganglien. In: *Primatologia. Handbuch der Primatenkunde, Lieferung 8, Vol. 2.* Hofer, H., Schultz, A. H., Starck, D., eds. Basel: S. Karger

Fischer, W., Gage, F.H. and Björklund, A. (1989): Degenerative changes in forebrain cholinergic nuclei correlate with cognitive impairments in aged rats. *Eur. J. Neurosci.* 1:34-45

Fischer, W., Wictorin, K., Björklund, A., Williams, L.R., Varon, S. and Gage, F.H. (1987): Amelioration of cholinergic neuron atrophy and spatial memory impairment in aged rats by nerve growth factor. *Nature* 329:65-68

Foix, C.E. and Nicolesco, J. (1925): Anatomie Cerebrale. *Les Noiyaux Gris Centraux et la Region Mesencephalo-sous-optique*. Paris: Masson

Francis, P.T., Palmer, A.M., Sims, N.R., Bowen, D.M., Davison, A.N., Esiri, M.M., Neary, D., Snowden, J.S. and Wilcock, G.K. (1985): Neurochemical studies of early-onset Alzheimer's disease: possible influence on treatment. *N. Engl. J. Med.* 313:7-11

Freund, T.F. and Antal, M. (1988): GABA-containing neurons in the septum control inhibitory interneurons in the hippocampus. *Nature* 36:170-173

Frotscher, M. and Léránth, C. (1985): Cholinergic innervation of the rat hippocampus as revealed by choline acetyltransferase immunocytochemistry: a combined light and electron microscopic study. *J. Comp. Neurol.* 239:237-246

Frotscher, M. and Léránth, C. (1986): The cholinergic innervation of the rat fascia dentata: identification of target structures on granule cells by combining choline acetyltransferase immunocytochemistry and Golgi impregnation. *J. Comp. Neurol.* 243:58-70

Fukada, K. (1985): Purification and partial characterization of a cholinergic neuronal differentiation factor. *Proc. Natl. Acad. Sci. USA* 82:8795-8799

Gage, F.H., Armstrong, D.M., Williams, D.R. and Varon, S. (1988): Morphological response of axotomized septal neurons to nerve growth factor. *J. Comp. Neurol.* 269:147-155

Gnahn, H., Hefti, F., Heumann, R., Schwab, M.E. and Thoenen, H. (1983): NGF-mediated increase of choline acetyltransferase (ChAT) in the neonatal rat forebrain: evidence for a physiological role of NGF in the brain? *Dev. Brain Res.* 9:45-52

Golgi, C. (1873): Sulla sostanza grigia del corvello. *Gaz. Med. Ital. Lombardia.* 6:244-246

Golgi, C. (1885): Sulla fina anatomia delgi organi centrale del sistema nervoso. *Riv. Sper. Freniat. Meg. Leg. Alien. Ment.* 11:72-123, 193-220

Gorry, J. D. (1963): Studies on the comparative anatomy of the ganglion basale of Meynert. *Acta. Anat.* 55:51-104

Grant, S.J. and Aston-Jones, G. (1986): Discharge properties of cortically projecting nucleus basalis neurons in behaving animals. *Soc. Neurosci. Abstr.* 12:572

Groenewegen, H.J. and Russchen, F.T. (1984): Organization of the efferent projections of the nucleus accumbens to pallidal, hypothalamic, and mesencephalic structures: a tracing and immunohistochemical study in the cat. *J. Comp. Neurol.* 223:347-367

Growdon, J.H. (in press): Biological therapies for Alzheimer's disease. In: *Dementia*. Whitehouse, P.J., ed. Philadelphia: FA Davis

Grove, E.A. (1988a): Efferent connections of the substantia innominata in the rat. *J. Comp. Neurol.* 277:347-364

Grove, E.A. (1988b): Neural associations of the substantia innominata in the rat: afferent connections. *J. Comp. Neurol.* 277:315-346

Grove, E.A., Domesick, V.B. and Nauta, W.J.H. (1986): Light microscopic evidence of striatal input to intrapallidal neurons of cholinergic cell group Ch4 in the rat: a study employing the anterograde tracer *Phaseolus vulgaris* leucoagglutinin (PHA-L). *Brain Res.* 367:379-384

Grünthal, E. (1932): Vergleichend anatomische Untersuchungen über den Zellbau des Globus pallidus und Nucleus basalis der Säuger und des Menschen. *J. Psychol. Neurol.* (Leipzig) 44:403-428

Grünthal, E. (1933): Neuere Ergebnisse vergleichend anatomischer Untersuchungen des Zwischenhirns der Säuger und das spezifisch Menschliche in seinem Bau. *Naturwissenschaften* 28:521-525

Haga, T., Haga, K., Berstein, G., Nishiyama, T., Uchiyama, H. and Ichiyama, A. (1988): Molecular properties of muscarinic receptors. *Trends Pharmacol. Sci.* 9 (Suppl):12-18

Hallanger, A.E., Levey, A.I., Lee, H.J., Rye, D.B. and Wainer, B.H. (1987): The origins of cholinergic and other subcortical afferents to the thalamus in the rat. *J. Comp. Neurol.* 262:105-124

Hammer, R., Berrie, C.P., Birdsall, N.J.M., Burgen, A.S.V. and Hulme, E.C. (1989): Pirenzepine distinguishes between different subclasses of muscarinic receptors. *Nature* 283:90-92

Hammond, D.N., Wainer, B.H., Tonsgard, J.H. and Heller, A. (1986): Neuronal properties of clonal hybrid cell lines derived from central cholinergic neurons. *Science* 234:1237-1240

Haroutunian, V., Kanof, P.D. and Davis, K.L. (1986): Partial reversal of lesion-induced deficits in cortical cholinergic markers by nerve growth factor. *Brain Res.* 396:397-399

Hawkins, R.D., Clark, G.A. and Kandel, E.R. (1987): Cell biological studies of learning in simple vertebrate and invertebrate systems. In: *Handbook of Physiology, Section 1: The Nervous System, Vol. V, Higher Functions of the Brain, Part 1.* Mountcastle V.B., ed. Bethesda, Maryland: American Physiological Society

Hedreen, J.C., Bacon, S.J., Cork, L.C., Kitt, C.A., Crawford, G.D., Salvaterra, P.M. and Price, D.L. (1983): Immunocytochemical identification of cholinergic neurons in the monkey central nervous system using monoclonal antibodies against choline acetyltransferase. *Neurosci. Lett.* 43:173-177

Hedreen, J.C., Struble, R.G., Whitehouse, P.J. and Price, D.L. (1984): Topography of the magnocellular basal forebrain system in human brain. *J. Neuropathol. Exp. Neurol.* 43:1-21

Hedreen, J.C., Uhl, G.R., Bacon, S.J., White, C.L. III, Price, D.L. and Fambrough, D.M. (1982): A fiber network in monkey cerebral cortex revealed by acetylcholinesterase immunocytochemistry. *Soc. Neurosci. Abstr.* 8:212

Hefti, F., (1986): Nerve growth factor promotes survival of septal cholinergic neurons after fimbrial transections. *J. Neurosci.* 6:2155-2162

Hefti, F., Dravid, A. and Hartikka, J. (1984): Chronic intraventricular injections of nerve growth factor elevate hippocampal choline acetyltransferase activity in adult rats with partial septo-hippocampal lesions. *Brain Res.* 293:305-311

Hefti, F., Hartikka, J., Salvatierra, A., Weiner, W.J., and Mash, D.C. (1986): Localization of nerve growth factor receptors in cholinergic neurons of the human basal forebrain. *Neurosci. Lett.* 69:37-41

Heimer, L., Alheid, G.F. and Záborszky, L., (1989): Basal forebrain and substantia innominata. In: *Neuroscience Year, Supplement 1 to the Encyclopedia of Neuroscience.* Adelman, G., ed. Boston: Birkhäuser

Hersh, L.B., Kong, C.F., Dyer, S., Strauss, W., Lorenz, M. and Hilt, D. (1989): Isolation of a genomic clone of human choline acetyltransferase. *Soc. Neurosci. Abstr.* 15:63

Higgins, G.A. and Mufson, E.J., (1989): NGF receptor gene expression is decreased in the nucleus basalis in Alzheimer's disease. *Exp. Neurol.* 106:222-235

Honegger, P. and Lenoir, D. (1982): Nerve growth factor (NGF) stimulation of cholinergic telencephalic neurons in aggregating cell cultures. *Dev. Brain Res.* 3:229-238

Ingham, C.A., Bolam, J.P. and Smith, A.D. (1988): GABA-immunoreactive synaptic boutons in the rat basal forebrain: comparison of neurons that project to the neocortex with pallidosubthalamic neurons. *J. Comp. Neurol.* 273:263-282

Irle, E. and Markowitsch, H.J. (1987): Basal forebrain-lesioned monkeys are severely impaired in tasks of association and recognition memory. *Ann. Neurol.* 22:735-743

Jacobowitz, D. and Palkovits, M. (1974): Topographic atlas of catecholamine and acetylcholinesterase-containing neurons in the rat brain. I. Forebrain (telencephalon, diencephalon). *J. Comp. Neurol.* 157:13-28

Jasper, H.H. and Tessier, J. (1971): Acetylcholine liberation from cerebral cortex during paradoxical (REM) sleep. *Science* 172:601-602

Johnson, D., Lanahan, A., Buck, C.R., Sehgal, A., Morgan, C., Mercer, E., Bothwell, M. and Chao, M. (1986): Expression and structure of the human NGF receptor. *Cell* 47:545-554

Johnston, M.V., McKinney, M., and Coyle, J.T. (1979): Evidence for a cholinergic projection to neocortex from neurons in basal forebrain. *Proc. Natl. Acad. Sci. USA* 76:5392-5396

Johnston, M.V., McKinney, M., and Coyle, J.T. (1981): Neocortical cholinergic innervation: a description of extrinsic and intrinsic components in the rat.

Exp. Brain Res. 43:159-172

Jones, B.E. and Moore, R.Y. (1977): Ascending projections of the locus coeruleus in the rat. II. Autoradiographic study. *Brain Res.* 127:23-53

Jones, E.G., Burton, H., Saper, C.B. and Swanson, L.W. (1976): Midbrain, diencephalic and cortical relationships of the basal nucleus of Meynert and associated structures in primates. *J. Comp. Neurol.* 167:385-420

Jope, R.S. (1979): High affinity choline transport and acetylCoA production in brain and their roles in the regulation of acetylcholine synthesis. *Brain Res. Rev.* 1:313-344

Kanai, T. and Szerb, J.C. (1965): Mesencephalic reticular activating system and cortical acetylcholine output. *Nature* 205:80-82

Kelley, A.E., Domesick, V.B. and Nauta, W.J.H. (1982): The amygdalostriatal projection in the rat: an anatomical study by anterograde and retrograde tracing methods. *Neurosci.* 7:615-630

Kievit, J. and Kuypers, H.G.J.M. (1975): Basal forebrain and hypothalamic connections to frontal and parietal cortex in the rhesus monkey. *Science* 187:660-662

Kimura, H., McGeer, P. L., Peng J.H. and McGeer E.G. (1981): Mapping of cholinergic systems in rostral forebrain of the rodent. In: *Cholinergic Mechanisms. Phylogenetic Aspects, Central and Peripheral Synapses, and Clinical Significance. Advances in Behavioral Biology, Vol. 25.* Pepeu, G., Ladinsky, H., eds. New York: Plenum Press

Kodama, S. (1926a): Über die sogenannten Basalganglien. (Morphogenetische und pathologisch-anatomische Untersuchungen). *Schweiz. Arch. Neurol. Psychiatr.* 18:179-246

Kodama, S. (1926b): Über die sogenannten Basalganglien. (Morphogenetische und pathologisch-anatomische Untersuchungen). D. Zusammenfassung und Schlussbetrachtungen. *Schweiz. Arch. Neurol. Psychiatr.* 19:152-177

Kodama, S. (1927): Über die sogenannten Basalganglien. (Morphogenetische und pathologisch-anatomische Untersuchungen). Pathologisch-anatomische Untersuchungen mit Bezug auf die sogenannten Basalganglien und ihre Adnexe. *Schweiz. Arch. Neurol. Psychiatr.* 20:209-261

Kodama, S. (1928a): Über die sogenannten Basalganglien. (Morphogenetische und pathologisch-anatomische Untersuchungen). Pathologisch-anatomische Untersuchungen mit Bezug auf die sogenannten Basalganglien und ihre Adnexe. B. über die Faserverbindungen zwischen den Basalganglien und ihren Adnexen, sowie den übrigen subkortikalen Kerngebieten beim Menschen, nebst einigen experimentellen Mitteilungen. *Schweiz. Arch. Neurol. Psychiatr.* 23:38-100

Kodama, S. (1928b): Über die sogenannten Basalganglien. (Morphogenetische und pathologisch-anatomische Untersuchungen). Pathologisch-anatomische Untersuchungen mit Bezug auf die sogenannten Basalganglien und ihre Adnexe. B. über die Faserverbindungen zwischen den Basalganglien und ihren Adnexen, sowie den übrigen subkortikalen Kerngebieten beim Menschen, nebst einigen experimentellen Mitteilungen. Kritische Betrachtungen. *Schweiz. Arch. Neurol. Psychiatr.* 23:179-259

Koelle, G.B. (1963): Cytological distributions and Physiological functions of cholinesterases. In: *Handb. exp. Pharmak., Vol. 15*. Eichle, O., Farah, A., eds. Heidelberg: Springer-Verlag

Koelle, G.B. (1987): Acetylcholine. In: *Encyclopedia of Neuroscience, Vol. I*. Adelman G., ed. Boston: Birkhäuser

Koelle, G.B. and Friedenwald, J.S. (1949): A histochemical method for localizing cholinesterase activity. *Proc. Soc. Exp. Biol. Med.* 70:617-622

Koh, S., Oyler, G.A. and Higgins, G.A. (1989): Localization of nerve growth factor receptor messenger RNA and protein in the adult rat brain. *Exp. Neurol.* 106:209-221

Köhler, C. and Chan-Palay, V. (1983): Distribution of gamma aminobutyric acid containing neurons and terminals in the septal area. *Anat. Embryol.* 167:53-65

Köhler, C., Chan-Palay, V. and Wu, J-Y. (1984): Septal neurons containing glutamic acid decarboxylase immunoreactivity project to the hippocampal region in the rat brain. *Anat. Embryol.* 169:41-44

Koliatsos, V.E. and Price, D.L. (submitted for publication): Organization of basal forebrain projections to the telencephalon: a reinvestigation with emphasis on limbic efferents

Koliatsos, V.E., Applegate, M.D., Kitt, C.A., Walker, L.C., DeLong, M.R. and Price, D.L. (1989): Aberrant phosphorylation of neurofilaments accompanies transmitter-related changes in rat septal neurons following transection of the fimbria-fornix. *Brain Res.* 482:205-218

Koliatsos, V.E., Applegate, M.D., Knüsel, B., Junard, E., Burton, L.E., Mobley, W.C., Hefti, F.F. and Price, D.L. (submitted for publication): Recombinant human nerve growth factor prevents retrograde degeneration of axotomized basal forebrain cholinergic neurons in the rat

Koliatsos, V.E., Martin, L.J., and Price, D.L. (in press, a): Efferent organization of the mammalian basal forebrain. In: *Brain Cholinergic Systems,* Steriade, M., Biesold, D., eds. Oxford: Oxford University Press

Koliatsos, V. E., Martin, L. J., Walker, L. C., Richardson, R. T., DeLong, M.R. and Price, D.L. (1988): Topographic, non-collateralized basal forebrain projections to amygdala, hippocampus, and anterior cingulate cortex in the rhesus monkey. *Brain Res.* 463:133-139

Koliatsos, V.E., Nauta, H.J.W., Clatterbuck, R.E., Holztman, D.M., Mobley, W.C. and Price, D.L. (in press, b): Mouse nerve growth factor prevents degeneration of axotomized basal forebrain cholinergic neurons in monkey. *J. Neurosci.*

Koo, E.K. and Price, D.L. (in press): The neurobiology of dementia. In: *Dementia*. Whitehouse, P.J., ed. Philadelphia: F.A. Davis

Korsching, S., Auburger, G., Heumann, R., Scott, J. and Thoenen, H. (1985): Levels of nerve growth factor and its mRNA in the central nervous system of the rat correlate with cholinergic innervation. *EMBO. J.* 4:1389-1393

Kordower, J.H. and Mufson, E.J. (in press): Galanin-like immunoreactivity within the primate basal forebrain: differential staining patterns between humans and monkeys. *J. Comp. Neurol.*

Kordower, J.H., Bartus, R.T., Bothwell, M., Schatteman, G. and Gash, D.M. (1988): Nerve growth factor receptor immunoreactivity in the nonhuman primate (*Cebus apella*): distribution, morphology, and colocalization with cholinergic enzymes. *J. Comp. Neurol.* 277:465-486

Krettek, J.E. and Price, J.L. (1978): Amygdaloid projections to subcortical structures within the basal forebrain and brainstem in the rat and cat. *J. Comp. Neurol.* 178:225-254

Krnjević, K. and Ropert, N. (1982): Electrophysiological and pharmacological characteristics of facilitation of hippocampal population spikes by stimulation of the medial septum. *Neurosci.* 7:2165-2183

Kromer, L.F. (1987): Nerve growth factor treatment after brain injury prevents neuronal death. *Science* 235:214-216

Kurosawa, M., Sato, A. and Sato, Y. (1989): Stimulation of the nucleus basalis of Meynert increases acetylcholine release in the cerebral cortex in rats. *Neurosci. Lett.* 98:45-50

Lacombe, P., Sercombe, R., Verrecchia, C., Philipson, V., MacKenzie, E.T. and Seylaz, J. (1989): Cortical blood flow increases induced by stimulation of the substantia innominata in the unanesthetized rat. *Brain Res.* 491:1-14

Larson, J., Wong, D. and Lynch, G. (1986): Patterned stimulation at the theta frequency is optimal for the induction of hippocampal long-term potentiation. *Brain Res.* 368:347-350

Lehmann, J., Nagy, J.I., Atmadja, S. and Fibiger, H.C. (1980): The nucleus basalis magnocellularis: the origin of a cholinergic projection to the neocortex of the rat. *Neurosci.* 5:1161-1174

Leontovich, T.A. and Zhukova, G.P. (1963): The specificity of the neuronal structure and topography of the reticular formation in the brain and spinal cord of carnivora. *J. Comp. Neurol.* 121:347-379

Léránth, C. and Frotscher, M. (1987): Cholinergic innervation of hippocampal GAD- and somatostatin-immunoreactive commissural neurons. *J. Comp. Neurol.* 261:33-47

Léránth, C. and Frotscher, M. (1989): Organization of the septal region in the rat brain: cholinergic-GABAergic interconnections and the termination of hippocampo-septal fibers. *J. Comp. Neurol.* 289:304-314

Léránth, C., MacLusky, N.J., Shanabrough, M. and Naftolin, F. (1988): Catecholaminergic innervation of luteinizing hormone-releasing hormone and glutamic acid decarboxylase immunopositive neurons in the rat medial preoptic area: an electron-microscopic double immunostaining and degeneration study.

Neuroendocrinol. 48:591-602

Levey, A.I., Armstrong, D.M., Atweh, S.F., Terry, R.D. and Wainer, B.H. (1983): Monoclonal antibodies to choline acetyltransferase: production, specificity, and immunohistochemistry. *J. Neurosci.* 3:1-9

Levey, A.I., Hallanger, A.E. and Wainer, B.H. (1987): Cholinergic nucleus basalis neurons may influence the cortex via the thalamus. *Neurosci. Lett.* 74:7-13

Levey, A.I., Simonds, W.F., Spiegel, A.M. and Brann, M.R. (1989): Characterization of muscarinic receptor subtype-specific antibodies. *Soc. Neurosci. Abstr.* 15:64

Levi-Montalcini, R. (1987): The nerve growth factor 35 years later. *Science* 237:1154-1162

Levi-Montalcini, R. and Hamburger, V. (1951): Selective growth stimulating effects of mouse sarcoma on the sensory and sympathetic nervous system of the chick embryo. *J. Exp. Zool.* 116:321-361

Levi-Montalcini, R. and Hamburger, V. (1953): A diffusible agent of mouse sarcoma, producing hyperplasia of sympathetic ganglia and hyperneurotization of viscera in the chick embryo. *J. Exp. Zool.* 123:233-287

Lewis, P.R. and Shute, C.C.D. (1967): The cholinergic limbic system: projections to hippocampal formation, medial cortex, nuclei of the ascending cholinergic reticular system, and the subfornical organ and supra-optic crest. *Brain* 90:521-540

Lindstrom, J., Schoepfer, R. and Whiting, P. (1987): Molecular studies of the neuronal nicotinic acetylcholine receptor family. *Mol. Neurobiol.* 1:281-338

Lister, T. and Ray, D.E. (1988): The role of basal forebrain in the primary cholinergic vasodilation in rat neocortex produced by systemic administration of cismethrin. *Brain Res.* 450:364-368

Loewi, O. (1921): Über humorale Übertragbarkeit der Herznervenwirkung. I. Mitteilung. *Pflügers Arch. Physiol.* 189:239-242

Luiten, P.G.M., Gaykema, R.P.A., Traber, J. and Spencer, D.G. Jr. (1987): Cortical projection patterns of magnocellular basal nucleus subdivisions as revealed by anterogradely transported *Phaseolus vulgaris* leucoagglutinin. *Brain Res.* 413:229-250

Mahanthappa, N.K., Gage, F.H. and Patterson, P.H. (in press): Adrenal chromaffin cells as multipotential neurons for autografts. *Prog. Brain Res.*

Mann, D.M.A., Yates, P.O. and Marcyniuk, B. (1984): Alzheimer's presenile dementia, senile dementia of Alzheimer type and Down's syndrome in middle age form an age related continuum of pathological changes. *Neuropathol. Appl. Neurobiol.* 10:185-207

Martínez-Murillo, R., Blasco, I., Alvarez, F.J., Villalba, R., Solano, M.L., Montero-Caballero, M.I. and Rodrigo, J. (1988): Distribution of enkephalin-immunoreactive nerve fibres and terminals in the region of the nucleus basalis magnocellularis of the rat: a light and electron microscopic study. *J. Neurocytol.* 17:361-376

Massoulié, J. and Bon, S. (1982): The molecular forms of cholinesterase and acetylcholinesterase in vertebrates. *Ann. Rev. Neurosci.* 5:57-106

Mautner, H.G. (1977): Choline acetyltransferase. *CRC Crit. Rev. Biochem.* 4:341-370

McCormick, D.A. (1989): Acetylcholine: distribution, receptors, and actions. *Sem. Neurosci.* 1:91-101

McGeer, P.L., McGeer, E.G., and Peng, J.H. (1984a): Choline acetyltransferase: purification and immunohistochemical localization. *Life Sci.* 34:2319-2338

McGeer, P.L., McGeer, E.G., Suzuki, J. and Norman, M. (1984b): Cholinergic and noradrenergic systems in aging, Alzheimer's disease and Down's syndrome. *Soc. Neurosci. Abstr.* 10:995

McGeer, P.L., McGeer, E.G., Suzuki, J., Dolman, C.E. and Nagai, T. (1984c): Aging, Alzheimer's disease, and the cholinergic system of the basal forebrain. *Neurol.* 34:741-745

Meier, R., Becker-André, M., Götz, R., Heumann, R., Shaw, A. and Thoenen, H. (1986): Molecular cloning of bovine and chick nerve growth factor (NGF): delineation of conserved and unconserved domains and their relationship to the biological activity and antigenicity of NGF. *EMBO. J.* 5:1489-1493

Melander, T. and Staines, W.A. (1986): A galanin-like peptide coexists in putative cholinergic somata of the septum-basal forebrain complex and in acetylcholinesterase containing fibers and varicosities within the hippocampus in the owl monkey (Aotus trivirgatus). *Neurosci. Lett.* 68:17-22

Melander, T., Staines, W.A., Hökfelt, T., Rökaeus, A., Eckenstein, F., Salvaterra, P.M. and Wainer, B.H. (1985): Galanin-like immunoreactivity in cholinergic neurons of the septum-basal forebrain complex projecting to the hippocampus of the rat. *Brain Res.* 360:130-138

Mesulam, M.-M., (1985): Patterns in behavioral neuroanatomy: association areas, the limbic system, and hemispheric specialization. In: *Principles of Behavioral Neurology.* Mesulam, M.-M, ed. Philadelphia: F. A. Davis, 1985, pp 1-70

Mesulam, M.-M., and Geula, C. (1988a): Acetylcholinesterase-rich pyramidal neurons in the human neocortex and hippocampus: absence at birth, development during the life span, and dissolution in Alzheimer's disease. *Ann. Neurol.* 24:765-773

Mesulam, M.-M., and Geula, C. (1988b): Nucleus basalis (Ch4) and cortical cholinergic innervation in the human brain: observations based on the distribution of acetylcholinesterase and choline acetyltransferase. *J. Comp. Neurol.* 275:216-240

Mesulam, M.-M., and Geula, C. (1990): Shifting patterns of cortical cholinesterases in Alzheimer's disease: implications for treatment, diagnosis, and pathogenesis. In: *Alzheimer's Disease. Advances in Neurology, Vol. 51.* Wurtman, R. J., Corkin, S., Growdon, J. H., Ritter-Walker, E., eds. New York: Raven Press

Mesulam, M.-M., and Mufson, E.J. (1984): Neural inputs into the nucleus basalis of the substantia innominata (Ch4) in the rhesus monkey. *Brain* 107:253-274

Mesulam, M.-M., and Van Hoesen, G.W. (1976): Acetylcholinesterase-rich projections from the basal forebrain of the rhesus monkey to neocortex. *Brain Res.* 109:152-157

Mesulam, M.-M., Mufson, E.J., and Wainer, B.H. (1986): Three-dimensional representation and cortical projection topography of the nucleus basalis (Ch4) in the macaque: concurrent demonstration of choline acetyltransferase and retrograde transport with a stabilized tetramethylbenzidine method for horseradish peroxidase. *Brain Res.* 367:301-308

Mesulam, M.-M., Mufson, E.J., Levey, A.I., and Wainer, B.H. (1984): Atlas of cholinergic neurons in the forebrain and upper brainstem of the macaque based on monoclonal choline acetyltransferase immunohistochemistry and acetylcholinesterase histochemistry. *Neurosci.* 12:669-686

Mesulam, M.-M., Mufson, E.J., Levey, A.I., and Wainer, B. H. (1983a): Cholinergic innervation of cortex by the basal forebrain: cytochemistry and cortical connections of the septal area, diagonal band nuclei, nucleus basalis (substantia innominata), and hypothalamus in the rhesus monkey. *J. Comp. Neurol.* 214:170-197

Mesulam, M.-M., Mufson, E.J., Wainer, B.H. and Levey, A.I. (1983b): Central cholinergic pathways in the rat: an overview based on an alternative nomenclature (Ch1-Ch6). *Neurosci.* 10:1185-1201

Metherate, R., Tremblay, N., and Dykes, R.W. (1987): Acetylcholine permits long-term enhancement of neuronal responsiveness in cat primary somatosensory cortex. *Neurosci.* 22:75-81

Mettler, F.A. (1942): *Neuroanatomy.* St. Louis: C.V. Mosby

Meynert, T. (1872): Vom Gehirn der Saugetiere. In: *Handbuch der Lehre von den Geweben des Menschen und Thiere, Vol. 2.* Stricker, S., ed. Leipzig: Engelmann

Miller, F.R., Stavraky, G.W. and Woonton, G.A. (1940): Effects of eserine, acetylcholine and atropine on the electrocorticogram. *J. Neurophysiol.* 3:131-138

Mishkin, M. and Appenzeller, T. (1987): The anatomy of memory. *Sci. Amer.* 80-89

Miyamoto, M., Kato, J., Narumi, S. and Nagaoka, A. (1987): Characteristics of memory impairment following lesioning of the basal forebrain and medial septal nucleus in rats. *Brain Res.* 419:19-31

Mobley, W.C., Neve, R.L., Prusiner, S.B. and McKinley, M.P. (1988): Nerve growth factor induces gene expression for prion- and Alzheimer's beta-amyloid proteins. *Proc. Natl. Acad. Sci. USA* 85:9811-9815

Mobley, W.C., Rutkowski, J.L., Tennekoon, G.I., Buchanan, K. and Johnston, M.V. (1985): Choline acetyltransferase activity in striatum of neonatal rats increased by nerve growth factor. *Science* 229:284-287

Mobley, W.C., Rutkowski, J.L., Tennekoon, G.I., Gemski, J., Buchanan, K. and

Johnston, M.V. (1986): Nerve growth factor increases choline acetyltransferase activity in developing basal forebrain neurons. *Mol. Brain Res.* 1:53-62

Mora, F., Rolls, E.T., and Burton, M.J. (1976): Modulation during learning of the responses of neurons in the lateral hypothalamus to the sight of food. *Exp. Neurol.* 53:508-519

Mori, N., Itoh, N. and Salvaterra, P.M. (1987): Evolutionary origin of cholinergic macromolecules and thyroglobulin. *Proc. Natl. Acad. Sci. USA* 84:2813-2817

Nachmansohn, D. and Machado, A.L. (1943): The formation of acetylcholine: a new enzyme: "choline acetylase." *J. Neurophysiol.* 6:397-403

Nagai, T., Satoh, K., Imamoto, K. and Maeda, T. (1981): Divergent projections of catecholamine neurons of the locus coeruleus as revealed by fluorescent retrograde double labeling technique. *Neurosci. Lett.* 23:117-123

Nathanson, N.M. (1987): Molecular properties of the muscarinic acetylcholine receptor. *Ann. Rev. Neurosci.* 10:195-236

Nicolesco, I. and Nicolesco, M. (1929): Quelques données sur les centres végétatifs de la région infundibulo-tubérienne et de la frontière diencéphalo-télencéphalique. *Rev. Neurol.* 2:289-317

Nissl, F. (1894): Der gegenwärtige Stand der Nervenzellenanatomie und irhe nächsten Ziele. *Neurol. Centralbl.* 14:66-75

Nissl, F. (1895): Der gegenwärtige Stand der Nervenzellenanatomie und irhe nächsten Ziele. *Neurol. Centralbl.* 14:104-110

Olton, D.S. and Wenk, G.L. (1987): Dementia: animal models of the cognitive impairments produced by degeneration of the basal forebrain cholinergic system. In: *Psychopharmacology: The Third Generation of Progress.* Meltzer, H.Y., ed. New York: Raven Press, pp 941-953

Ottersen, O.P. (1980): Afferent connections to the amygdaloid complex of the rat and cat: II. Afferents from the hypothalamus and the basal telencephalon. *J. Comp. Neurol.* 194:267-289

Papez, J.W. and Aronson, L.R. (1934): Thalamic nuclei of Pithecus (Macacus) rhesus. I. Ventral thalamus. *Arch. Neurol. Psychiatry* 32:1-26

Parent, A., Boucher, R. and O'Reilly-Fromentin, J. (1981): Acetylcholinesterase-containing neurons in cat pallidal complex: morphological characteristics and projection towards the neocortex. *Brain Res.* 230:356-361

Parent, A., Gravel, S. and Olivier, A. (1979): The extrapyramidal and limbic systems' relationship at the globus pallidus level: a comparative histochemical study in the rat, cat, and monkey. In: *Advances in Neurology, Vol. 24.* Poirier, L. J., Sourkes, T. L., Bedard, P. J., eds. New York: Raven Press

Parent, A., Poirier, L.J., Boucher, R. and Butcher, L.L. (1977): Morphological characteristics of acetylcholinesterase-containing neurons in the CNS of DFP-treated monkeys. Part 2. Diencephalic medial telencephalic structures. *J. Neurol. Sci.* 32:9-28

Parent, A., Poitras, D. and Dubé, L. (1984): Comparative anatomy of central monoaminergic systems. In: *Classical Transmitters in the CNS, Part I, Handbook of Chemical Neuroanatomy, Vol. 2*. Björklund A, Hökfelt T, eds. Amsterdam: Elsevier

Parnavelas, J.G., Kelly, W. and Burnstock, G. (1985): Ultrastructural localization of choline acetyltransferase in vascular endothelial cells in rat brain. *Nature* 316:724-725

Pavlides, C., Greenstein, Y.J., Grudman, M. and Winson, J. (1988): Long-term potentiation in the dentate gyrus is induced preferentially on the positive phase of θ-rhythm. *Brain Res.* 439:383-387

Paxinos, G. and Watson, C. (1986): *The Rat Brain in Stereotaxic Coordinates*, second edition. Sydney: Academic Press

Pearson, R.C.A., Gatter, K.C. and Powell, T.P.S. (1983a): Retrograde cell degeneration in the basal nucleus in monkey and man. *Brain Res.* 261:321-326

Pearson, R.C.A., Sofroniew, M.V., Cuello, A.C., Powell, T.P.S., Eckenstein, F., Esiri, M.M. and Wilcock, G.K. (1983b): Persistence of cholinergic neurons in the basal nucleus in a brain with senile dementia of the Alzheimer's type demonstrated by immunohistochemical staining for choline acetyltransferase. *Brain Res.* 289:375-379

Peng, J.H., Kimura, H., McGeer, P.L. and McGeer, E.G. (1981): Anti-choline acetyltransferase fragments antigen binding (Fab) for immunohistochemistry. *Neurosci. Lett.* 21:281-285

Peralta, E.G., Winslow, J.W., Ashkenazi, A., Smith, D.H., Ramachandran, J. and Capon, D.J. (1988): Structural basis of muscarinic acetylcholine receptor subtype diversity. *Trends Pharmacol. Sci.* 9:6-11

Perry, E. K., Gibson, P. H., Blessed, G., Perry, R. H. and Tomlinson, B. E. (1977): Neurotransmitter enzyme abnormalities in senile dementia. *J. Neurol. Sci.* 34:247-265

Perry, E. K., Tomlinson, B.E., Blessed, G., Bergmann, K., Gibson, P.H. and Perry, R.H. (1978): Correlation of cholinergic abnormalities with senile plaques and mental test scores in senile dementia. *Br. Med. J.* 2:1457-1459

Perry, R.H., Candy, J.M., Perry, E.K., Irving, D., Blessed, G., Fairbairn, A.F. and Tomlinson, B.E. (1982): Extensive loss of choline acetyltransferase activity is not reflected by neuronal loss in the nucleus of Meynert in Alzheimer's disease. *Neurosci. Lett.* 33:311-315

Phelps, C.H., Gage, F.H., Growdon, J.H., Hefti, F., Harbaugh, R., Johnston, M.V., Khachaturian, Z.S., Mobley, W.C., Price, D.L., Raskind, M., Simpkins, J., Thal, L.J. and Woodcock, J. (1989): Potential use of nerve growth factor to treat Alzheimer's disease. *Neurobiol. Aging* 10:205-207

Pilleri, G. (1962): Über die Verbindungen des Nucleus basalis Meynert mit der Temporalhirnrinde. *Acta Anat.* 50:389

Pilleri, G. (1966a): The Kluver-Bucy syndrome in man. A clinico-anatomical contribution to the function of the medial temporal lobe structures. *Psychiatr.*

Neurol. (Basel)152:65-103

Pilleri, G. (1966b): Weitere Beobachtung zur Frage der Projektion des Ganglion basale Meynert (Nucleus ansae lenticularis) beim Menschen. *Acta Anat.* 65:138-145

Pilleri, G. (1966c): Zur Frage der Verbindungen des Ganglion basale von Meynert (Nucleus ansae lenticularis) mit der Temporalrinde beim Menschen. *J. Hirnforsch.* 8:343-357

Pope, A., Hess, H.H. and Lewin, E. (1964): Microchemical pathology of the cerebral cortex in pre-senile dementias. *Trans. Am. Neurol. Assoc.* 89:15-16

Price, D.L., Cork, L.C., Struble, R.G., Whitehouse, P.J., Kitt, C.A. and Walker, L.C. (1985): The functional organization of the basal forebrain cholinergic system in primates and the role of this system in Alzheimer's disease. *Ann. N. Y. Acad. Sci.* 444:287-295

Price, D.L., Koo, E.H., Wagster, M.V., Walker, L.C., Wenk, G.L., Applegate, M.D., Kitt, C.A. and Cork, L.C. (1990): Behavioral, cellular, and molecular biological studies of aged nonhuman primates. In: *Alzheimer's Disease. Advances in Neurology, Vol. 51.* Wurtman, R.J., Corkin, S., Growdon, J.H., Ritter-Walker, E., eds. New York: Raven Press

Price, D. L., Martin, L. J., Koo, E. H., Sisodia, S. S., Koliatsos, V.E. and Cork, L.C. (in press): Alzheimer's disease and animal models. In: *Molecular Mechanisms of Aging.* Schettler, G., Beyreuther, K., eds. Berlin: Springer-Verlag

Price, J.L. and Amaral, D.G. (1981): An autoradiographic study of the projections of the central nucleus of the monkey amygdala. *J. Neurosci.* 1:1242-1259

Price, J.L. and Stern, R. (1983): Individual cells in the nucleus basalis-diagonal band complex have restricted axonal projections to the cerebral cortex in the rat. *Brain Res.* 269:352-356

Ramón y Cajal, S. (1928): *Degeneration and Regeneration of the Nervous System, Vol. II.* May, R. M., ed. and transl. London: Oxford University Press

Ramón y Cajal, S. (1911): *Histologie du Système Nerveux de l'Homme et des Vertébrés,* Tome II. Paris: A Maloine

Ramon-Moliner, E. and Nauta, W.J.H. (1966): The isodendritic core of the brain stem. *J. Comp. Neurol.* 126:311-336

Rao, M., Landis, S.C. and Patterson, P.H. (1989): Comparison of three factors inducing cholinergic properties in cultured sympathetic neurons. *Soc. Neurosci. Abstr.* 15:1362

Reichert, C. B. (1861): *Der Bau Des Menschlichen Gehirns.* Leipzig: Verlag von Wilhelm Engelmann

Reil, J.C. (1809): Untersuchungen über den Ban des grossen Gehirns in Mehschen. a. Das Hirnschenkel-System oder die Hirnschenkel-Organisation im grossen Gehirn. *Arch. Physiol.* 9:147-171

Richardson, R.T. and DeLong, M.R. (1986): Nucleus basalis of Meynert neuronal activity during a delayed response task in monkey. *Brain Res.* 399:364-368

Richardson, R.T. and DeLong, M.R. (1988): A reappraisal of the functions of the nucleus basalis of Meynert. *Trends Neurosci.* 11:264-267

Richardson, R.T., Mitchell, S.J., Baker, F.H. and DeLong, M.R. (1988): Responses of nucleus basalis of Meynert neurons in behaving monkeys. In: *Cellular Mechanisms of Conditioning and Behavioral Plasticity.* Woody, C.D., Alkon, D.L., McGaugh, J.L., eds. New York: Plenum Publishing Corporation

Riley, H.A. (1943): *An Atlas of the Basal Ganglia, Brain Stem and Spinal Cord.* Based on Myelin-Stained Material. Baltimore: Williams & Wilkins

Rinne, J.O., Paljärvi, L. and Rinne, U.K. (1987): Neuronal size and density in the nucleus basalis of Meynert in Alzheimer's disease. *J. Neurol. Sci.* 79:67-76

Rogers, J.D., Brogan, D. and Mirra, S.S. (1985): The nucleus basalis of Meynert in neurological disease: a quantitative morphological study. *Ann. Neurol.* 17:163-170

Rosenberg, M.B., Friedmann, T., Robertson, R.C., Tuszynski, M., Wolff, J.A., Breakefield, X.O. and Gage, F.H. (1988): Grafting genetically modified cells to the damaged brain: restorative effects of NGF expression. *Science* 242: 1575-1581

Rossor, M.N. (1981): Parkinson's disease and Alzheimer's disease as disorders of the isodendritic core. *Br. Med. J.* 283:1588-1590

Rossor, M.N. (1982): Dementia. *Lancet* 2:1200-1204

Russchen, F.T., Amaral, D.G. and Price, J.L. (1985): The afferent connections of the substantia innominata in the monkey, Macaca fascicularis. *J. Comp. Neurol.* 242:1-27

Rye, D.B., Wainer, B.H., Mesulam, M.-M., Mufson, E.J., and Saper, C.B. (1984): Cortical projections arising from the basal forebrain: a study of cholinergic and noncholinergic components employing combined retrograde tracing and immunohistochemical localization of choline acetyltransferase. *Neurosci.* 13:627-643

Saadat, S., Sendtner, M. and Rohrer, H. (1989): Ciliary neurotrophic factor induces cholinergic differentiation of rat sympathetic neurons in culture. *J. Cell Biol.* 108:1807-1816

Salvaterra, P.M. (1987): Molecular biology and neurobiology of choline acetyltransferase. *Mol. Neurobiol.* 1:247-280

Saper, C.B. (1984): Organization of cerebral cortical afferent systems in the rat. I. Magnocellular basal nucleus. *J. Comp. Neurol.* 222:313-342

Saper, C.B. (1987): Diffuse cortical projection systems: anatomical organization and role in cortical function. In: *Handbook of Physiology, Section 1: The Nervous System, Vol. V, Higher Functions of the Brain, Part 1.* Mountcastle VB, ed. Bethesda, Maryland: American Physiological Society

Saper, C.B., Swanson, L.W. and Cowan, W.M. (1976): The efferent connections of the ventromedial nucleus of the hypothalamus of the rat. *J. Comp. Neurol.* 169:409-442

Schatteman, G.C., Gibbs, L., Lanahan, A.A., Claude, P. and Bothwell, M. (1988): Expression of NGF receptor in the developing and adult primate central nervous system. *J. Neurosci.* 8:860-873

Schwab, M.E., Otten, U., Agid, Y. and Thoenen, H. (1979): Nerve growth factor (NGF) in the rat CNS: absence of specific retrograde axonal transport and tyrosine hydroxylase induction in locus coeruleus and substantia nigra. *Brain Res.* 168:473-483

Segal, M. (1978): The acetylcholine receptor in the rat hippocampus; nicotinic, muscarinic or both? *Neuropharmacol.* 17:619-623

Seiler, M. and Schwab, M.E. (1984): Specific retrograde transport of nerve growth factor (NGF) from neocortex to nucleus basalis in the rat. *Brain Res.* 300:33-39

Semba, K., Reiner, P.B., McGeer, E.G., and Fibiger, H.C. (1988a): Brainstem afferents to the magnocellular basal forebrain studied by axonal transport, immunohistochemistry, and electrophysiology in the rat. *J. Comp. Neurol.* 267:433-453

Semba, K., Reiner, P.B., McGeer, E.G., and Fibiger, H.C. (1988b): Morphology of cortically projecting basal forebrain neurons in the rat as revealed by intracellular iontophoresis of horseradish peroxidase. *Neurosci.* 2:637-651

Shelton, D.L. and Reichardt, L.F. (1986): Studies on the expression of the nerve growth factor (NGF) gene in the central nervous system: level and regional distribution of NGF mRNA suggest that NGF functions as a trophic factor for several distinct populations of neurons. *Proc. Natl. Acad. Sci. USA* 83:2714-2718

Shute, C.C.D. and Lewis, P.R. (1967): The ascending cholinergic reticular system: neocortical, olfactory and subcortical projections. *Brain* 90:497-520

Sillito, A.M. and Kemp, J.A. (1983): Cholinergic modulation of the functional organization of the cat visual cortex. *Brain Res.* 289:143-155

Simon, H., LeMoal, M. and Calas, A. (1979): Efferents and afferents of the ventral tegmental-A10 region studied after local injection of [^{3}H]leucine and horseradish peroxidase. *Brain Res.* 178:17-40

Smith, Y. and Parent, A. (1984): Distribution of acetylcholinesterase-containing neurons in the basal forebrain and upper brainstem of the squirrel monkey (Saimiri sciureus). *Brain Res. Bull.* 12:95-104

Snider, W.D. and Johnson, E.M. Jr. (1989): Neurotrophic molecules. *Ann. Neurol.* 26:489-506

Sofroniew, M.V. and Isacson, O. (1988): Distribution of degeneration of cholinergic neurons in the septum following axotomy in different portions of the fimbria-fornix: a correlation between degree of cell loss and proximity of neuronal somata to the lesion. *J. Chem. Neuroanat.* 1:327-337

Sofroniew, M.V., Pearson, R.C.A., Eckenstein, F., Cuello, A.C. and Powell, T.P.S. (1983): Retrograde changes in cholinergic neurons in the basal forebrain of the rat following cortical damage. *Brain Res.* 289:370-374

Stephan, H. and Andy, O.J. (1962): The septum. (A comparative study on its size in insectivores and primates.) *J. Hirnforsch.* 9:229-244

Stephan, H. and Andy, O.J. (1964): Cytoarthitectonics of the septal nuclei in old world monkeys (Cercopithecus and Colobus). *J. Hirnforsch.* 7:1-23

Steriade, M., Parent, A., Paré, D. and Smith, Y. (1987): Cholinergic and non-cholinergic neurons of cat basal forebrain project to reticular and mediodorsal thalamic nuclei. *Brain Res.* 408:372-376

Sterman, A.B. and Schaumburg, H.H. (1980): Neurotoxicity of selected drugs. In: *Experimental and Clinical Neurotoxicology.* Spencer, P. S., Schaumburg, H. H., eds. Baltimore: Williams & Wilkins

Stewart, D.J., MacFabe, D.F. and Vanderwolf, C.H. (1984): Cholinergic activation of the electrocorticogram: role of the substantia innominata and effects of atropine and quinuclidinyl benzilate. *Brain Res.* 322:219-232

Strömberg, I., Wetmore, C.J., Ebendal, T., Ernfors, P., Persson, H. and Olson, L. (1990): Rescue of basal forebrain cholinergic neurons after implantation of genetically modified cells producing recombinant NGF. *J. Neurosci. Res.* 25:405-411

Struble, R.G., Lehmann, J., Mitchell, S.J., McKinney, M., Price, D.L., Coyle, J.T. and DeLong, M.R. (1986): Basal forebrain neurons provide major cholinergic innervation of primate neocortex. *Neurosci. Lett.* 66:215-220

Sugiura, Y., Lee, C.L. and Perl, E.R. (1986): Central projections of identified, unmyelinated (C) afferent fibers innervating mammalian skin. *Science* 234:358-361

Swanson, L.W. (1976): An autoradiographic study of the efferent connections of the preoptic region in the rat. *J. Comp. Neurol.* 167:227-256

Swanson, L.W. and Cowan, W.M. (1979): The connections of the septal region in the rat. *J. Comp. Neurol.* 186:621-655

Swanson, L.W., Simmons, D.M., Whiting, P.J. and Lindstrom, J. (1987): Immunohistochemical localization of neuronal nicotinic receptors in the rodent central nervous system. *J. Neurosci.* 7:3334-3342

Szerb, J.C. (1967): Cortical acetylcholine release and electroencephalographic arousal. *J. Physiol.* 192:329-343

Tagliavini, F., Pilleri, G., Bouras, C. and Constantinidis, J. (1984): The basal nucleus of Meynert in patients with progressive supranuclear palsy. *Neurosci. Lett.* 44:37-42

Tagliavini, F. and Pilleri, G. (1983): Neuronal counts in basal nucleus of Meynert in Alzheimer disease and in simple senile dementia. *Lancet* 1:469-470

Taylor, P. (1985): Cholinergic agonists. In: *The Pharmacological Basis of Therapeutics,* seventh edition. Gilman, A.G., Goodman, L.S., Rall, T.W., Murad, F., eds. New York: Macmillan Publishing Company

Taylor, P. and Brown, J.H. (1989): Acetylcholine. In: *Basic Neurochemistry: Molecular, Cellular, and Medical Aspects,* fourth edition. Siegel, G.J. et al., eds. New York: Raven Press

Thal, L.J., Fuld, P.A., Masur, D.M. and Sharpless, N.S. (1983): Oral physostigmine and lecithin improve memory in Alzheimer disease. *Ann. Neurol.* 13: 491-496

Tuček, S. (1982): The synthesis of acetylcholine in skeletal muscles of the rat. *J. Physiol.* 322:53-69

van der Kooy, D. and Hattori, T. (1980): Dorsal raphe cells with collateral projections to the caudate-putamen and substantia nigra: a fluorescent retrograde double labeling study in the rat. *Brain Res.* 186:1-7

Vertes, R.P. and Martin, G.F. (1988): Autoradiographic analysis of ascending projections from the pontine and mesencephalic reticular formation and the median raphe nucleus in the rat. *J. Comp. Neurol.* 275:511-54

von Buttlar-Brentano, K. (1952): Pathohistologische Feststellungen am Basalkern Schizophrener. *J. Nerv. Ment. Dis.* 116:646-653

von Kölliker, A. (1896): *Handbuch der Gewebelehre des Menschen, Vol. 2* 6th edition. Leipzig: Engelmann

Wada, E., Wada, K., Boulter, J., Deneris, E., Heinemann, S., Patrick, J. and Swanson, L.W. (1989): Distribution of alpha2, alpha3, alpha4, and beta2 neuronal nicotinic receptor subunit mRNAs in the central nervous system: a hybridization histochemical study in the rat. *J. Comp. Neurol.* 284:314-335

Walker, L.C., Kitt, C.A., DeLong, M.R. and Price, D.L. (1985): Noncollateral projections of basal forebrain neurons to frontal and parietal neocortex in primates. *Brain Res. Bull.* 15:307-314

Walker, L.C., Koliatsos, V.E., Kitt, C.A., Richardson, R.T., Rökaeus, A. and Price, D.L. (1989a): Peptidergic neurons in the basal forebrain magnocellular complex of the rhesus monkey. *J. Comp. Neurol.* 280:272-282

Walker, L.C., Price, D.L. and Young, W.S. III (1989b): GABAergic neurons in the primate basal forebrain magnocellular complex. *Brain Res.* 499:188-192

Walker, L.C., Price, D.L. and Young, W.S. III (1989c): Galanin mRNA in the primate nucleus basalis of Meynert. *Soc. Neurosci. Abstr.* 15:407

Wenk, H., Bigl, V. and Meyer, U. (1980): Cholinergic projections from magnocellular nuclei of the basal forebrain to cortical areas in rats. *Brain Res. Rev.* 2:295-316

Wenk, G.L., Cribbs, B. and McCall, L. (1984): Nucleus basalis magnocellularis: optimal coordinates for selective reduction of choline acetyltransferase in frontal neocortex by ibotenic acid injections. *Exp. Brain Res.* 56:335-340

Whitehouse, P.J., Hedreen, J.C., White, C.L. III and Price, D.L. (1983): Basal forebrain neurons in the dementia of Parkinson disease. *Ann. Neurol.* 13:243-248

Whitehouse, P.J., Price, D.L., Clark, A.W., Coyle, J.T. and DeLong, M.R. (1981): Alzheimer disease: evidence for selective loss of cholinergic neurons in the nucleus basalis. *Ann. Neurol.* 10:122-126

Whitehouse, P.J., Price, D.L., Struble, R.G., Clark, A.W., Coyle, J.T. and DeLong, M.R. (1982): Alzheimer's disease and senile dementia: loss of neurons in the basal forebrain. *Science* 215:1237-1239

Whitlock, D.G. and Nauta, W.J.H. (1956): Subcortical projections from the temporal neocortex in macaca mulatta. *J. Comp. Neurol.* 106:183-212

Whittemore, S.R., Holets, V.R. and Levy, D.J. (1989): Transplantation of a hippocampal, NGF-secreting, temperature-sensitive cell line into adult rats with fimbria-fornix lesions spares cholinergic septal neurons. *Mol. Neurobiol. Neuropharmacol.* 9:85

Will, B. and Hefti, F. (1985): Behavioural and neurochemical effects of chronic intraventricular injections of nerve growth factor in adult rats with fimbria lesions. *Behav. Brain Res.* 17:17-24

Williams, L.R., Varon, S., Peterson, G.M., Wictorin, K., Fischer, W., Björklund, A. and Gage, F.H. (1986): Continuous infusion of nerve growth factor prevents basal forebrain neuronal death after fimbria fornix transection. *Proc. Natl. Acad. Sci. USA* 83:9231-9235

Wong, V. and Kessler, J.A. (1987): Solubilization of a membrane factor that stimulates levels of substance P and choline acetyltransferase in sympathetic neurons. *Proc. Natl. Acad. Sci. USA* 84:8726-8729

Woody, C.D., Swartz, B.E. and Gruen, E. (1978): Effects of acetylcholine and cyclic GMP on input resistance of cortical neurons in awake cats. *Brain Res.* 158:373-395

Woolf, N.J. and Butcher, L.L. (1982): Cholinergic projections to the basolateral amygdala: a combined Evans Blue and acetylcholinesterase analysis. *Brain Res. Bull.* 8:751-763

Woolf, N.J., Eckenstein, F. and Butcher, L. L. (1984): Cholinergic systems in the rat brain: I. Projections to the limbic telencephalon. *Brain Res. Bull.* 13:751-784

Wurtman, R.J., Blusztajn, J. K., Ulus, I.H., Lopez, G., Coviella, I., Buyukuysal, R.L., Growdon, J.H. and Slack, B.E. (1990): Choline metabolism in cholinergic neurons: implications for the pathogenesis of neurodegenerative diseases. In: *Alzheimer's Disease. Advances in Neurology, Vol. 51.* Wurtman, R.J., Corkin, S., Growdon, J.H., Ritter-Walker, E., eds. New York: Raven Press

Záborszky, L. (1989): Afferent connections of the forebrain cholinergic projection neurons, with special reference to monoaminergic and peptidergic fibers. In: *Central Cholinergic Synaptic Transmission.* Frotscher, M., Misgeld, U., eds. Basel: Birkhäuser

Záborszky, L., and Cullinan, W.E. (1989): Hypothalamic axons terminate on forebrain cholinergic neurons: an ultrastructural double-labeling study using PHA-L tracing and ChAT immunocytochemistry. *Brain Res.* 479:177-184

Záborszky, L., Carlsen, J., Brashear, H.R. and Heimer, L. (1986a): Cholinergic and GABAergic afferents to the olfactory bulb in the rat with special emphasis on the projection neurons in the nucleus of the horizontal limb of the diagonal band. *J. Comp. Neurol.* 243:488-509

Záborszky, L., Heimer, L., Eckenstein, F. and Léránth, C. (1986b): GABAergic input to cholinergic forebrain neurons: an ultrastructural study using retrograde tracing of HRP and double immunolabeling. *J. Comp. Neurol.* 250:282-295

Záborszky, L., Léránth, C. and Heimer, L. (1984): Ultrastructural evidence of amygdalofugal axons terminating on cholinergic cells of the rostral forebrain. *Neurosci. Lett.* 52:219-225

Behavioral Neuroanatomy of Cholinergic Innervation in the Primate Cerebral Cortex

M.-Marsel Mesulam*

Central cholinergic pathways have been implicated in the regulation of extrapyramidal motor function, arousal, sleep, mood and especially memory (Karczmar, 1975). In keeping with the diversity of these behavioral affiliations, cholinergic pathways reach all levels of the neuraxis but also display a strict topographical arrangement. Modern methods for axonal tracing and immunohistochemistry have led to the accumulation of considerable information on the anatomical organization of these pathways.

The cholinergic innervation of the striatal complex is predominantly intrinsic and originates from cholinergic interneurons (Woolfe and Butcher, 1981). In contrast, the cholinergic innervation of the cerebral cortex, amygdaloid nuclei, olfactory bulb, thalamus and mesencephalic tectum is almost exclusively extrinsic, at least in the adult primate. The hippocampal formation receives its major cholinergic innervation from the medial septal nucleus (the cholinergic neurons of which are also designated as Chl) and the vertical limb nucleus of the diagonal band (Ch2); the olfactory bulb from the horizontal limb nucleus of the diagonal band (Ch3); the cerebral cortex and amygdaloid nuclei from the nucleus basalis (Ch4); the thalamus from the pedunculopontine (Ch5) and laterodorsal tegmental nuclei (Ch6); the interpeduncular nucleus from the medial habenula (Ch7) and the superior colliculus from the parabigeminal nucleus (Ch8) (Mesulam et al., 1983a, b; Mufson et al., 1986).

---

* This paper appeared in slightly different form in *Central Cholinergic Synaptic Transmission*, in Frotscher, M. and Misgeld, U., eds. ©1989 Birkhäuser Verlag.

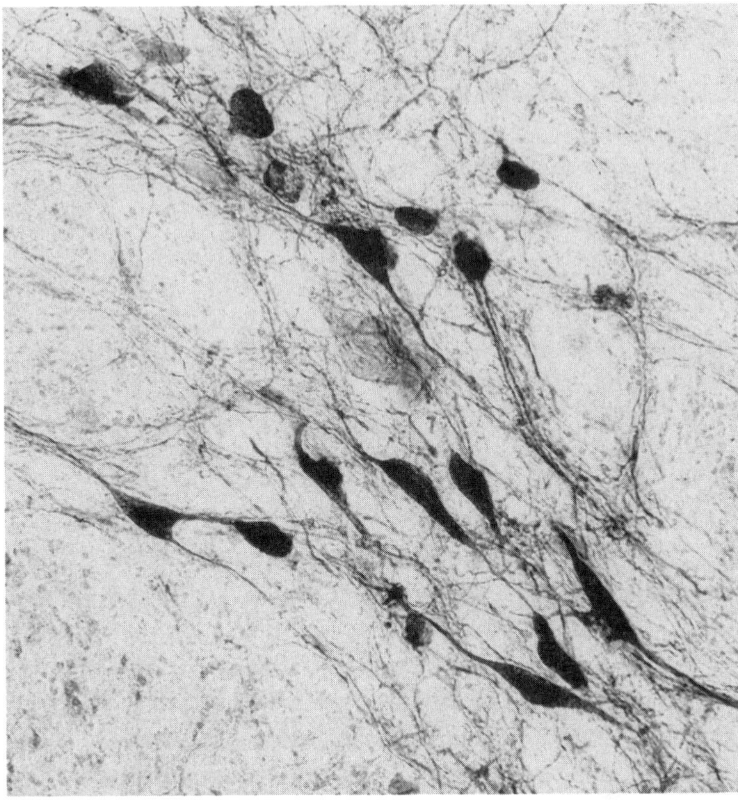

Figure 1. Choline acetyltransferase immunoreactive cholinergic neurons of the human Ch4 complex.

The cholinergic nature of the nucleus basalis (NB) neurons has been demonstrated in a large number of animal species by showing the presence of an AChE-rich and ChAT-positive staining pattern (Wainer et al., 1984). In both man and monkey, more than 90% of the magnocellular NB neurons are also ChAT-positive (Mesulam et al., 1983a; Mesulam and Geula, 1988). These observations justify the designation of this cell group as the NB-Ch4 complex. We use the term Ch4 (sensu strictu) when referring exclusively to the ChAT-positive (cholinergic) neurons and the term NB-Ch4 when referring to the entire NB complex. The neurochemical properties of the ChAT-negative NB neurons remain to be determined. Some of these are NADPH and/or somatostatin-positive (Candy et al., 1985; Ellison et al., 1987).

Two types of observations have shown that the NB-Ch4 complex is the major source of cortical cholinergic innervation. First, retrogradely transported tracers injected into cortical areas always label substantial numbers of cholinergic NB-Ch4 neurons (Mesulam et al., 1983a, b). Second, lesions involving Ch4 cause a major reduction of cortical ChAT levels and cholinergic fiber staining (Johnston et al., 1979; Mufson et al., 1987). This type of evidence is not available for the human brain. However, indirect support has been gathered from patients with Alzheimer's disease in whom cell loss of the NB-Ch4 complex is almost always associated with a corresponding depletion of cortical ChAT (Etienne et al., 1986).

The human NB-Ch4 extends from the level of the olfactory tubercle to that of the anterior hippocampus, spanning a distance of 13–14 mm in the sagittal plane. It attains its greatest medio-lateral width of 18 mm within the substantia innominata (subcommissural gray). Arendt et al. (1985) have estimated that the human NB-Ch4 complex contains 200,000 neurons in each hemisphere. Thus, the NB-Ch4 is about 10 times larger than the nucleus locus coeruleus which contains approximately 15,000 neurons in the adult human brain (Vijayashankar and Brody, 1979). The human NB-Ch4 can be subdivided into six subsectors: anteromedial (NB-Ch4am), anterolateral (NB-Ch4al), anterointermediate (NB-Ch4ai), intermediodorsal (NB-Ch4id), intermedioventral (NB-Ch4iv) and posterior (NB-Ch4p) (Mesulam and Geula, 1988).

Gorry (1963) has pointed out that the NB displays a progressive evolutionary trend, becoming more and more extensive and differentiated in more highly evolved species, especially in primates and cetacea. Our observations in the brains of turtles, mice, rats, squirrel monkeys, rhesus monkeys and humans are consistent with this general view and show that the primate NB-Ch4 is a highly differentiated and relatively large structure. Although many morphological features of the human NB-Ch4 are similar to those described for the rhesus monkey, there is also a sense of increased complexity and differentiation.

The NB-Ch4 complex has been designated as an "open" nucleus. There is a certain overlap with surrounding cell groups such as the olfactory tubercle, preoptic area, hypothalamic nuclei, striatal structures, nuclei of the diagonal band, amygdaloid nuclei and globus pallidus. There is no strict delineation between nuclear aggregates and passing fiber tracts. Many NB-Ch4 neurons, for example, are embedded within (or abut upon) the internal capsule, the diagonal bands of Broca, the anterior commissure, the ansa peduncularis (inferior thalamic peduncle) and the ansa lenticularis. In fact, previous designations for the nucleus basalis used terms such as the "nucleus of the ansa peduncularis" and the "nucleus of thc ansa lenticularis." The physiological implication of this intimate association with fiber bundles is unknown. Conceivably, the NB-Ch4 complex could monitor and perhaps influence the electrical activity along those fiber tracts. In addition to this open nuclear structure, the neurons of NB-Ch4 are heteromorphic in shape and have an isodendritic morphology with overlapping dendritic fields. These characteristics, also present in the nuclei of the brainstem reticular formation, have led to the suggestion that the NB-Ch4 complex could be conceptualized as a telencephalic extension of the brainstem reticular core (Ramon-Moliner and Nauta, 1966).

Experimental neuroanatomical methods in the monkey brain have shown that different cortical areas receive their major cholinergic input from different subsectors of the NB-Ch4 complex. Thus, Ch4am provides the major source of cholinergic input to medial cortical areas including the cingulate gyrus; Ch4al to frontal and parietal opercular regions and the amygdaloid nuclei; Ch4i to lateral frontal, parietal, peristriate and temporal regions; and Ch4p to superior temporal and temporopolar areas (Mesulam et al., 1983a, 1986a). The experimental methods that have been used to reveal this topographic arrangement cannot be used in the human brain. However, indirect evidence for a topographical arrangement can be gathered from disease states that selectively affect individual sectors of Ch4 or only parts of the cortical cholinergic innervation. For example, we described two cases with Alzheimer's disease in which extensive loss of cholinergic fibers in temporopolar but not frontal opercular cortex was associated with marked cell loss in Ch4p but not in Ch4a. This relationship is consistent with the topography of these projections in the monkey brain (Mesulam and Geula, 1988). Many additional cases will bc necessary in order to unravel the complete topography of the corticopetal cholinergic projections of the NB-Ch4 complex in the human brain. The two cases that we have reported indicate that this projection is not diffuse and that it obeys a pattern that may well parallel the overall organization described in the rhesus monkey.

The AChE-rich fibers of the human cortex can be visualized in great detail with the help of recently developed and highly sensitive modifications of the Karnovsky-Roots procedure (Tago et al., 1986; Mesulam et al., 1987). Several lines of evidence indicate that these AChE-rich fibers are essentially identical to the cholinergic axons originating from Ch4 (see Mesulam et al., 1984; Mufson et al., 1987 for discussion). The laminar organization and regional density of AChE-rich (putatively cholinergic) fibers varies from one cortical area to another. Histochemical and neurochemical studies in the rhesus monkey have shown that limbic and paralimbic areas receive the most intense cholinergic input, whereas the primary sensory-motor and isocortical association ares have a much less intense input. These differences are quite marked and may be as high as seven-fold (Mesulam et al., 1984, 1986b). Observations in the human brain show an almost identical pattern, including a close adherence to cytoarchitectonic boundaries (Mesulam and Geula, 1988).

Regional variations in the cholinergic innervation of the cerebral cortex suggest that sensory information about extrapersonal events (especially those that are motivationally relevant) is likely to come under progressively greater cholinergic influence as it is conveyed along the multisynaptic pathways leading to limbic structures (Mesulam et al., 1986b). We speculated that these cholinergic pathways may provide a gating mechanism for regulating the access of sensory information into the limbic system.

Neuroanatomical experiments in the monkey show that the reciprocal connectivity between the NB-Ch4 complex and the cerebral cortex is highly skewed (Mesulam and Mufson, 1984; Russchen et al., 1985). Although this nucleus projects to all cortical areas, it receives input only from a handful of regions, all of which belong to the limbic and paralimbic parts of the brain (i.e., piriform, orbitofrontal, insular, temporopolar, parahippocampal and probably cingulate regions). Additional input comes from other limbic structures such as the amygdala, hypothalamus, septum and nucleus accumbens (or ventral globus pallidus). Our preliminary observations based on silver staining of 2 brains with circumscribed lesions suggests that the cingulate gyrus and the medial temporal region in the human brain send projections to the NB-Ch4 complex. Whether the skewed connectivity pattern described in the monkey will also be found to exist in the human brain must await many additional cases that lend themselves to neuroanatomical investigation. In the human brain, catecholaminergic fibers (probably originating from the nucleus locus coeruleus) have also been shown to reach the region of the NB-Ch4 (Gaspar et al., 1985).

The skewed connectivity between NB-Ch4 and the cerebral cortex suggests that most cortical areas (primary sensory, motor and high order association areas) have no direct feedback control upon the cholinergic input that they receive, whereas a handful of limbic and paralimbic areas can have direct control over the cholinergic input that they receive as well as over the cholinergic input that reaches all other parts of the cerebral cortex. Thus, the NB-Ch4 complex is in a position to act as a cholinergic relay for rapidly modulating the activity of the entire cortical surface according to the prevailing motivational conditions as reflected by the limbic system. This skewed organization, which is probably also found in the nucleus locus coeruleus, the brainstem raphe nuclei and the substantia nigra is well suited for modulating behavioral states (Mesulam, 1987).

Physiological experiments indicate that the acetylcholine (ACh) released by cortical cholinergic axons has two effects upon pyramidal neurons: a rapid and inhibitory effect probably mediated by GABAergic interneurons, and a more prolonged excitatory effect probably reflecting the direct effect of ACh upon postsynaptic cholinergic receptors located on pyramidal neurons (McCormick and Prince, 1985). The latter effect is caused by a reduction of potassium conductance in the membrane of the cholinoceptive neuron (Krnjevic, 1981). The excitatory nature and prolonged time course of this effect have led to the designation of ACh as an excitatory neuromodulator of cortical pyramidal neurons.

The ubiquitous distribution of cholinergic innervation indicates that virtually all cortical regions, and therefore all realms of behavior, are likely to be influenced by cholinergic transmission. In fact, even the neuronal response of primary somatosensory cortex to simple tactile stimulation can be modulated by the local application of ACh (Metherate et al., 1987). On the other hand, the preferential concentration of cholinergic pathways in limbic and paralimbic areas also explains why NB-Ch4 lesions (or systemically administered cholinoactive drugs) have their greatest impact on learning and memory, behaviors that are closely associated with the limbic system.

The behavioral specializations of the NB-Ch4 complex have been investigated in a number of animal species with the help of single unit recordings and focal ablations. In the awake and behaving rhesus monkey, these neurons are responsive to the sight and taste of food in a manner that appears to reflect the degree of hunger and even the desirability of the food object (Rolls et al., 1979). This contrasts sharply with the response contingencies of immediately adjacent globus pallidus neurons which fire mostly in conjunction with specific movements (DeLong, 1971). It appears that the NB-Ch4 neurons are important for encoding the existence of rewarding events. This may explain why electrical stimulation in this general area in some patients has elicited reports of a pleasurable sensation (Heath, 1959) and perhaps also why this region sustains self-stimulation in animals (Olds and Milner, 1954).

In the absence of entirely selective cholinotoxins, it is difficult to interpret experiments based on electrolytic or excitotoxin-induced lesions of the NB-Ch4 complex. Such lesions almost certainly include additional damage to adjacent structures. However, some experiments include two types of controls that increase the specificity of the findings. First, they show that the degree of behavioral deficit correlates with the extent of cortical ChAT depletion. Secondly, they show that the behavioral deficits are reversible by the administration of cholinoactive agents. The most closely studied behaviors in these types of experiments have been in the area of memory and learning. In a number of species, including rodents and primates, NB-Ch4 lesions have impaired the acquisition and retention of new tasks and also the relearning of discriminations that had been mastered in the presurgical period (Flicker et al., 1983; Ridley et al., 1986; Dunnett et al., 1987).

Additional ablation experiments (in rats and cats) have suggested that the NB-Ch4 complex is responsible for mediating the low voltage fast cortical EEG activity that is induced by cholinergic drugs (Steward et al., 1984) and the cortical vasodilation that is elicited by cerebellar stimulation (Iadecola et al., 1983). Unilateral lesions in Ch4 have also led to a decrease, at least transiently, of glucose utilization in the ipsilateral cerebral cortex (Orzi et al., 1986). Furthermore, the ability of cats to maintain non-REM sleep is impaired by lesions that appear to include the NB-Ch4 complex (Szymusiak and McGinty, 1986).

Degenerative changes in the NB-Ch4 complex have been reported in a surprisingly large number of neurological diseases. This rapidly growing list now includes Alzheimer's disease, Down's Syndrome, Parkinson's disease, olivopontocerebellar atrophy, Pick's disease, supranuclear ophthalmoplegia and even schizophrenia (for review see Averback, 1981; Casanova et al., 1985; Rogers et al., 1985; Tagliavini and Pilleri,

1985). It remains to be determined to what extent the involvement in NB-Ch4 contributes to the mental state alteration that exists in each of these conditions. The most extensive observations have been reported in conjunction with Alzheimer's and Parkinson's diseases. These conditions involve a substantial loss of NB-Ch4 neurons and an associated loss of cortical ChAT and cholinergic fibers.

The suggestion had been advanced that the cholinergic loss constitutes the central feature of Alzheimer's disease in a manner that may parallel the relationship between Parkinson's disease and the loss of dopaminergic nigrostriatal projections. The loss of cortical cholinergic innervation in Alzheimer's disease is marked, consistent and significantly correlated with the extent of mental state deficit (Perry et al., 1978). It is likely that the loss of cortical cholinergic pathways contributes to the severity of the memory loss and perhaps to the other features of the dementia. However, in view of the many additional pathological features of this disease (especially the great number of cortical neurofibrillary tangles, neuritic plaques and neuronal loss) it is doubtful that the cholinergic lesion is the pivotal feature or the prime mover in Alzheimer's disease. It is not even known if the loss of cholinergic cortical innervation in Alzheimer's disease represents a primary involvement of the perikarya in the NB-Ch4 complex or if the primary lesion is in the cortical fibers, resulting in a retrograde degeneration within NB-Ch4 (Mesulam, 1986). It has been shown that the survival of the NB-Ch4 neurons is dependent on the retrograde transport of nerve growth factor (NGF) from the cerebral cortex. Conceivably, the severe cortical pathology in Alzheimer's disease may interfere with the availability and uptake of NGF and other trophic factors necessary for the upkeep of the NB-Ch4 perikarya (Hefti and Weiner, 1986). In other conditions such as Parkinson's disease where cortical involvement is much less consistent, the involvement of NB-Ch4 may begin at the level of the perikarya and proceed in a corticopetal direction (Bloxam et al., 1984). The pathophysiological mechanism for the involvement of NB-Ch4 in neurodegenerative conditions may thus vary from one disease to another.

A good deal of attention has also been directed to the age-related changes in the NB-Ch4 complex. The most extensive studies have been done in the rodent and show that these neurons display an age-related decrease in volume but probably not in number. A similar situation may exist in the human brain. The age-related shrinkage of NB-Ch4 neurons could be responsible for the relatively minor alterations of memory abilities characteristic of advanced age (see Hornberger et al., 1985; Mesulam et al., 1987b for review).

In summary, the NB-Ch4 complex is highly developed in the primate brain and provides the origin of one of the most important transmitter systems of the forebrain. Anatomical, physiological and behavioral experiments are only beginning to unravel some of the mechanisms that link this nucleus to complex behavior, aging and neurodegenerative diseases.

ACKNOWLEDGMENTS

I want to thank Leah Christie for expert secretarial assistance. Supported in part by a Javits Neuroscience Investigator Award of the NINCDS and the Alzheimer's Disease and Related Disorders Association. This review contains paraphrases and quotations from Mesulam and Geula (1988).

REFERENCES

Arendt, T., Bigl, V., Tennstedt, A. and Arendt, A. (1985): Neuronal loss in different parts of the nucleus basalis is related to neuritic plaque formation in cortical target areas in Alzheimer's disease. *J. Neurosci. Ann. Neurol.* 14: 1-14

Averback, P. (1981): Lesions of the nucleus ansae peduncularis in neuropsychiatric disease. *Arch. Neurol.* 38:230-235

Bloxam, C.A., Perry, E.K., Perry, R.H. and Candy, J.M. (1984): Neuropathological and neurochemical correlate of Alzheimer-type and Parkinsonian dementia. In: *Advances in Basic Research and Therapies.* Wurtman, R.J., Corkin, S.H., and Growdon, J.H., eds. Alzheimer's Disease: Center for Brain Sciences and Metabolism Charitable Trust, Cambridge, MA, pp. 39-52

Candy, J.M., Perry, R.H., Thompson, J.E., Johnson, M., Oakley, A.E. and Edwardson, J.A. (1985): The current status of the cortical cholinergic system in Alzheimer's disease and Parkinson's disease. *J. Anat.* 140:309-327

Casanova, M.F., Walker, L.C., Whitehouse, P.J. and Price D.L. (1985): Abnormalities of the nucleus basalis in Down's Syndrome. *Ann. Neurol.* 18: 310-313

DeLong, M.R. (1971): Activity of pallidal neurons during movement. *J. Neurophysiol.* 34:414-427

Dunnett, S.B., Whishaw, I.Q., Jones, G.H., and Bunch, S.T. (1987): Behavioral, biochemical and histochemical effects of different neurotoxic amino acids injected into nucleus basalis magnocellularis of rats. *J. Neurosci.* 20:653-669

Ellison, D.W., Kowall, N.W. and Martin, J.B. (1987): Subset of neurons characterized by the presence of NADPH-diophorase in human substantia innominata.

J. Comp. Neurol. 260:233-245

Etienne, P., Robitaille, Y., Wood, P., Gauthier, S., Nair, N.P.V. and Quirion, R. (1986): Nucleus basalis neuronal loss, neuritic plaques and choline acetyltransferase activity in advanced Alzheimer's disease. *J. Neurosci.*19:1279-1291

Flicker, C., Dean, R.L., Watkins, D.L., Fisher, S.K., and Bartus, R.T. (1983): Behavioral and neurochemical effects following neurotoxic lesions of a major cholinergic input to the cerebral cortex in the rat. *Pharmac. Biochem. Behav.* 18:973-981

Gaspar, P., Berger, B., Alvarex, C., Vigny, A. and Henry, J. P. (1985): Catecholaminergic innervation of the septal area in man: immunocytochemical study using TH and DBH antibodies. *J. Comp. Neurol.* 214:12-33

German, D.C., Bruce, G., and Hersh, L.B. (1985): Immunohistochemical staining of cholinergic neurons in the human brain using a polyclonal antibody to human choline acetyltransferase. *Neurosci. Lett.* 61:1-5

Gorry, J.D. (1963) Studies on the comparative anatomy of the ganglion basale of Meynert. *Acta. Anat.* 55:51-104

Heath, R.G. (1959): *Studies in Schizophrenia.* Harvard University Press, Cambridge, MA.

Hefti, F. and Weiner, W.J. (1986): Nerve growth factor and Alzheimer's disease. *Ann. Neurol.* 20:275-281

Hornberger, J.C., Buell, S.J., Flood, D.G. (1985): Stability of numbers but not size of forebrain cholinergic neurons to 53 months. *Neurobiol. Aging* 6:269-275

Iadecola, C., Mraovitch, S., Meeley, M.P. and Reis, D.J. (1983): Lesions of the basal forebrain in rat selectively impair vasodilation elicited from cerebellar fastigial nucleus. *Brain Res.* 279:41-52

Johnston, M.V., McKinney, M. and Coyle, J.T. (1979): Evidence for a cholinergic projection to neocortex from neurons in basal forbrain. *Proc. Natl. Acad. Sci.* 76:5392-5396

Karczmar, A.G. (1975): Cholinergic influences on behavior. In: *Cholinergic Mechanisms.* Waser, P.G., ed. Raven Press, New York, pp. 501-529

Krnjević, K. (1981): Acetylcholine as a modulator of amino-acid-mediated synaptic transmission. In: *The Role of Peptides and Amino Acids as Neurotransmitters.* A. Liss, New York, pp. 124-141

McCormick, D.A., and Prince, D.A. (1985): Two types of muscarinic responses to acetylcholine in mammalian cortical neurons. *Proc. Natl Acad. Sci. USA* 82:6344-6348

Mesulam, M.-M. (1986): Alzheimer's plaques and cortical cholinergic innervation. *Neurosci.* 17:275-276

Mesulam, M.-M. (1987a): Asymmetry of neural feedback in the organization of behavioral states. *Science* 237:537-538

Mesulam, M.-M. and Geula, C. (1988): Nucleus basalis (Ch4) and cortical cholinergic innervation in the human brain. *J. Comp. Neurol.* 275:216-240

Mesulam, M.-M. and Mufson, E.J. (1984): Neural inputs into the nucleus basalis of the substantia innominata (Ch4) in the rhesus monkey. *Brain* 107:253-274

Mesulam, M.-M., Mufson, E.J., Levey, A.I. and Wainer, B.H. (1983a): Cholinergic innervation of cortex by the basal forebrain: cytochemistry and cortical connections of the septal area, diagonal band nuclei, nucleus basalis (substantia innominata) and hypothalamus in the rhesus monkey. *J. Comp. Neurol.* 214:170-197

Mesulam, M.-M., Mufson, E.J. and Rogers, J. (1987b): Age-related shrinkage of cortically projecting cholinergic neurons: a selective effect. *Ann. Neurol.* 22:31-36

Mesulam, M.-M., Mufson, E.J. and Wainer, B.H. (1986a): Three-dimensional representation and cortical projection topography of the nucleus basalis (Ch4) in the macaque: concurrent demonstration of choline acetyltransferase and retrograde transport with a stabilized tetramethylbenzidine method for HRP. *Brain Res.* 367:301-308

Mesulam, M.-M., Mufson, E.J., Wainer, B.H. and Levey, A.I. (1983b): Central cholinergic pathways in the rat: an overview based on an alternative nomenclature (Ch1-Ch6). *Neurosci.* 10:1185-1201

Mesulam, M.-M., Rosen, A.D. and Mufson, E.J. (1984): Regional variations in cortical cholinergic innervation: chemoarchitectonics of acetylcholinesterase-containing fibers in the macaque brain. *Brain Res.* 311:245-258

Mesulam, M.-M., Volicer, L., Marquis, J.K. Mufson, E.J. and Green, R.C. (1986b): systematic regional differences in the cholinergic innervation of the primate cerebral cortex: distribution of enzyme activities and some behavioral implications. *Ann. Neurol.* 19:144 -151

Metherate, R., Tremblay, N. and Dykes, R.W. (1987): Acetylcholine permits long-term enhancement of neuronal responsiveness in cat primary somatosensory cortex. *Neurosci.* 22:75-81

Mufson, E.J., Kehr, A.D., Wainer, B.H. and Mesulam, M.-M. (1987): Cortical effects of neurotoxic damage to the nucleus basalis in rats: persistent loss of extrinsic cholinergic input and lack of transsynaptic effect upon the number of somatostatin-containing, cholinesterase-positive and cholinergic cortical neurons. *Brain Res.* 417:385-388

Mufson, E.J., Martin, T.L., Mash, D.C., Wainer, B.H. and Mesulam, M.-M. (1986): Cholinergic projections from the parabigemenal nucleus (Ch8) to the superior colliculus in the mouse: a combined analysis of HRP transport and choline acetyltransferase immunohistochemistry. *Brain Res.* 370:144-148

Nagai, T., McGeer, P.L., Peng, J.H., McGeer, E.G. and Dolman, C.E. (1983): Choline acetyltransferase immunohistochemistry in brains of Alzheimer's disease patients and controls. *Neurosci. Lett.* 36:195-199

Olds, J. and Milner, P. (1954): Positive reinforcement produced by electrical stimulation of septal area and other regions of the rat brain. *J. Comp. Physiol. Psychol.* 47:419-427

Orzi, F., Diana, G., Palombo, E., Lenzi, G.L., Bracco, L. and Fieschi, C. (1986): Effects of unilateral lesion of the nucleus basalis on local cerebral glucose utilization in the rat. In: *Neuroendocrine System and Aging*. Vezzadini, P., Facchini, A., and Labo, G., eds. Eurage, pp. 259-264

Pearson, R.C.A., Sofroniew, M.V., Cuello, A.C., Powell, T.P.S., Eckenstein, F., Esiri, M. M. and Wilcock G.K. (1984): Persistence of cholinergic neurons in the basal nucleus in a brain with senile dementia of the Alzheimer's type demonstrated by immunohistochemical staining for choline acetyltransferase. *Brain Res.* 289:375-379

Perry, E.K., Tomlinson, B.E., Blessed, G., Bergmann, K., Gibson, P.H. and Perry, R.H. (1978): Correlation of cholinergic abnormalities with senile plaques and mental test scores in senile dementia. *Br. Med. J.* 2:1457-1459

Ramon-Moliner, E. and Nauta, W.J.H. (1966): The isodendritic core of the brain stem. *J. Comp. Neurol.* 126:311

Ridley, R.M., Murray, T.K., Johnson, J.A. and Baker, H.F. (1986): Learning impairment following lesion of the basal nucleus of Meynert in the marmoset: modification by cholinergic drugs. *Brain Res.* 376:108-116

Rogers, J.D., Brogan, D. and Mirra, S.S. (1985): The nucleus basalis of Meynert in neurological disease: a quantitative morphological study. *Ann. Neurol.* 17:163-170

Rolls, E.T., Sanghera, M.K. and Rober-Hall, A. (1979): The latency of activation of neurons in the lateral hypothalamus and substantia innominata during feeding in the monkey. *Brain Res.* 164:121-135

Russchen, F.T., Amaral, D.G. and Price, J.L. (1985): The afferent connections of the substantia innominata in the monkey, Macaca fascicularis. *J. Comp. Neurol.* 24:1-27

Saper, C.B. and Chelimsky, T.C. (1984): A cytoarchitectonic and histochemical study of nucleus basalis and associated cell groups in the normal human brain. *Neurosci.* 13:1023-1037

Steward, D.J., MacFabe, D.F. and Vanderwolf, C.N. (1984): Cholinergic activation of the electrocorticogram: role of the substantia innominata and effects of atropine and quinuclidinyl benzylate. *Brain Res.* 322:219-232

Szymusiak, R. and McGinty, D. (1986): Sleep suppression following kainic acid-induced lesions of the basal forebrain. *Exp. Neurol.* 94:598-614

Tagliavini, F. and Pilleri, G. (1985): Neuronal loss in the basal nucleus of Meynert in a patient with olivopontocerebellar atrophy. *Acta. Neuropath.* 66:127-133

Tago, H., Kimura, H. and Maeda, T. (1986): Visualization of detailed acetylcholinesterase fiber and neuron staining in rat brain by a sensitive histochemical procedure. *J. Histochem. Cytochem.* 34: 1431-1438

Vijayashankar, N. and Brody, H. (1979): A quantitative study of the pigmented neurons in the nuclei locus coeruleus and sub coeruleus in man as related to aging. *J. Neuropath. Exp. Neurol.* 38:490-497

Wainer, B.H., Levey, A.I., Mufson, E.J. and Mesulam, M.-M. (1984): Cholinergic systems in mammalian brain identified with antibodies against choline acetyltransferase. *Neurochem. Int.* 6:163-182

Woolfe, N. J. and Butcher, L.L. (1981) Cholinergic neurons in the caudate-putamen complex proper are intrinsically organized: a combined Evans Blue and acetylcholinesterase analysis. *Brain Res.* 7:487-507

Input/Output Relations of the Magnocellular Nuclei of the Basal Forebrain

J.L. Price and K.M. Carnes

The magnocellular nuclei of the basal forebrain (MNBF) consist of several groups of cholinergic and non-cholinergic cells scattered through the septum, substantia innominata, peripallidum and preoptic region. Although anatomically confusing, this distribution is understandable if it is realized that all of the groups are situated within and along the major fiber pathways of the ventral forebrain. Thus, the nuclei of the diagonal band and the medial septal nucleus are arrayed along the vertical and horizontal limbs of the diagonal band (of Broca), and continue back into the rostral part of the medial forebrain bundle. The nucleus basalis is partially situated along the medial forebrain bundle, but is also related to the ventral amygdalofugal pathway, the ansa lenticularis and (in primates) the medullary laminae of the globus pallidus. As seen with the Golgi method, all these nuclei are made up of multipolar cells with long radiating, spine-free dendrites that extend across the fiber bundles, apparently receiving synaptic inputs from a large number of fibers. Thus, based on their anatomical configuration, cells throughout the MNBF appear to have the capacity to sample and integrate diverse information passing between structures such as the orbito-medial prefrontal cortex, septum, amygdaloid complex, hypothalamus and brainstem. This information may be presumed to shape the functional outputs that the MNBF sends to the cerebral cortex and other telencephalic structures.

INPUTS

The afferent projections to the MNBF have been analyzed in rats and monkeys by several research groups using both anterograde and retrograde axonal tracing methods (e.g., Mesulam and Mufson, 1984; Saper, 1984; Russchen et al., 1985; Grove, 1988; Carnes et al., 1990). These will be summarized by region.

Limbic Forebrain

One of the densest inputs to the MNBF arises in the amygdaloid nuclei and adjacent structures such as the entorhinal and piriform cortex (Mesulam and Mufson, 1984; Russchen et al., 1985; Irle and Markowitsch, 1986; Haring and Wang, 1986; Grove, 1988; Carnes et al., 1990). The subiculum also projects to the rostromedial part of the MNBF (Irle and Markowitsch, 1986; Carnes et al., 1990), and there appears to be a lighter projection from cells in hippocampal fields CA1, CA3 and the hilus of the dentate gyrus (Carnes et al., 1990). In the amygdala, the cells that project to the MNBF are distributed in relatively specific patterns. For example, cells labeled from injections of retrograde axonal tracers in the substantia innominata of the monkey (involving the nucleus of the horizontal diagonal band and the major part of the nucleus basalis) are concentrated in the ventral, parvicellular part of the basal nucleus, and in the accessory basal and central nuclei (Figs. 1,2). In contrast, there are surprisingly few such cells in the lateral nucleus or the dorsal, magnocellular part of the basal nucleus. The lack of a strong projection from the magnocellular basal amygdaloid nucleus is particularly interesting since this part of the nucleus receives the densest cholinergic projection of any forebrain structure (e.g., Hellendall et al., 1985).

Anterograde tracer experiments indicate that the fibers from the amygdala and entorhinal cortex sweep through the MNBF on their course to other parts of the brain, especially to the diencephalon and brainstem (Russchen et al., 1985). Therefore, it might be suggested that these fibers are merely "passing through" the MNBF, and do not synapse there. However, visualization of these fibers with the lectin tracer *Phaseolus vulgarus* leucoagglutinin (PHA-L) shows that they bear bouton-like varicosities along their length, indicating that they form boutons-en-passant throughout the substantia innominata (Fig. 3; Russchen et al., 1985; Grove 1988). In the rat, electron microscopic examination of amygdaloid fibers also demonstrates that they form synapses with cholinergic cells of the MNBF (Záborszky et al., 1985).

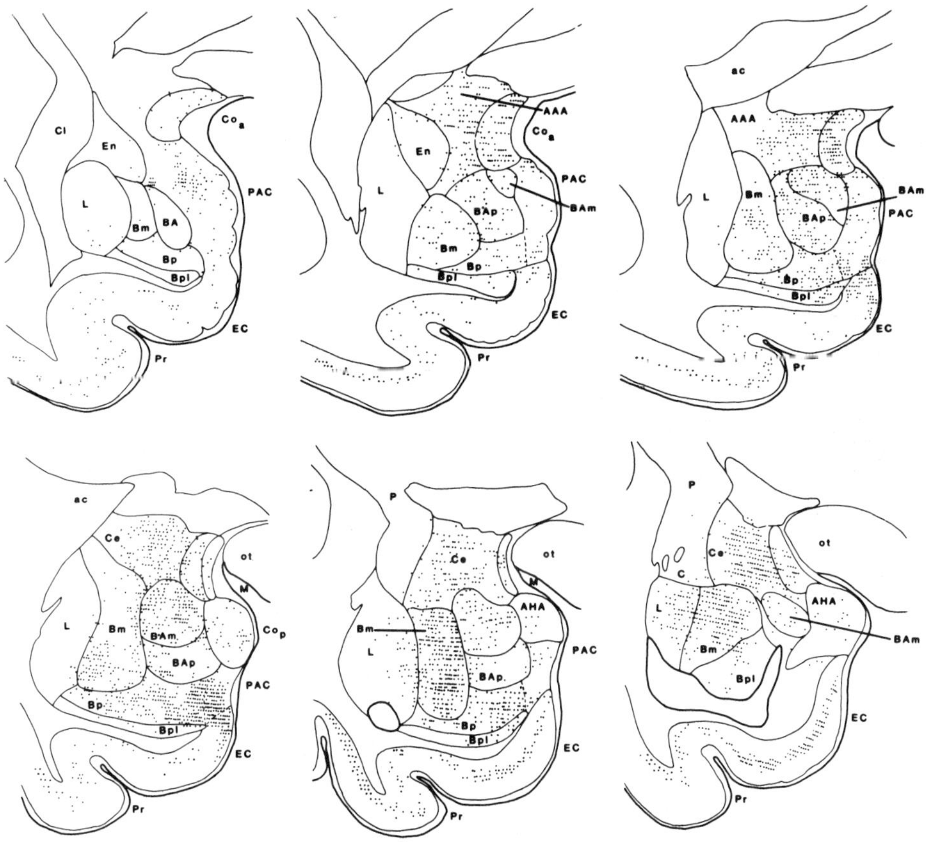

Figure 1. The distribution of cells in the amygdala and adjacent areas (including the periamygdaloid and entorhinal cortex) that project to the nucleus basalis, retrogradely labeled from an injection of WGA-HRP into the basal forebrain. Note the absence of cells in the most dorsal part of the basal amygdaloid nucleus. Reprinted with permisssion of the authors and Alan R. Liss, Inc. from Russchen et al., (1985): The afferent connections of the substantia innominata in the monkey, Macaca fascicularis, *J. Comp. Neurol.* 242:1-27.

Cortex

While the MNBF send axons to all parts of the cerebral cortex, most of the available evidence in the monkey, cat and rat indicates that the bulk (at least) of the neocortical projection to the MNBF originates in areas of the prefrontal, anterior insular and anterior temporal cortical areas that are closely interconnected to the amygdala and other limbic structures (Fig. 4; Mesulam and Mufson, 1984; Saper, 1984; Russchen et al., 1985; Irle and

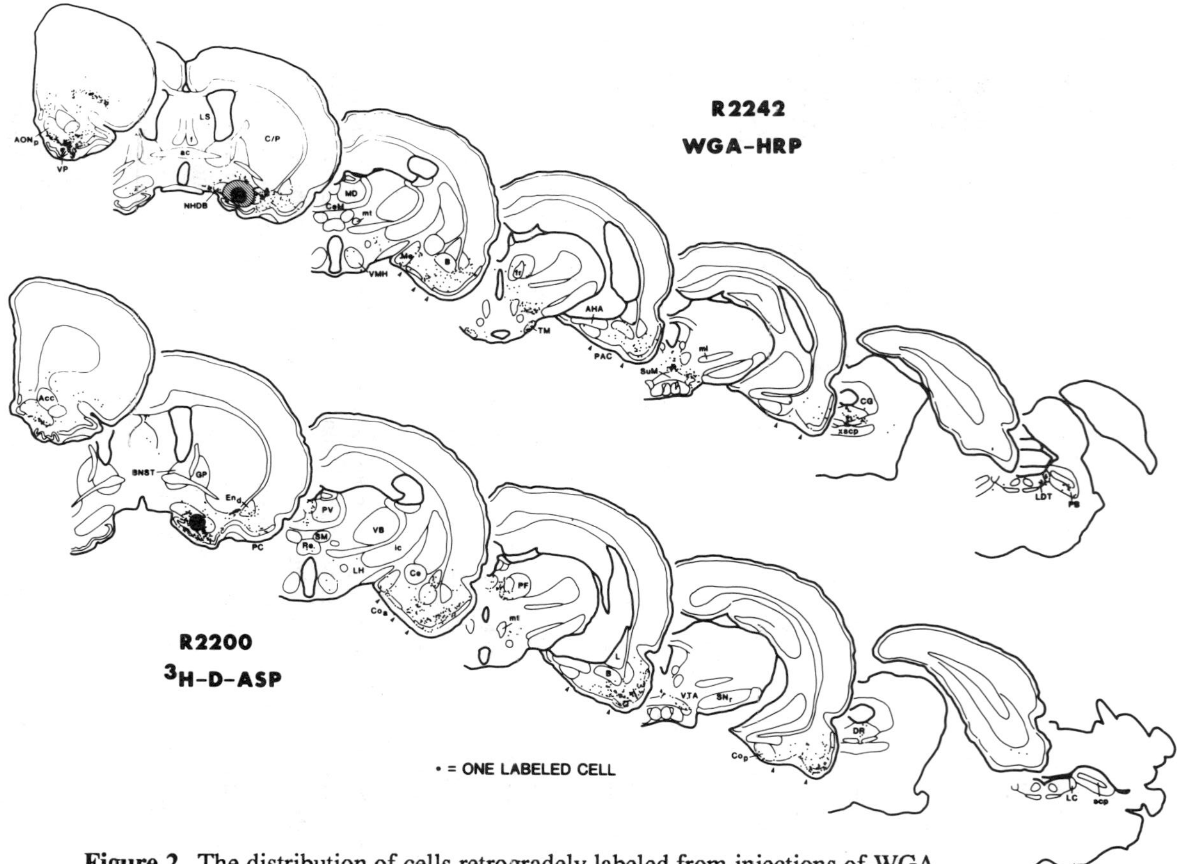

Figure 2. The distribution of cells retrogradely labeled from injections of WGA-HRP (R2242, above) and the "transmitter-specific" tracer ^{3}H-D-aspartate (R2200, below), into the nucleus of the horizontal diagonal band. Note that cells are labeled in the midbrain and dorsal pons with WGA-HRP, but not with ^{3}H-D-aspartate. Adapted from Carnes et al. (1990): *J. Comp Neurol.* 302:824-852

Markowitsch, 1986; Haring and Wang, 1986; Grove, 1988; Carnes et al., 1990). Within the prefrontal cortex the major input is from the posterior orbital and mesial areas. In the rat the caudal, peripallidal part of the MNBF may also receive input from the dorsolateral frontal cortex and the cingulate cortex (Saper, 1984; Haring and Wang, 1986).

Other Forebrain Subcortical Structures

Injections of retrograde axonal tracers into the MNBF also label cells in the lateral septum, the bed nucleus of the stria terminalis, ventral parts of the striatum, the midline thalamic nuclei, and the contralateral MNBF (Figs. 2, 5; Russchen et al., 1985; Grove, 1988; Carnes et al., 1990). Of these, the bed nucleus of the stria terminalis is closely associated with the amygdala, and its projections may be considered similar to those of the amygdala itself. Similarly, the lateral septum receives a strong input

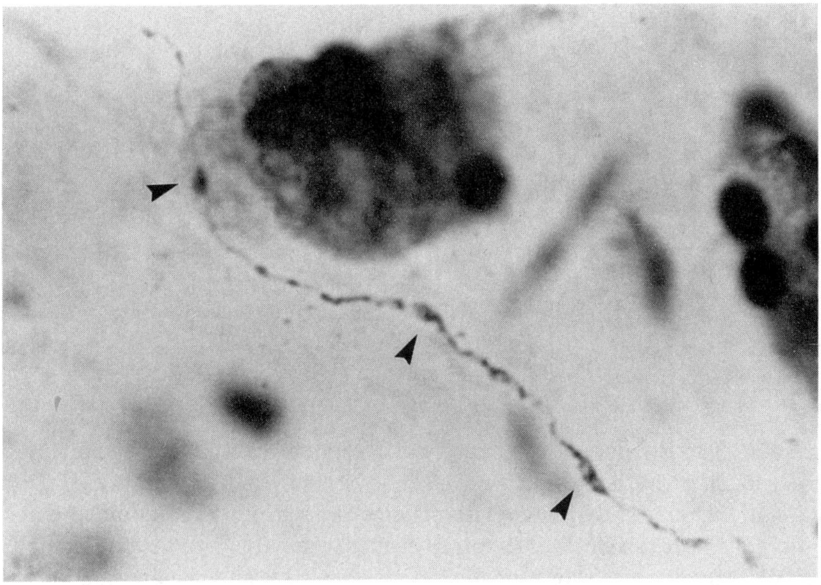

Figure 3. A fiber in the nucleus basalis, labeled with PHA-L injected into the central nucleus of the amygdala. The arrowheads indicate varicosities, which are probably synaptic boutons. Reprinted with permisssion of the authors and Alan R. Liss, Inc. from Russchen et al., (1985): The afferent connections of the substantia innominata in the monkey, Macaca fascicularis, *J. Comp. Neurol.* 242:1-27.

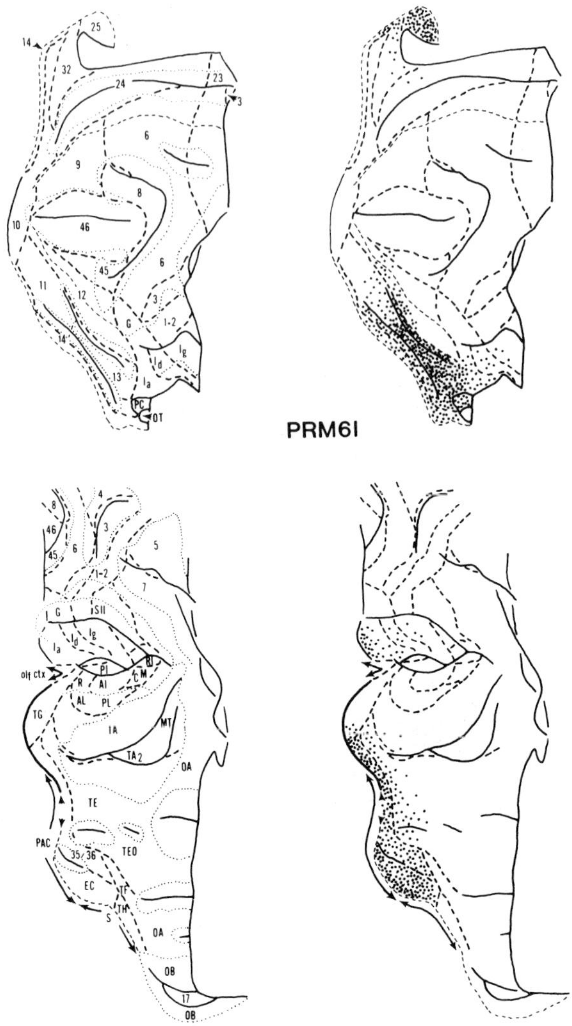

Figure 4. The distribution of cells in the cerebral cortex of the monkey that project to the nucleus basalis, retrogradely labeled from an injection of WGA-HRP into the substantia innominata. The cells are plotted on unfolded maps of the frontal cortex (above) and temporal-insular cortex (below); the designations of cytoarchitectonic areas shown on the left are adapted from the maps of Brodmann, Walker and Bonin and Bailey (see Amaral and Price, 1984). Note that the cells are restricted to the orbital and medial prefrontal cortex (areas 11, 12, 13, 14, 25 and 32), the rostral temporal cortex (areas 35 and 36, the edge of areas TG and TE, and the entorhinal cortex, EC), and rostral insular areas (areas Ia and Id). Reprinted with permisssion of the authors and Alan R. Liss, Inc. from Russchen et al., (1985): The afferent connections of the substantia innominata in the monkey, Macaca fascicularis, *J. Comp. Neurol.* 242:1-27.

from the hippocampal formation, and may be expected to relay this to the MNBF; the septal fibers terminate primarily in the rostromedial components of the MNBF (Carnes et al., 1990). Since the ventral striatum and midline thalamus also project heavily to ventral striato-pallidal areas that are closely associated with the MNBF, it is difficult to be certain that fibers from those structures end on cells of the magnocellular nuclei. However, Grove and her colleagues have provided electron microscopic evidence that cholinergic cells within the region of overlap between the MNBF and the globus pallidus receive synaptic input from striatal axons (Grove and Ingham, 1986).

The projection from the contralateral MNBF is particularly interesting anatomically because it connects homotopic regions of the MNBF on the two sides, and because the fibers take an unusual course through the stria medullaris and habenular commissure (Price and Powell, 1970b; Semba et al., 1988; Carnes et al., 1990). The transmitter used by the fibers is not known. Double labeling experiments with retrograde axonal tracers combined with choline acetyltransferase immunohistochemistry indicate that the projection is not cholinergic, and further experiments with the "transmitter specific" tracer ^{3}H-D-aspartate indicate that they are not glutamatergic (Semba et al., 1988a; Carnes et al., 1990). Similar experiments with ^{3}H-GABA as a retrograde tracer also failed to provide evidence that the cells are GABAergic, but negative evidence with this tracer may be less reliable.

Organization and Transmitters

There is some degree of organization in the cortical input to the MNBF, at least in the rat (Saper, 1984; Carnes et al., 1990). The more rostromedial nuclei (i.e., the medial septal nucleus and the nucleus of the vertical diagonal band) receive fibers primarily from the medial prefrontal cortex, while progressively more lateral and caudal nuclei (the nucleus of the horizontal diagonal band and the nucleus basalis) receive their major cortical inputs from progressively more lateral orbital and insular areas.

The amygdaloid projection is less obviously organized, but fibers from different nuclei show differential patterns of termination within the MNBF. For example, although both the basal and central amygdaloid nuclei in the monkey project throughout the nucleus basalis, the fibers from the central nucleus tend to be concentrated in patches, while those from the basal nucleus are more evenly distributed (Fig. 6; Russchen et al., 1985). In the rat it also appears that different parts of the amygdala project to different parts of the substantia innominata (Grove, 1988).

The great majority of the forebrain projections to the MNBF can be labeled with the "transmitter-specific" retrograde tracer ^{3}H-D-aspartate, and may be presumed to utilize glutamate and/or aspartate as their transmitter (Fig. 2; Carnes et al., 1990). The major exception is the projection

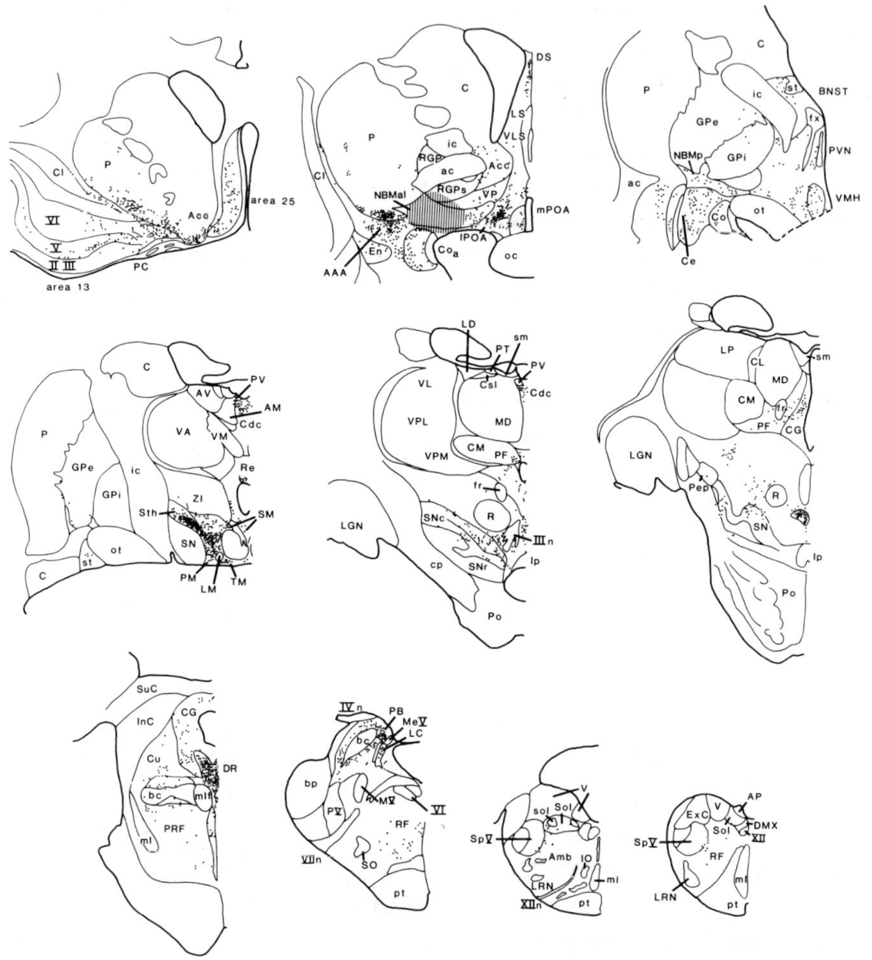

Figure 5. Cells labeled with WGA-HRP in subcortical areas of the monkey, after an injection into the nucleus basalis (indicated by shaded area). Reprinted with permisssion of the authors and Alan R. Liss, Inc. from Russchen et al., (1985): The afferent connections of the substantia innominata in the monkey, Macaca fascicularis, *J. Comp. Neurol.* 242:1-27.

from hippocampal fields CA1 and CA3, and the hilus of the dentate gyrus. Alonso and Kohler (1982) also indicate that this projection may originate from non-pyramidal cells, whereas the putatively glutamatergic projection from the subiculum arises from pyramidal cells. As described above, the crossed projection from the homotopic part of the contralateral MNBF apparently does not utilize glutamate, GABA or acetylcholine as transmitters.

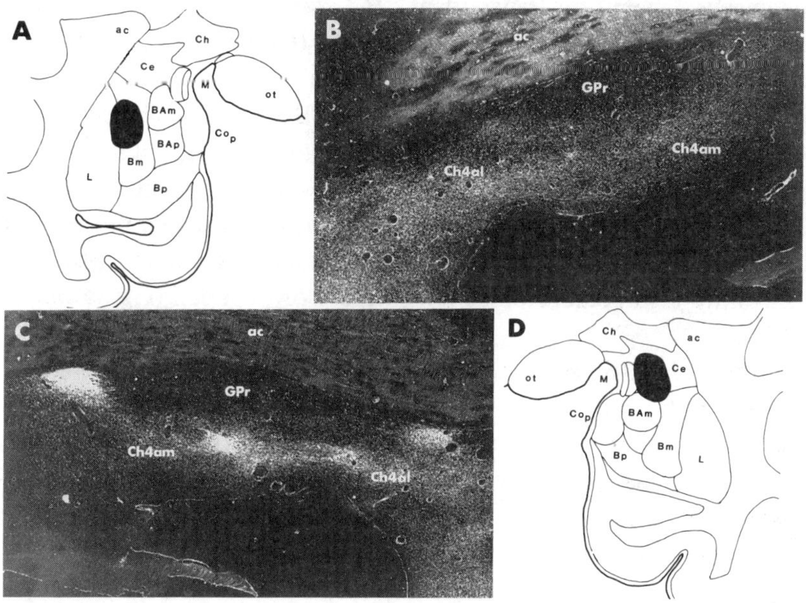

Figure 6. Differential patterns of labeled amygdaloid fibers in the nucleus basalis and adjacent areas in the monkey, after injections of ^{3}H-leucine into the basal amygdaloid nucleus (A & B) and the central amygdaloid nucleus (C & D).

Hypothalamus and Brainstem

In addition to the forebrain inputs described above, there are extensive ascending projections to the MNBF from the hypothalamus and brainstem (Figs. 2, 5; Russchen et al., 1985; Vertes, 1986; Semba et al., 1988b; Grove, 1988; Carnes et al., 1990). These arise from cells scattered through the preoptic area, the medial and lateral hypothalamus (including the ventromedial, supramammillary and tuberomammillary nuclei), the ventral midbrain (including the ventral tegmental area and the pedunculopontine tegmental nucleus), the dorsal and median raphe nuclei, the dorsal pons (including the laterodorsal tegmental nucleus and the parabrachial nuclei) and much of the mesencephalic, pontine and medullary reticular formation. A few cells are even found as far caudal as the nucleus of the solitary tract.

While the scattered distribution of these cells makes it difficult to group them into distinct groups, many of them can be classified by the transmitter they use. The cells of the preoptic area and medial hypothalamus can be labeled by transport of ^{3}H-D-aspartate, and putatively use glutamate and/or aspartate as their transmitter (Carnes et al., 1990). However, only a fraction of the cells of the lateral hypothalamus that can be labeled by WGA-HRP injections into the MNBF are also labeled by comparable injections of ^{3}H-D-aspartate; and almost none of the more caudal brainstem cells can be labeled with ^{3}H-D-aspartate. It is not known what transmitter the cells of the lateral hypothalamus may use, although other studies indicate that the tuberomammillary nucleus cells are histaminergic, and may also contain other transmitters or peptides (e.g., Kohler et al., 1986).

Further caudally, as Semba and her colleagues have shown, many cells in the pedunculopontine and laterodorsal tegmental nuclei that send axons to the MNBF can also be stained immunohistochemically for choline acetyltransferase and are presumed to be cholinergic (Semba et al., 1988b). Similarly, the cells of the ventral tegmental area that project to the basal forebrain double label with antibodies to tyrosine hydroxylase (TH), and may be presumed to be dopaminergic. A further observation from the same group is that most (but not all) of the MNBF projecting cells in the dorsal and median raphe nuclei label for either serotonin or TH. The transmitter used by the substantial projection to the MNBF from the parabrachial nucleus is not known, but other projections from this nucleus have been shown to the peptidergic (e.g., Fulwiler and Saper, 1984; Yamano et al., 1988).

OUTPUTS

Cerebral Hemisphere

It is well established that the MNBF collectively project to all parts of the cerebral cortex (including the hippocampus and olfactory cortex), as well as to other telencephalic structures such as the amygdala and olfactory bulb (Daitz and Powell, 1954; Price and Powell, 1970a; Divac,

1975; Swanson and Cowan, 1979; Amaral and Cowan, 1980; Macrides et al., 1981; Luskin and Price, 1982; Mesulam et al., 1983; Saper, 1984; Eckenstein et al., 1988). In fact, the corpus striatum appears to be the only telencephalic structure that does not receive axons from the MNBF.

The projections to limbic structures (olfactory bulb and cortex, amygdala and hippocampus) are at least as substantial and distinctive as those to the neocortex. For example, the cholinergic projection to the amygdala from the NMBF is highly patterned; the basal amygdaloid nucleus receives the densest projection of any forebrain structure, while the central and medial nuclei receive little if any projection (Fig. 7; Hellendall et al., 1985). The fibers to both the olfactory bulb and the hippocampus have very specific, laminar patterns of termination (e.g. Macrides et al., 1981; Swanson et al., 1987; Nickell and Shipley, 1988).

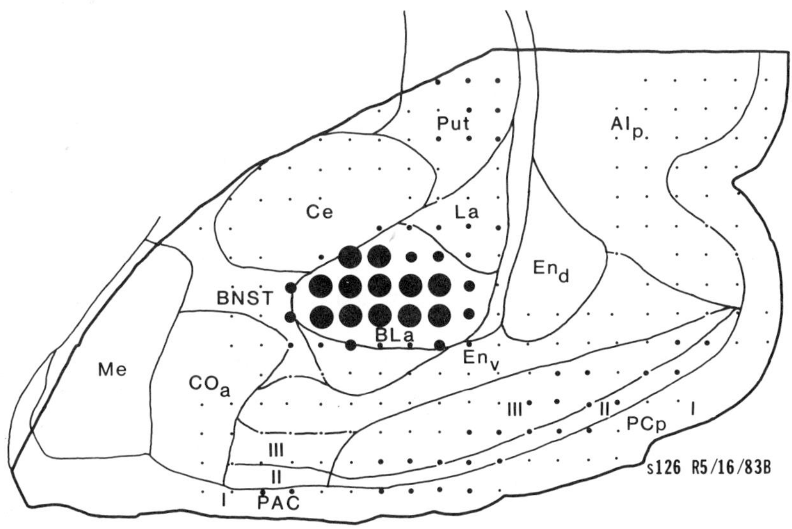

Figure 7. The distribution of choline acetyltransferase activity in the amygdala of the rat, measured as umol/kg dry weight/min from samples microdissected out of freeze dried sections. No dot represents 0–400 umol/kg/min, the smallest dots 401–800 umol/kg/min, the next largest dots 801–1600 umol/kg/min, the next largest 1601–3200 umol/kg/min, and the largest dots 3201-6400 umol/kg/min. Reprinted with permission of the authors and Alan R. Liss, Inc. from Hellendall et al., (1985): The distribution of choline acetyltransferase in the rat amygdaloid complex and adjacent cortical areas as determined by quantitative micro-assay and immunohistochemistry, *J. Comp. Neurol.* 249:486-498.

There is a considerable degree of organization within the overall projection from the MNBF (Fig. 8; Mesulam et al., 1983; Price and Stern, 1983; Saper, 1984; Rye et al., 1984; Eckenstein et al., 1988). In general, more medial areas of the cerebral hemisphere receive the heaviest part of their input from anteromedial parts of the MNBF; the hippocampus, which can be considered phylogenetically to be the most medial part of the cortex, receives fibers from the medial septal nucleus and the nucleus of the vertical diagonal band. More lateral areas of the cortex tend to receive fibers from more caudolateral part of the MNBF; the major projection to the temporal cortex arises from the posterior part of the nucleus basalis, near the caudal edge of the globus pallidus. Ventral structures such as the amygdala and the olfactory bulb and cortex receive fibers from the horizontal diagonal band and adjacent cells.

On the other hand, the organization is not precise. For example, Mesulam et al. (1983) found that while the greatest proportion of the cells that project to the hippocampus are situated in the vertical diagonal band nucleus, lower numbers of cells are scattered through all other parts of the MNBF, including the most caudal part of the nucleus basalis. Similarly, at least a few cells projecting to the temporal cortex are found in anterior parts of the MNBF.

This somewhat imprecise and overlapping organization of projections from the MNBF initially gave rise to suggestions that the projection from individual cells might be relatively widespread, with individual axons branching to innervate a large part of the cortex (e.g., McKinney et al., 1983). However, other experiments using fluorescent "double" retrograde tracers have indicated that individual cells in fact project to relatively restricted areas of cortex, approximately 1 to 1.5 mm in diameter (Bigl et al., 1982; Price and Stern, 1983). For example, injections of two fluorescent dyes into the cortex double labeled less than 1% of the cells labeled in the basal forebrain unless the injections were placed within 1.5 mm of each other, or involved the white matter in such a way as to label fibers of passage from the other area (Fig. 8). Similarly, Eckenstein et al. (1988) noted that, following small lesions of the MNBF, the area of depletion of choline acetyltransferase (ChAT) positive fibers is sharply separated from the area of normal fiber density, with a border of no more than 400 um in width.

In order to visualize the fibers from the MNBF more definitively, individual fibers to the frontal cortex of the rat have been labeled by

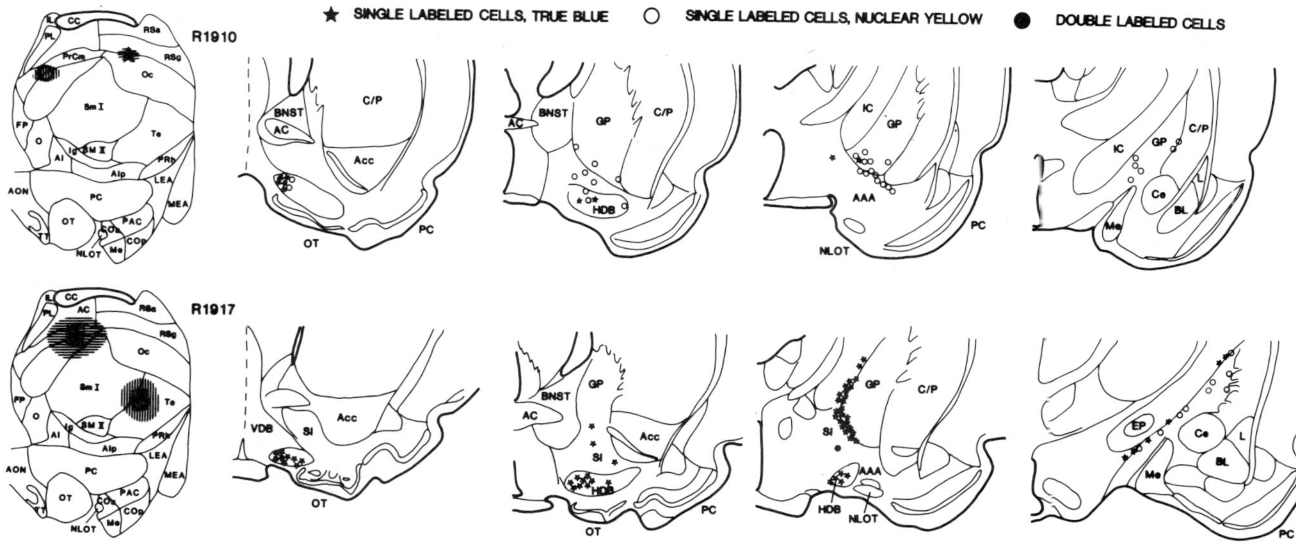

Figure 8. The distribution of cells labeled in the MNBF from injections of the fluorescent dyes true blue and nuclear yellow into different areas of cortex. The injection sites are shown on unfolded maps of the rat cortex, with the corpus callosum at the top and the olfactory areas at the bottom. Reprinted with permission of the authors and Elsevier Science Publishers, B.V. from Price and Stern, (1983): Individual cells in the nucleus basalis-diagonal band complex have restricted axonal projections to the cerebral cortex in the rat, *Brain Res.* 269:352-356.

small injections of the anterograde tracer PHA-L into the basal forebrain. Very small injections (*ca.* 500 um in diameter) labeled few enough fibers so that an individual fiber could be selected in the depth of the cortex, and then followed in successive serial sections as it ramified through the cortical layers (Fig. 9; Carnes and Price, 1988). Four such fibers have been reconstructed; from these, two different types of fibers have been identified. Three of the fibers ramify extensively in layers 3 to 5 of the cortex, while the fourth fiber has a substantial ramification in layer I, but few branches in the cellular layers. This matches the distribution of ChAT positive fibers, which have a high density in both layer I and layer V (Eckenstein et al., 1988). Importantly, all of the fibers are largely restricted to an area 1.0 to 1.5 mm in diameter (the distal fiber segments extend another 0.5 mm in two cases).

Thalamus and Brainstem

In addition to the projections to the cerebral hemisphere, cholinergic (and possibly also non-cholinergic) fibers from the caudal part of the MNBF have recently been found to the reticular nucleus of the thalamus in the rat (Steriade et al., 1987; Asanuma, 1989). These ramify around both the neuronal somata and dendrites of nucleus (Asanuma, 1989). Since the reticular nucleus interacts with all of the principal thalamic nuclei, the input from the MNBF may alter the general activity level of the thalamus. This, in turn, would provide another mechanism by which the MNBF could affect cortical function, by altering the transmission of information reaching the cortex through the thalamus.

Other cells of the basal forebrain also project to the medial, magnocellular part of the mediodorsal thalamic nucleus, and to portions of the intralaminar nuclei near the midline. However, few of these fibers are cholinergic (Young et al., 1984; Steriade et al., 1987). Indeed, most of the cells that project to the medial thalamus from the basal forebrain are not located within the magnocellular nuclei, but are in the ventral pallidum and polymorph zone of the olfactory tubercle, or, in the monkey, in the substantia innominata outside the magnocellular cell groups (Price and Slotnick, 1983; Russchen et al., 1987). The medial part of the mediodorsal nucleus has a very low concentration of acetylcholinesterase, compared to the lateral part or to other thalamic nuclei, suggesting that it receives very few cholinergic fibers from any source (e.g., Russchen et al., 1987).

The basal forebrain also projects to the lateral hypothalamus and several brainstem areas, including the ventral tegmental area and substantia nigra, the midbrain reticular formation and the parabrachial nucleus (Fig. 10; Carnes and Price, 1988). However, many of these may arise in the pallidal areas instead of the magnocellular nuclei, and it is unclear whether any are cholinergic.

Transmitters

Although most of the cells in the MNBF stain for both choline acetyltransferase and acetylcholinesterase, and may be presumed to be cholinergic, there are also non-cholinergic magnocellular neurons within the same cell groups. Indeed, double labeling studies have shown that a high proportion of the cells projecting to the hippocampus and olfactory bulb do not stain for choline acetyltransferase (e.g., Mesulam et al., 1983). Many of these non-cholinergic cells have been shown to be GABAergic (Kohler et al., 1984; Záborszky et al., 1986). In the case of the cells projecting to the olfactory bulb, the GABAergic cells tend to be located in the lateral part of the horizontal diagonal band, whereas the cholinergic cells are in the medial part. This suggests that they may be influenced by different inputs, although the nature of these has not been defined. As mentioned above, the commissural projection between a portion of the MNBF on the two sides is apparently neither cholinergic nor glutamatergic (Semba et al., 1988a; Carnes et al., 1990).

FUNCTION

Although the anatomical connections of the MNBF do not in themselves provide direct evidence on the function of these nuclei, a few points that are implicit in the anatomy can be noted (see the above discussion for references to anatomical papers). Since the cells of the MNBF all tend to have long dendrites that radiate across the major fiber systems that run through the ventral forebrain, they can be expected to integrate influences from a variety of sources. The inputs can be generally divided into two groups: (1) those from the hypothalamus and lower brainstem, and (2) those from limbic areas such as the amygdala and entorhinal cortex, and from related cortical areas in the orbital and medial frontal

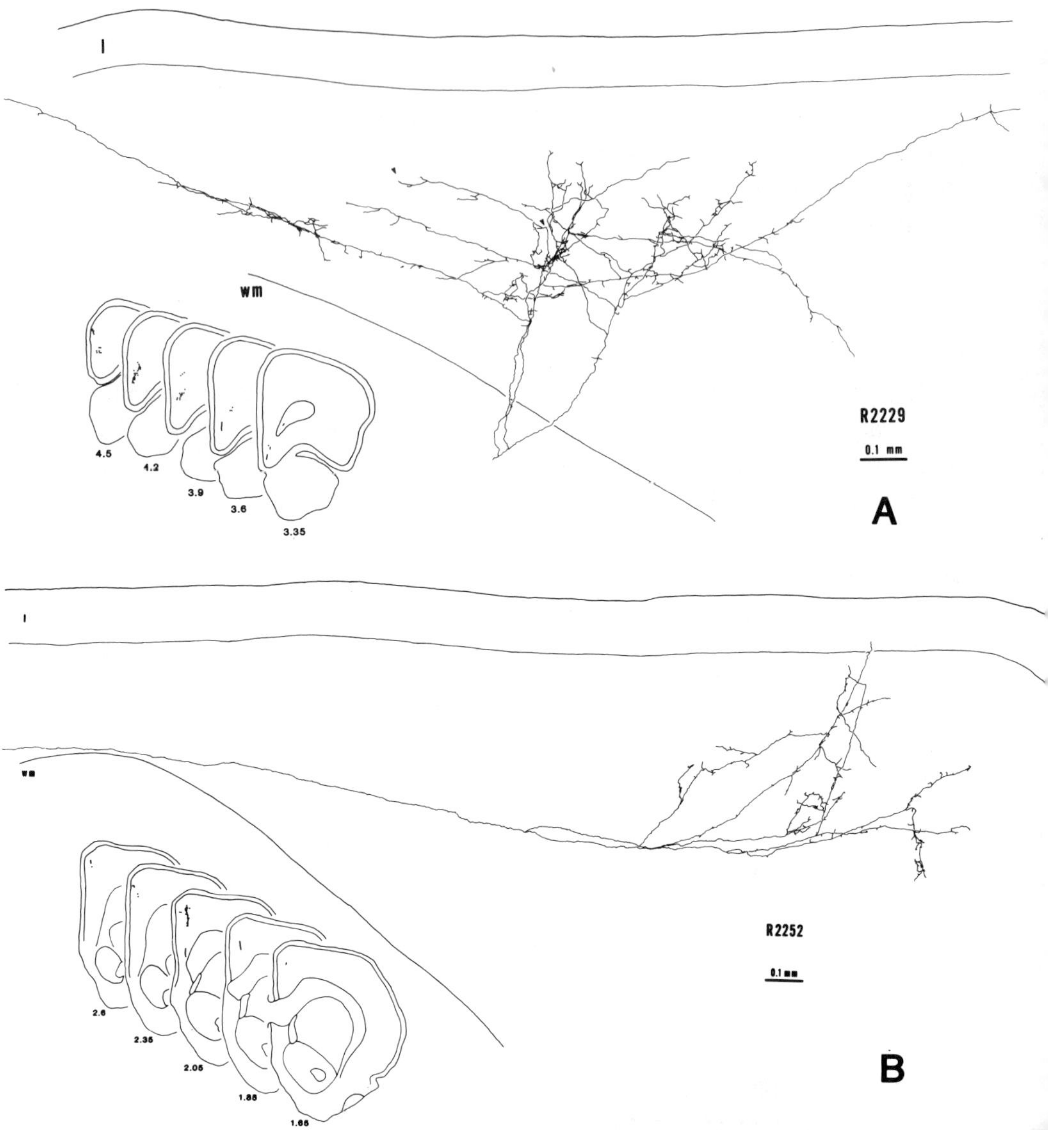

Figure 9a,b,c,d. Four axons labeled by small injection of PHA-L into the MNBF of the rat, and reconstructed from serial sections of the frontal cortex. Note that the fibers ramify through several layers of cortex, but are restricted to an area about 1.5mm in diameter.

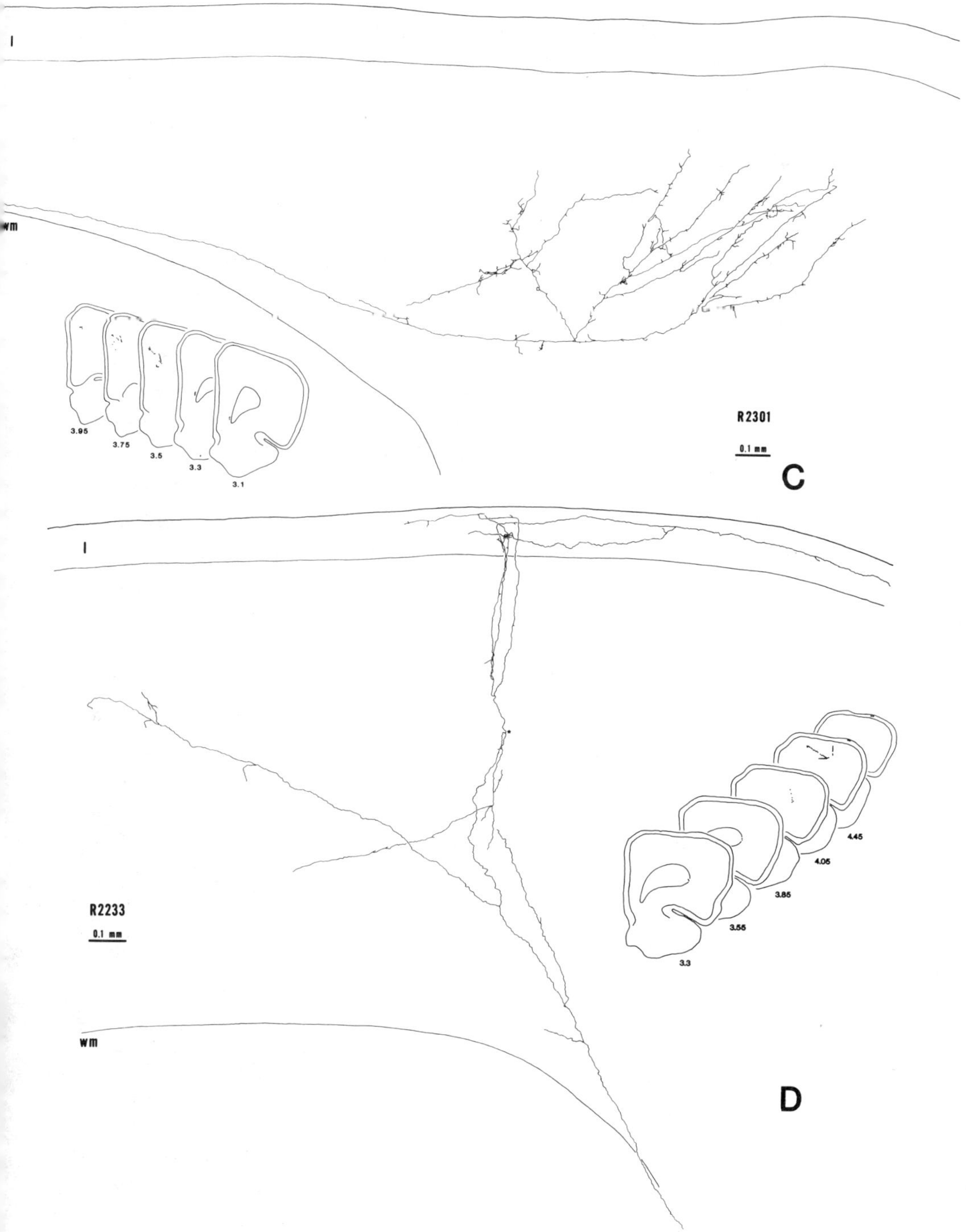
I
wm
3.95
3.75
3.5
3.3
3.1
R2301
0.1 mm
C
I
R2233
0.1 mm
4.45
4.05
3.85
3.55
3.3
wm
D

lobe, the rostral insula and the rostral temporal lobe. Although these two groups of areas are themselves linked by an extensive set of ascending and descending connections, they can be expected to provide different drives or modulatory influences on the MNBF, which would combine to determine the output of the complex.

Brainstem Inputs

Many of the brainstem inputs appear to link the MNBF with the ascending activation or arousal system. In recent years projections from the lateral dorsal tegmental nucleus and other cell groups in the dorsal pons have been shown to control the level of excitability of the thalamus, and the transition between states of sleep and wakefulness. This is done both through actions on the thalamic reticular nucleus, and by direct projections to the other thalamic nuclei (e.g., Steriade and Deschenes, 1988). The MNBF are closely related to this mechanism of thalamic activation, for they not only receive inputs from the same brainstem nuclei, but they also contribute to the cholinergic input of the thalamic reticular nucleus. Of course, the MNBF also presumably contributes to brainstem arousal of the cortex by relaying the ascending signals from the brainstem directly to the cortex.

Another role that has been shown to be associated with the MNBF and its ascending brainstem input is the elicitation of rhythmic slow activity in the hippocampus (theta rhythm) and elsewhere (see Bland, 1986, and Vertes, 1986 for recent reviews and references). Thus, cells of the medial septal nucleus can be shown to fire in rhythmic bursts which match theta frequencies (e.g., Gogolak et al., 1967; Wilson et al., 1976), and stimulation of the medial septum/diagonal band drives hippocampal theta (e.g., McNaughton et al., 1977). Conversely, lesions of the medial septal nucleus/diagonal band can abolish the hippocampal theta rhythm

---

Figure 10. The distribution of axons labeled by an injection of PHA-L into the peripallidal region of the MNBF (black area on the fifth section). Reprinted with permission of Kluwer Academic Publishers, from Carnes and Price (1988): Demonstration of individual fibers from the substantia innominata to the frontal cortex of the rat, using *Phaseolus vulgaris* leucoagglutinin (PHA-L). In: *Neurobiology of Amino Acids, Peptides and Trophic Factors*, Ferrendelli, J.A., Collins, R.C., Johnson, E.M., eds. *See page 105*

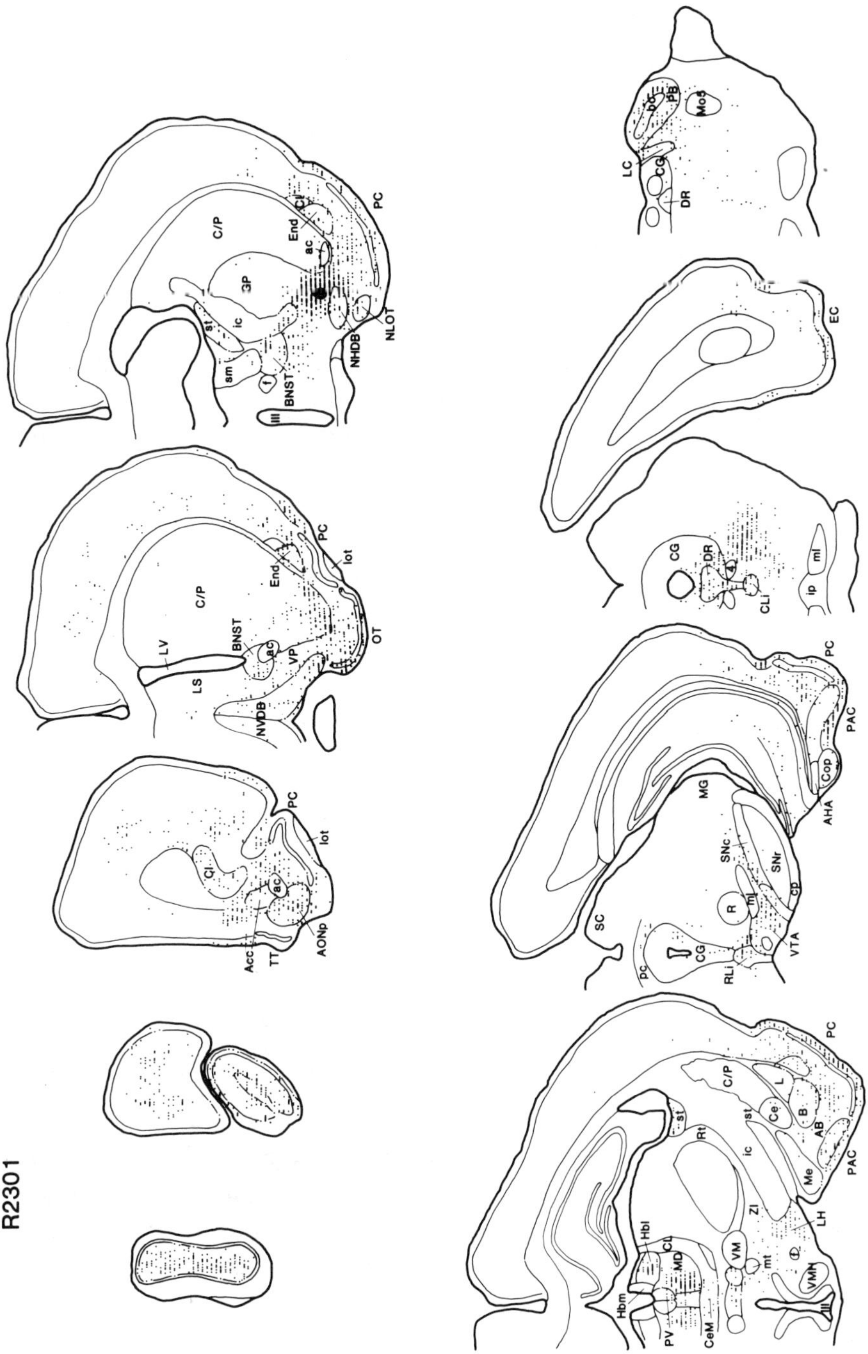
R2301
Cl
ac
Acc
TT
AONp
lot
PC
LV
LS
BNST
VP
NVDB
End
C/P
OT
st
sm
f
III
ic
GP
NHDB
NLOT
Hbm
Hbl
PV
CeM
CL
MD
VM
mt
VMH
ZI
LH
Rt
Me
PAC
AB
B
Ce
L
RLi
CG
pc
SC
VTA
R
ml
cp
SNr
SNc
MG
AHA
Cop
CLi
ip
DR
EC
LC
MoS
PB

(e.g., Bland, 1986). The theta rhythm can also be elicited by stimulating the ascending projections to the MNBF from the brainstem (Vertes, 1986). Stimulation of the pontine reticular formation is particularly effective in producing theta, while stimulation of the median raphe nucleus may have the effect of desynchronizing theta. In addition to direct projections from these areas to the MNBF, there may be relays through the supramammillary nucleus and other hypothalamic areas.

Although the functional significance of the theta rhythm and other rhythmic slow activity is not clear, there is evidence that it may reflect a "timing" signal that allows correlation of activity in different parts of the brain. For example, when a rat is actively sampling an odor as part of an odor discrimination task, there is a tendency for the hippocampal theta rhythm to come into phase with the sniff cycle, and thereby with discharge patterns of cells in the olfactory bulb (Macrides et al., 1982; Eichenbaum et al., 1987). A similar correlation is found between theta and other rhythmic sensorimotor activity, such as whisker movement in rodents (Komisaruk, 1970, 1977). This suggests that a common area, possibly in the pons, controls and synchronizes both the theta rhythm (and other similar slow rhythmic activity) and sensorimotor activity. Since it has also been shown that long term potentiation is best produced in the hippocampus by stimulation at theta frequencies (Larson et al., 1986; Greenstein et al., 1988), the effect of this correlation of sensory responses and the theta rhythm may be to produce long lasting enhancement of appropriately synchronized signals. Vertes (1986) suggests that the theta rhythm serves as a "natural tetanizer"). Indeed, the correlation between the theta rhythm and the sniff cycle is greatest in the period just before the animal reaches criteria in learning an odor discrimination task (Macrides et al., 1982).

Forebrain Inputs

The amygdala, entorhinal cortex and related areas in the prefrontal, insular and temporal cortex provide the major telencephalic inputs to the MNBF. Together these limbic structures form a tightly interconnected neuronal system that receives multimodal inputs from association sensory cortical areas, and may have the general behavioral role of attaching significance to ongoing sensory experience. For example, in the classical Kluver-Bucy syndrome, which involves bilateral destruction of much of the rostral temporal lobe, monkeys are unable to recognize the behavioral significance of objects (e.g., they become tame to normally fearful stimuli such as snakes or humans, and they cannot discriminate food and non-food items; Kluver and Bucy, 1939). Similarly, stimulation of the amygdala and hippocampus in human patients undergoing surgery for epilepsy most frequently evokes sensations of fear and anxiety (Gloor et al., 1980), and positron emission tomography (PET) studies of patients undergoing "panic attacks" indicate there is unusual activity in the cortex of the temporal pole (Reiman et al., 1989). In addition, lesion studies have indicated that most of the structures, especially the entorhinal cortex, amygdala and orbitomedial prefrontal cortex, are critically involved along with the hippocampal formation in object recognition memory (e.g., Mishkin, 1982; Bachevalier and Mishkin, 1986; Murray and Mishkin, 1986; Zola-Morgan et al., 1989).

Recordings from the amygdala (e.g., Leonard et al., 1985; Nishijo et al., 1988) and the orbitofrontal cortex (e.g., Thorpe et al., 1983; Fuster, 1989) in awake, behaving monkeys indicate that cells in these areas carry relatively specific multimodal sensory information, often firing selectively in response to complex stimuli (e.g., the sight and taste of watermelon, but not of apple, or of salted watermelon). Many cells also appear to signal the affective nature of the stimulus, responding differentially to reward vs. aversive stimuli, or to novel vs. familiar stimuli. In addition, cells are found in the prefrontal cortex that fire in relation to a delayed response task during the delay period between stimulus and response, suggesting that they are involved in short term memory during the trial (Fuster, 1989). This information is presumably transferred to the MNBF. For example, Richardson and DeLong (1986) have shown that some MBF neurons significantly alter their discharge rate during the performance of a delayed response task, and that most of these responses occur during the choice and reward periods of the task. Other groups have also demonstrated MBF neurons that responded differentially to rewarding stimuli (e.g., Wilson and Rolls, 1985; Rigdon and Pirch, 1986).

Outputs

The function of the MNBF is usually considered in terms of the cholinergic projections to the cerebral cortex. However, the prominent inputs to the MNBF from limbic structures are matched by equally prominent cholinergic and non-cholinergic projections from the basal forebrain to the amygdala, hippocampus, olfactory cortex and related neocortical areas. That is, the basal forebrain exerts substantial influence over the limbic system, just as it receives inputs from it. Bilateral lesions of the MNBF produce deficits in recognition memory similar to those seen with lesions of the limbic structures themselves (e.g., Aigner et al., 1984, 1987). This could be attributed to either the loss of basal forebrain inputs to the limbic structures or to loss of cholinergic inputs to the cortex.

The organization of the MNBF projection to the cerebral cortex, and the observation that individual cells project to an area of cortex only about 1.0 to 1.5 mm in diameter, indicate that neurons in the MNBF have the potential to differentially modulate relatively restricted cortical areas. Assuming that the input to the MNBF itself is sufficiently organized so that individual cells can be activated differentially, the system might provide a mechanism whereby specific cortical functions represented in small regions of cortex could be enhanced selectively. Alternatively, the activity of mosaics or constellations of small cortical zones could be modulated in concert. This could underlie such mechanisms as selective attention, or the coordination of diverse elements into a multimodal sensation or memory.

REFERENCES

Aigner, T., Mitchell, S., Aggleton, J., DeLong, M., Struble, R., Wenk, G., Price, D. and Mishkin, M. (1984): Recognition deficit in monkeys following neurotoxic lesions of the basal forebrain. *Neurosci. Abstr.* 10:386

Aigner, T.G., Mitchell, S.J., Aggleton, J.P., DeLong, M.R., Struble, R.G., Wenk, G.L., Price, D.L. and Mishkin, M. (1987): Effects of scopolamine and physostigmine on recognition memory in monkeys with ibotenic-acid lesions of the nucleus basalis of Meynert. *Psychopharmacol.* 92:292-300

Alonso, A. and Kohler, C. (1982): Evidence for separate projections of hippocampal pyramidal and non-pyramidal neurons to different parts of the septum in the rat brain. *Neurosci. Lett.* 31:209-214

Amaral, D.G. and Cowan, W.M. (1980): Subcortical afferents to the hippocampal formation in the monkey. *J. Comp. Neurol.* 189:573-591

Amaral, D.G. and Price, J.L. (1984): Amygdalo-cortical projections in the monkey. *J. Comp. Neurol.* 230:465-496

Asanuma, C. (1989): Axonal arborizations of a magnocellular basal nucleus input and their relation to the neurons in the thalamic reticular nucleus of rats. *Proc. Natl. Acad. Sci.* 86:4746-4750

Bachevalier, J. and Mishkin, M. (1986): Visual recognition impairment follows ventromedial but not dorsolateral prefrontal lesions in monkeys. *Behav. Brain Res.* 20:249-261

Bigl, S.J., Woolf, N. J. and Butcher, L.L. (1982): Cholinergic projections from the basal forebrain to frontal, parietal, temporal, occipital, and cingulate cortices: a combined fluorescent tracer and acetylcholinesterase analysis. *Brain Res.* 8:727-749

Bland, B.H. (1986): The physiology and pharmacology of hippocampal formation theta rhythms. *Prog. in Neurobiol.* 26:1-54

Carnes, K.M. and Price, J.L. (1988): Demonstration of individual fibers from the substantia innominata to the frontal cortex of the rat, using *Phaseolus vulgaris* leucoagglutinin (PHA-L). In: *Neurobiology of Amino Acids, Peptides and Trophic Factors*. Ferrendelli, J.A., Collins, R.C., Johnson, E.M., eds. Kluwer Academic Publishers, pp 215-218

Carnes, K.M., Fuller, T.A. and Price, J.L. (1990): Sources of presumptive glutamatergic/aspartatergic afferents to the magnocellular basal forebrain in the rat. *J. Comp. Neurol.* 302:824-852

Daitz, H.M. and Powell, T.P.S. (1954): Studies on the connexions of the fornix system. *J. Neurol. Neurosurg. Psychiat.* 17:75-82

Divac, I. (1975): Magnocellular nuclei of the basal forebrain project to neocortex, brain stem, and olfactory bulb: review of some functional correlates. *Brain Res.* 93:385-398

Eckenstein, F.P., Baughman, R.W. and Quinn, J. (1988): An anatomical study of cholinergic innervation in rat cerebral cortex. *Neurosci.* 25:457-474

Eichenbaum, H., Kuperstein, M., Fagan, A. and Nagode, J. (1987): Cue-sampling and goal-approach correlates of hippocampal unit activity in rats performing an odor-discrimination task. *J. Neurosci.* 7:716-732

Fulwiler, C.E. and Saper, C.B. (1984): Subnuclear organization of the efferent connections of the parabrachial nucleus in the rat. *Brain Res.* 319:229-59

Fuster, J.M. (1989): *The Prefrontal Cortex*. New York: Raven Press

Gloor, P., Oliver, A., Quesney, L.F., Andermann, F. and Horowitz, S. (1980): The role of the limbic system in experiential phenomena of temporal lobe epilepsy. *Ann. Neurol.* 12:129-144

Gogolak, G., Petsche, H., Sterc, J. and Stumpf, C. (1967): Septum cell activity in the rabbit under reticular stimulation. *Brain Res.* 5:508-510

Greenstein, Y.J., Pavlides, C. and Winson, J. (1988): Long-term potentiation in the dentate gyrus is preferentially induced at theta rhythm periodicity. *Brain Res.* 438:331-334

Grove, E.A. (1988): Neural associations of the substantia innominata in the rat: afferent connections. *J. Comp. Neurol.* 277:315-346

Grove, E.A. and Ingham, C.A. (1986): Electron microscopic evidence of striatal input to intrapallidal neurons of cholinergic cell group Ch4 in the rat. *Neurosci. Abstr.* 12:1328

Haring, J.H. and Wang, R.Y. (1986): The identification of some sources of afferent input to the rat nucleus basalis magnocellularis by retrograde transport of horseradish peroxidase. *Brain Res.* 366:152-158

Hellendall, R.P., Godfrey, D.A., Ross, C.D., Armstrong, D.M. and Price, J.L. (1985): The distribution of choline acetyltransferase in the rat amygdaloid complex and adjacent cortical areas as determined by quantitative micro-assay and immunohistochemistry. *J. Comp. Neurol.* 249:486-498

Irle, E. and Markowitsch, H.J. (1986): Afferent connections of the substantia innominata/basal nucleus of Meynert in carnivores and primates. *J. Hirnforsch* 27:343-367

Kluver, H. and Bucy, P.C. (1939): Preliminary analysis of functions of the temporal lobe in monkeys. *Arch. Neurol.* 42:979-1000

Kohler, C., Chan-Palay, V. and Wu, J. (1984): Septal neurons containing glutamic acid decarboxylase immunoreactivity project to the hippocampal region in the rat brain. *Anat. Embryol.* 169:41-44

Kohler, C., Ericson, L., Watanabe, T., Polak, J. and Palay, S. (1986): Galanin-immunoreactivity is present in hypothalamic histamine neurons: further evidence for multiple chemical messengers in the tuberomammillary nucleus. *J. Comp. Neurol.* 250:58-65

Komisaruk, B. R. (1970): Synchrony between limbic system theta activity and rhythmical behavior in rats. *J. Comp. Physiol. Psychol.* 70:482-492

Komisaruk, B. R. (1977): The role of rhythmical brain activity in sensorimotor integration. In: *Progress in Psychobiology and Physiological Psychology, Vol 7*. Sprague, J.M., Epstein, A.N., eds. New York: Academic Press, pp 55-90

Larson, J., Wong, D. and Lynch, G. (1986): Patterned stimulation at the theta frequency is optimal for the induction of hippocampal long-term potentiation. *Brain Res.* 368:347-350

Leonard, C.M., Rolls, E.T., Wilson, F.A. and Baylis, G.C. (1985): Neurons in the amygdala of the monkey with responses selective for faces. *Behav. Brain Res.* 15:159-176

Luskin, M.B. and Price, J. L. (1982): The distribution of axon collaterals from the olfactory bulb and the nucleus of the diagonal band to the olfactory cortex, demonstrated by double retrograde labeling techniques. *J. Comp. Neurol.* 209:249-263

Macrides, F., Davis, B.J., Youngs, W.M., Nadi, N.S. and Margolis, F.F. (1981): Cholinergic and catecholaminergic afferents to the olfactory bulb in the hamster: a neuroanatomical biochemical and histochemical investigation. *J. Comp. Neurol.* 203:495-514

Macrides, F., Eichenbaum, H.B. and Forbes, W.B. (1982): Temporal relationship between sniffing and the limbic theta rhythm during odor discrimination reversal learning. *J. Neurosci.* 2:1705-1717

McKinney, M., Coyle, J.T. and Hedreen, J.C. (1983): Topographic analysis of the innervation of the rat neocortex and hippocampus by the basal forebrain cholinergic system. *J. Comp. Neurol.* 217:103-121

McNaughton, N., James, D.T.D., Steward, J., Gray, J.A., Valero, I. and Drenowski, A. (1977): Septal driving of hippocampal theta rhythm as a function of frequency in the male rat: effect of drugs. *Neurosci.* 2:1019-1027

Mesulam, M.-M. and Mufson, E.J. (1984): Neural inputs into the nucleus basalis of the substantia innominata (Ch4) in the rhesus monkey. *Brain Res.* 107:253-274

Mesulam, M.-M., Mufson, E.J., Levey, A.I. and Wainer, B.H. (1983): Cholinergic innervation of cortex by the basal forebrain: cytochemistry and cortical connections of the septal area, diagonal band nuclei, nucleus basalis (substantia innominata), and hypothalamus in the rhesus monkey. *J. Comp. Neurol.* 214:170-197

Mishkin, M. (1982): A memory system in the monkey. *Phil. Trans. R. Soc. Lond. B.* 298:85-95

Murray, E.A. and Mishkin, M. (1986): Visual recognition in monkeys following rhinal cortical ablations combined with either amygdalectomy or hippocampectomy. *J. Neurosci.* 6:1991-2003

Nickell, W.T. and Shipley, M.T. (1988): Two anatomically specific classes of candidate cholinoceptive neurons in the rat olfactory bulb. *J. Neurosci.* 8:4482-4491

Nishijo, H., Ono, T. and Nishino, H. (1988): Single neuron responses in amygdala of alert monkeys during complex sensory stimulation with affective significance. *J. Neurosci.* 8:3570-3583

Price, J.L. and Powell, T.P.S. (1970a): An experimental study of the origin and the course of the centrifugal fibers to the olfactory bulb in the rat. *J. Anat.* 107:215-237

Price, J.L. and Powell, T.P.S. (1970b): The afferent connexions of the nucleus of the horizontal limb of the diagonal band. *J. Anat.* 107:239-256

Price, J.L. and Slotnick, B.M. (1983): Dual olfactory representation in the rat thalamus: an anatomical and electrophysiological Study. *J. Comp. Neurol.* 215:63-77

Price, J.L. and Stern, R. (1983): Individual cells in the nucleus basalis-diagonal band complex have restricted axonal projections to the cerebral cortex in the rat. *Brain Res.* 269:352-356

Reiman, E.M., Raichle, M.E., Robins, E., Mintun, M.A., Fusselman, M. J., Fox, P.T., Price, J.L. and Hackman, K.A. (1989): Neuroanatomical correlates of a lactate-induced anxiety attack. *Arch. Gen. Psychiat.* 46:493-500

Richardson, R.T. and DeLong, M.R. (1986): Nucleus basalis of Meynert neuronal activity during a delayed response task in monkey. *Brain Res.* 399:364-368

Rigdon, G.C. and Pirch, J.H. (1986): Nucleus basalis involvement in conditioned neuronal reponses in the rat frontal cortex. *J. Neurosci.* 6:2535-2542

Russchen, F.T., Amaral, D.G. and Price, J.L. (1985): The afferent connections of the substantia innominata in the monkey, Macaca fascicularis. *J. Comp. Neurol.* 242:1-27

Russchen, F.T., Amaral, D.G. and Price, J.L. (1987): The afferent input to the magnocellular division of the mediodorsal thalamic nucleus in the monkey, Macaca fascicularis. *J. Comp. Neurol.* 256:175-210.

Rye, D.B., Wainer, B.H., Mesulam, -M.M., Mufson, E.J. and Saper, C.B. (1984): Cortical projections arising from the basal forebrain: a study of cholinergic and noncholinergic components employing combined retrograde tracing and immunohistochemical localization of choline acetyltransferase. *Neurosci.* 13:627-643

Saper, C.B. (1984): Organization of cerebral cortical afferent systems in the rat: I. Magnocellular basal nucleus. *J. Comp. Neurol.* 222:313-342

Semba, K., Reiner, P.B., McGeer, E.G. and Fibiger, H.C. (1988a): Non-cholinergic basal forebrain neurons project to the contralateral basal forebrain in the rat. *Neurosci. Lett.* 84:23-28

Semba, K., Reiner, P.B., McGeer, E.G. and Fibiger, H.C. (1988b): Brainstem afferents to the magnocellular basal forebrain studied by axonal transport, immunohistochemistry, and electrophysiology in the rat. *J. Comp. Neurol.* 267:433-453

Steriade, M., Parent, A., Pare, D. and Smith, Y. (1987): Cholinergic and non-cholinergic neurons of cat basal forebrain project to reticular and mediodorsal thalamic nuclei. *Brain Res.* 408:372-376

Steriade, M. and Deschenes, M. (1988): Intrathalamic and brainstem-thalamic networks involved in resting and alert states. In: *Cellular Thalamic Mechanisms*. Bentivoglio, M., Spreafico, R., eds. Amsterdam: Excerpta Medica, pp. 37-62

Swanson, L.W. and Cowan, W.M. (1979): The connections of the septal region in the rat. *J. Comp. Neurol.* 186:621-665

Swanson, L.W., Kohl, C. and Bjorklund, A. (1987): The limbic system. I: The septohippocampal system. In: *Handbook of Chemical Neuroanatomy Vol. 5, Integrated systems in the CNS, part I*, Björklund, A., Hökfelt, T., Swanson, L.W., eds. Amsterdam: Amsterdam, pp. 125-277

Thorpe, S.J., Rolls, E.T. and Maddison, S. (1983): The orbitofrontal cortex: neuronal activity in the behaving monkey. *Exp. Brain Res.* 49:93-115

Vertes, R.P. (1986): Brainstem modulations of the hippocampus: anatomy, physiology, and significance. In: *The Hippocampus, Vol. 4*. Isaacson, R.L., Pribram, K.H., eds. New York: Plenum Press, pp. 41-75

Wilson, C.L., Motter, B.C. and Lindsley, D.B. (1976): Influences of hypothalamic stimulation upon septal and hippocampal electrical activity in the cat. *Brain Res.* 107:55-68

Wilson, F.A.W. and Rolls, E.T. (1985): Reinforcement-related unit activity in the basal forebrain and amygdala. *Neurosci. Abstr.* 11:525

Yamano, M., Hillyard, C.J., Girgis, S., MacIntyre, I., Emson, P.C. and Tohyama, M. (1988): Presence of a substance P-like immunoreactive neuron system from the parabrachial area to the central amygdaloid nucleus of the rat with reference to coexistence with calcitonin gene-related peptide. *Brain Res.* 451:179-88

Young, W.S., Alheid, G.F. and Heimer, L. (1984): The ventral pallidal projection to the mediodorsal thalamus: a study with fluorescent retrograde tracers and immunohistofluorescence. *J. Neurosci.* 4:1626-1638

Záborszky, L., Carlsen, J., Brashear, H.R. and Heimer, L. (1986): Cholinergic and GABAergic afferents to the olfactory bulb in the rat with special emphasis on the projection neurons in the nucleus of the horizontal limb of the diagonal band. *J. Comp. Neurol.* 243:488-509

Zola-Morgan, S., Squire, L.R., Amaral, D.G. and Suzuki, W. A. (1989): Lesions of perirhinal and parahippocampal cortex that spare the amygdala and hippocampal formation produce severe memory impairment. *Neurosci.* 9:4355-4370

Role of the Basal Forebrain Cholinergic System in Cortical Activation and Arousal

György Buzsáki and Fred H. Gage

INTRODUCTION

A basic question about the physiology of the cerebral cortex concerns the activating afferents that keep the neocortex in the aroused or waking state. Imbedded in this question are several other questions: Why must the cerebral cortex be aroused in the first place in order to interact with the environment? Why is the brain not hard-wired exclusively for the information processing mode, as seen in computers? What is the biological significance of the dichotomy of the activated (open-loop) and non-activated (closed-loop) states of the cerebral hemispheres? And finally, what are the neurophysiological mechanisms involved in the switching between the diametrically opposite functional states? This last question, as we will discuss it in this chapter, is under intensive investigation and clarification, whereas little work or even speculation is appearing on the evolutionary advantage of the functional dichotomy of the brain (Buzsáki, 1989).

For the past four decades it has been generally accepted that the reticulo-thalamic system served as the structural basis of neocortical activation. Cholinergic (Shute and Lewis, 1967) and other neurons in the brainstem reticular formation were purported to excite the neocortical neurons directly (Krnjević et al., 1971; Phillis, 1980; Vanderwolf and Robinson, 1981) or indirectly, via the reticular nucleus of the thalamus (RT) (Jasper, 1949; Papez, 1956) and, later, via the intralaminar nuclei of the thalamus (Steriade, 1970). In turn, a diffuse projection from these thalamic nuclei to the cerebral cortex was thought to represent the final common pathway of the ascending reticular activating system (Moruzzi and Magoun, 1949).

In this chapter we will summarize data indicating that the reticulothalamic neocortical arousal model is no longer tenable and will suggest that the cholinergic nucleus basalis (NB) is the major anatomical substrate of neocortical activation. Furthermore, we will point out that functionally similar changes occur simultaneously in the thalamus and neocortex during behavioral activation, even though anatomically distinct pathways may be involved in this process. In addition, we will propose a unifying hypothesis for a physiological explanation of EEG and behavioral arousal.

DEFINITION OF AROUSAL: AN UPDATE

We suggest that the necessary and sufficient structural requirements for generalized activation of the thalamus and neocortex are that (a) a group of neurons innervate the entire thalamus and/or cortex, (b) the terminal arborization of the individual cells access the individual nuclei of the thalamus and cortical columns, and (c) importantly, these neurons must possess a transmitter that can enhance the effectiveness of the "specific" (sensory; thalamic, associational and commissural) inputs and motor outputs. From the *functional* point of view, activity of the neurons of the candidate arousal system(s) (a) should maintain similar activity levels spontaneously or in response to activation of their various afferents, and (b) their discharge rates should covary with thalamic and neocortical activation and behavioral arousal. In general, the arousal process serves to increase the *responsivity* of the projection neurons, but this operation does not necessarily imply excitation per se and depolarization in the traditional sense. Operationally, arousal is defined as a "stand-by" mode of neurons for the processing and transformation of afferent information and for efficient efferent commands.

Based on the above criteria, several systems may satisfy the structural requirements of the arousal mechanism. Several studies have examined the activity of locus coeruleus (LC) neurons in the unanesthetized rat, cat and monkey, and have reported that LC cells are most active in waking, discharge less during slow wave sleep, and are virtually quiescent in rapid eye movement (REM) sleep (Foote et al., 1980; Aston-Jones and Bloom, 1981). Serotoninergic median raphe cells have a very low spontaneous firing rate and, like LC neurons, discharge most during waking, at reduced rates during slow wave sleep, and at lowest levels in REM sleep (Trulson and Jacobs, 1979). However, the neocortex displays desynchronized (activated) activity not only during awake states but also during REM sleep. Obviously, these neurons contribute little, if any, to thalamic and neocortical activation during REM sleep. As will be discussed in this chapter, the discharge frequency of cholinergic nucleus basalis (NB) neurons during REM sleep is as high as in the awake animal. Thus, it appears that the ascending cholinergic system alone is capable of keeping the neocortex in its information processing mode. In this context it should be pointed out, however, that in the awake animal the brainstem aminergic afferents may have an important adjuvant effect in neocortical activation (Vanderwolf and Baker, 1986; Vanderwolf and Stewart, 1986; Vanderwolf, 1988), although the primary activating systems appear to be the cholinergic brainstem-thalamus and the NB-neocortical projections (Buzsáki et al., 1988b; Steriade and Buzsáki, 1989).

REEVALUATION OF THE RETICULO-THALAMIC-NEOCORTEX MODEL OF AROUSAL

There are several reasons why the exclusive role of the reticulo-thalamic-neocortex model should be reevaluated. First, anatomical evidence indicates that direct cholinergic reticulo-cortical and RT-neocortical projections are nonexistent (Fibiger, 1982; Mesulam et al., 1983; Jones, 1985). The only reticulo-thalamo-cortical path with the required diffuse projection has remained the intralaminar nuclei, which have widespread terminations in the neocortex and are innervated by cholinergic cell groups located in the midbrain (Hallanger et al., 1987). However, it has recently been suggested that the intralaminar nuclei are responsible for the induction of neocortical slow activity and not activation-related desynchronization (Fox and Armstrong-James, 1986). Second, a major cholinergic system originating in the basal forebrain with widespread cortical targets has been discovered (Divac, 1975; Jones et al., 1976; Mesulam and Van Hoesen, 1976) without any assigned physiological function. Third, increased power of slow delta EEG activity was reported in Alzheimer patients with severe loss of basal forebrain cholinergic neurons (Coben et al., 1985; Pentilla et al., 1985). Fourth, the neurotransmitter of thalamocortical neurons, including those of the intralaminar nuclei, is probably glutamate (Jones, 1985; Fox and Armstrong-James, 1986). Recent studies on the biophysical and pharmacological properties of cortical and thalamic cells (Llinas, 1988; Nicoll, 1988) indicate that glutamate alone is not capable of maintaining an efficient responding state in pyramidal cells or in thalamocortical projection neurons (see arguments below). Thus, while the brainstem cholinergic system is a prerequisite for thalamic arousal, the thalamic output alone is not capable of maintaining a "stand-by" mode of neocortical cells. Diffuse corticopetal afferents containing other than glutamate or aspartate are necessary for normal neocortical activation (Buzsáki et al., 1988).

NEOCORTICAL EEG AND ACTIVITY OF NB NEURONS

In the rat, three basic EEG patterns can be distinguished qualitatively. In the alert animal, the EEG consists of predominantly low voltage fast waves (desynchronized or arousal pattern). In the drowsy or sleeping rat, large-amplitude slow waves in the delta band (1 - 4 Hz) predominate (Longo, 1956; Vanderwolf, 1975, 1988). In the motionless but awake rat, an additional, highly synchronized pattern, characterized by large rhythmic spikes and waves (high voltage spindle, HVS), has also been described (Klingberg and Pickenhain, 1968). As we will discuss below, these distinct patterns reflect different degrees of functional isolation or interaction of the neocortex with thalamic and other subcortical structures. Therefore, isolating these respective patterns in the freely moving animal can give us a fairly precise picture of the degree of the brain's interaction with the environment.

In an attempt to reveal the role of the NB in neocortical activation, we investigated the correlation between neocortical EEG and cellular activity in the NB, thalamus and neocortex. We also studied the consequences of circumscribed ibotenic acid lesions of the NB, RT and other thalamic nuclei on neocortical electrical activity. Finally, we compared the power and spatial distribution of the EEG in both the young and aged rat.

An early suggestion that the basal forebrain might be responsible for the induction of sleep (McGinty and Sterman, 1968) was based mainly on experiments using lesions and electrical stimulation of this region. A wide range of stimulation frequencies was reported to slow the neocortical EEG and suppress ongoing behavior (Sterman and Clemente, 1962; Siegel and Wang, 1974). A major problem with this approach is the difficulty of revealing a causal relationship between the stimulation effects and the consequent behavioral and EEG changes. Electrical stimuli might simply have excited fiber tracts which passed through the NB or inhibitory afferents to the NB neurons. Alternatively, activation of the descending NB projections may have induced suppression of ongoing behavior, which in turn secondarily affected the EEG activity. In contrast to these reports, more recent experiments suggest that electrical stimulation of NB results in short-latency excitation of neocortical neurons in the frontal region (Funahashi, 1983; Stern and Pugh, 1984), long-lasting neocortical desynchronization (Belardetti et al., 1977) and release of acetylcholine (ACh) in the neocortex (Casamenti et al., 1986). A more selective activation or inhibition of neurons can be obtained by local microinjection of drugs. In immobilized rats, Rigdon and Pirch (1986) have reported that excitation of neocortical neurons by a conditioning stimulus was considerably decreased following injection of GABA into the NB.

To date, the majority of studies on NB neurons have been carried out in anesthetized animals, and relatively little is known of the physiological characteristics of these neurons.

Aston-Jones et al. (1984) observed that a portion of NB neurons exhibit multiple discrete antidromic latencies (see also Lamour et al., 1986). The latencies of antidromic activation of NB cells in the rat vary from 3.9 to 14.5 ms (Aston-Jones et al., 1984; Lamour et al., 1986; Reiner et al., 1987). In an elegant study by Reiner et al. (1987) and Semba et al. (1987), horseradish peroxidase was injected into physiologically characterized NB cells. Neurons with slow conduction velocity appeared to have a much greater number of dendritic spines than did fast conducting neurons.

Unfortunately, very little is known about the neurotransmitter properties of the physiologically characterized subgroups. Neurons have been characterized physiologically, marked anatomically, and stained for acetylcholinesterase in tissue culture (Nakajima et al., 1986) and *in vitro* slices (Griffith and Matthews, 1986) of the NB area. From these double labeling studies, it appears that cholinergic cells may fire Ca^{2+}- spikes with superimposed Na^+ spike-bursts followed by long-lasting afterhyperpolarizations.

Several earlier (DeLong, 1971; Rolls et al., 1979) and recent studies (Mitchell et al., 1987a, b) investigated the role of NB area neurons in learning and memory tasks in the awake monkey (for reviews see Richardson and DeLong, 1988; Richardson et al., 1988). In these studies it was found that cellular activity increased differentially to the presentation of food, but not to non-food stimuli. Since these stimuli were associated with different motor responses (movement and no movement) and different reward contingencies, a common denominator responsible for increased neuronal activity in these experiments may have been the motor performance and associated change of the arousal of the animals. This interpretation does not exclude the suggested role of NB neurons in positive reinforcement and appetitive conditioning, but point to the indirect role of the NB in these processes by allowing other (attention and memory) structures to carry out the required computation.

In our studies, the highest frequency activity of NB neurons was observed during running, followed by drinking and immobility. The decrease in the firing rate correlated with the increase in the power of slow activity in the neocortex (Fig. 1) (Buzsáki et al., 1988a). At least some of these neurons projected to the neocortex, as demonstrated by antidromic activation in response to neocortical volleys. A similar inverse correlation between NB neuronal discharge frequency and neocortical slow waves has been reported in urethane anesthetized rats (Detarí and Vanderwolf, 1987). In awake, but diazepam-sedated rats, three quarters of NB neurons exhibited robust increases in firing rates during the presentation of a conditioned tone cue (Rigdon and Pirch, 1986). Based on spontaneous firing repertories, Detarí et al. (1984) have distinguished five subgroups of neurons in the pallidal/peripallidal region of the cat. From 75 to 100 percent of cells in all groups had higher frequency discharge rates in the awake state and the paradoxical phase of sleep than in slow wave sleep. The majority of the neurons had higher than 10 Hz firing frequency, and neurons in three subgroups fired in "bursts" during slow wave sleep, and with single spikes during awake behaviors. A similar frequency increase with sleep-awake transitions was reported in another study (Szymusiak and McGinty, 1986).

From these studies it appears that the frequency changes of NB neurons correlate well with both behavioral and neocortical electrical arousal. Increased discharge frequency in NB neurons may therefore be considered a putative cause for neocortical desynchronization. The cholinergic nature of these NB neurons awaits further confirmation.

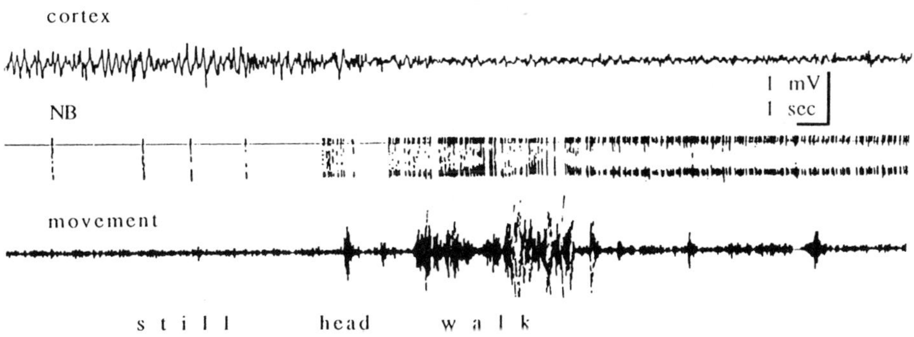

Figure 1. Relationship between firing of a NB neuron (magnocellular preoptic region, NB) and epidurally recorded EEG over the sensorimotor cortex (cortex) in the freely moving rat. Bottom trace: movement sensor. Note increased firing of the NB neurons and desynchronized neocortical EEG when the drowsy animal (still) was aroused by tapping on the cage. Head: orienting head movement; walk: following a pencil.

NUCLEUS BASALIS, THALAMIC LESIONS AND NEOCORTICAL ACTIVITY

It has been known for some time that cholinergic system(s) play a critical role in neocortical activation, since systemic injection of cholinolytics, such as atropine and scopolamine, can produce slow delta waves in the neocortex of all mammalian species tested (Wikler, 1952). Given the organization of the brainstem and basal forebrain cholinergic systems (see chapter by Mesulam), the most probable targets of these drugs are the postsynaptic sites of the cholinergic terminals in the thalamus and neocortex. Consequently, cholinolytics may interfere with behavioral arousal at two distinct levels: the thalamus and the cortex (both archicortex and neocortex).

The role of the brainstem cholinergic system in thalamic activation has been recently summarized (Steriade and Buzsáki, 1989). Considerably less information is available about the physiology of the NB-neocortical system. To date, only a few studies have examined neocortical EEG activity following damage of various parts of the basal forebrain cell groups. Lo Conte et al. (1982) used electrolytic lesions and reported that neocortical activity became "depressed". Stewart et al. (1984), using extensive kainic acid destruction of the NB, involving parts of the thalamus, found increased delta wave activity in the neocortex during immobility. Unfortunately, in this latter study the lesion also produced extensive damage to areas surrounding the NB, including the thalamus, and interpretation of the findings was not straightforward because of the distal cortical damage caused by kainic acid lesion (Arendash et al., 1987).

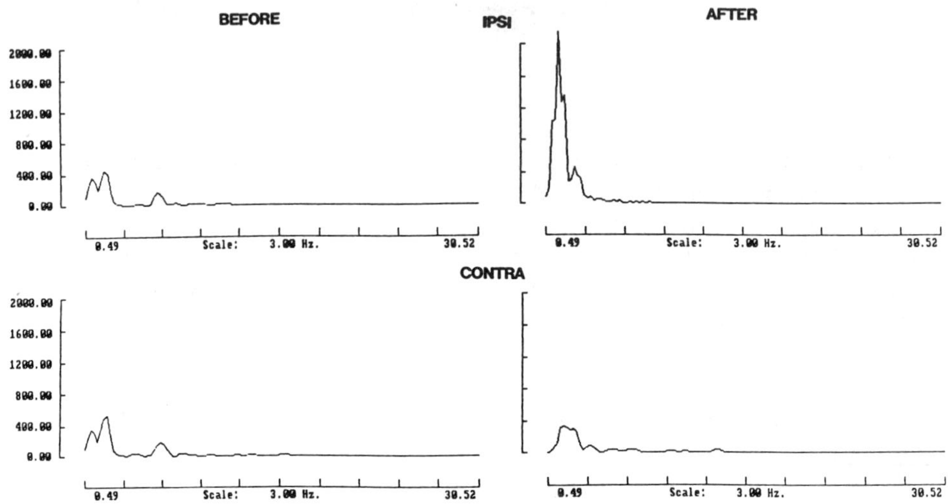

Figure 2. Power spectra of neocortical activity in sensorimotor cortex of the alert but immobile rat before and after ibotenic acid lesion of the right (ipsi) NB. Eight epidural electrodes were placed over the neocortex in each hemisphere. Only the maximum change at the site of the lesion and at the mirror site in the intact hemisphere (contra) are shown. Note substantial increase of delta power in the lesioned hemisphere after NB lesion. Ordinate: arbitrary units.

In our approach, we produced small, circumscribed lesions in the peripallidal or magnocellular preoptic regions of the NB using ibotenic acid. Because such small lesions were expected to affect only their target areas within a restricted region of the neocortex, we constructed power maps of the neocortical delta waves (Buzsáki et al., 1988a). Such small lesions resulted in increased power of delta activity under at least some of the epidural electrodes (delta focus) (Fig. 2). Subsequent histological evaluation of the brains revealed that the delta focus corresponded to neocortical areas where AChE-positive fiber density was mostly reduced (Buzsáki et al., 1988a). We have also shown that the asymmetric distribution of delta power in the lesioned rats could be reduced by scopolamine, indicating that the increased slow activity in the lesioned hemisphere was due mainly to the malfunctioning of the cholinergic NB projection (Buzsáki et al., 1988a). Large and small lesions of the thalamus, including the intralaminar nuclei, on the other hand, produced only a minor and transient effect on the neocortical slow waves but abolished HVS (Buzsáki, 1988a; Vanderwolf and Stewart, 1988). In summary, the intactness of the NB and its connections with the neocortex appear essential for normal neocortical activation.

CHOLINERGIC CONTROL OF NEOCORTICAL HIGH-VOLTAGE SPINDLES

A neocortical pattern that reliably reflects the presence and degree of thalamic oscillation in rats is HVS. HVS occur occasionally, while the rat is sitting motionless, with highest amplitude over the sensorimotor area. Depth profile measurements indicated that the laminar profiles of HVS and delta waves were different in the neocortex, and the depth profile of HVS fits the anatomical distribution of thalamic afferents to the neocortex. All neurons in the neocortex and thalamocortical nuclei fired exclusively during the spike component of the HVS. Neurons of the n. reticularis thalami, on the other hand, discharge with rhythmic burst dominantly during the wave portion of HVS. Several recent experiments support the notion that the interaction between neurons in the n. reticularis thalami and relay nuclei of the thalamus are intimately involved in the pattern generation of rhythmic neocortical patterns (Steriade and Deschenes, 1988; Steriade and Llinas, 1988; Buzsáki et al., 1990).

In connection with thalamic oscillation, we found that some neurons in the NB also fired rhythmically during the HVS. Importantly, an abrupt decrease in the firing of NB neurons often preceded or coincided with the onset of HVS (Buzsáki et al., 1988a). The hypothesized suppressive action of NB neurons on thalamic oscillation was further supported by lesion experiments. Bilateral lesions of the NB by ibotenic acid increased the incidence of HVS. Unilateral lesions often resulted in asymmetric distribution of HVS. While in the intact rat HVS occurred virtually synchronously over the two hemispheres, unilaterally occurring HVS were often encountered in the lesioned hemisphere, but not in the intact one (our unpublished findings). Small doses of the cholinolytic scopolamine increased the incidence but decreased the duration of the HVS episodes in young rats. Finally, in aged (24-28 mo) rats with shrunken NB neurons, the incidence and duration of HVS was four to eight times above the levels in young controls (Buzsáki et al., 1988b). Important in the present context is the discovery of a significant projection from the NB to the n. reticularis and other thalamic nuclei in rats, cats and monkeys (Hallanger et al., 1987; Steriade et al., 1987; Asanuma, 1989). Thus, it appears that the NB may exert a dual control over the neocortical activity: directly and indirectly via the thalamus.

CELLULAR GENERATION OF NEOCORTICAL DELTA WAVES: A HYPOTHESIS

Why is the neocortical activity desynchronized during aroused states and dominated by slow delta waves during drowsy and sleep states? What is the neurophysiological mechanism behind this strict correlation?

Depth profile measurements in the neocortex of the cat (Calvet et al., 1973; Ball et al., 1977), rabbit (Rappelsberger et al., 1981), and rat (Buzsáki et al., 1988a) revealed that surface negative-deep positive delta waves during slow wave sleep correlate with the suppression or cessation of discharges of layer V pyramidal neurons. Our studies indicate further that this suppression of neuronal firing is present in all cortical layers. The polarity reversal of delta waves occurred at the border of layers IV and V. In anesthetized animals the deep positive waves correlate with hyperpolarization of pyramidal cells (Creutzfeldt et al., 1966).

The depth profile of the slow delta waves and the observed field-unit relationship are compatible with the hypothesis that the extracellularly recorded delta waves reflect inhibition of pyramidal cells mediated by GABAergic interneurons (Ribak, 1978). GABA released at the somata of layer V pyramidal cells would open the Cl^-– channels and produce an active outward current whose extracellular spatial summation corresponds to deep positivity. A simultaneously occurring passive inward current at the distal dendrites would set up extracellular (surface) negativity. Indeed, with their widespread action, GABAergic interneurons may play an important role in affecting large numbers of pyramidal cells. Assuming that subcortical inputs terminate also on GABAergic interneurons (Somogyi et al., 1983), the subcortical afferents may globally affect the whole neocortical mantle.

An explicit prediction of the GABA-interneuron pyramidal cell model of slow wave generation is that GABAergic cells should fire maximally during the deep-positive delta waves. However, we have failed to find such a correlation in the rat neocortex. All putative, physiologically identified, neocortical interneurons decreased their firing rates during the deep-positive slow waves (Buzsáki et al., 1988a). Based on this finding and on the similar depth profiles of several different types of slow waves, we suggested that extracellular waves are not exclusively a result of synaptic activity, but may reflect summation of long-lasting afterhyperpolarizations (AHP) of layer V pyramidal neurons (Buzsáki et al., 1988a). A major part of the AHP is due to a Ca^{2+}-mediated K^+- conductance change. The K^+ current is outgoing at the level of the soma. The long-lasting nature of AHP favors the summation of outward currents of individual pyramidal cells, resulting in a large local field positivity in deep layers.

An attractive feature of the AHP hypothesis of slow-wave generation is that it is capable of explaining the correlation between EEG activity and behavioral arousal. ACh appears to block the Ca^{2+}- activated K^+ conductance underlying the long-lasting AHP. A further action of ACh is a blockade of the accommodation of the cell, that is, a decreased probability of the occurrence of action potentials in response to afferent excitation (Benardo and Prince, 1982; Cole and Nicoll, 1984; Madison and Nicoll, 1986; McCormick and Prince, 1986). Blockade of the AHP and accommodation by ACh will increase the fidelity of information transmission of the neuron by responding with action potentials to any depolarizing input with only a small effect upon the resting membrane potential, or responses to hyperpolarizing inputs. In this context, it is important to emphasize that several other subcortical neurotransmitters with widespread cortical projections, including histamine and noradrenaline, attenuate the AHP of pyramidal cells (Haas and Konnerth, 1983; Madison and Nicoll, 1986). We assume that behavioral arousal and neocortical desynchronization are linked by the blockade of AHP in pyramidal cells as a result of the increased activity of basal forebrain cholinergic and/or brainstem amine-containing neurons. Suppression of AHP will abolish synchronous extracellular current flow and the neocortex will display low-amplitude, desynchronized EEG. At the same time, the lack of long-lasting AHP and blockade of accommodation will allow the cortical cells to respond briskly and without failure to the specific information transmitted from the thalamus.

PHYSIOLOGICAL ROLE OF NB AND THE CONCEPT OF AROUSAL

The notion of activation is a Newtonian concept, implying the necessity of external sources to energize and set into motion an inert system. The sleeping or "non-aroused" brain, however, is clearly not inert. It is not active in the sense that the information-carrying capacity of both the afferent and efferent systems is at its minimum. The "non-aroused" nervous system is in a "closed-loop" state, but it is by no means inactive and without intrinsic activity. The dichotomy of open vs. closed-loop states appear to be present at all levels of the central nervous system (Table 1).

Table 1. Dichotomy of operations at different levels of neuronal organization.

level	activated	non-activated
behavior	aroused*	non-aroused
field (EEG)	desynchronized*	synchronized
population (network)	asynchronous	synchronous
cellular	continuous firing	burst firing
control	extrinsic	intrinsic
state	open-loop	closed-loop
function	information processing	memory formation

* REM sleep is regarded as an activated state at the thalamic and neocortical levels, although clearly no behavioral arousal is present.

Recent developments of recording techniques combined with *in vitro* techniques have offered new insights into the the operations of nerve cells and allowed us to begin to distinguish the intinsic biophysical characteristics of individual neurons from network-derived response properties. The majority of neurons in the mammalian brain have two basic modes of operation: steady firing and burst discharge. The burst discharge mode appears to be an intrinsic feature of several neuronal types, including thalamic and neocortical projection neurons (Llinas, 1988). Since the burst mode is an intrinsic property of neurons, the information transmitted by the cells to their respective targets will be rather independent of their inputs in this mode of discharge. In other words, the bursting mode of cell activity is probably the least optimal state for high fidelity information transfer. In contrast, sustained firing appears to be the characteristic neuronal pattern in the awake, behaviorally responsive animal. As discussed above and elsewhere (Steriade and Buzsáki, 1989), both thalamic and cortical neurons require transmitters extrinsic to these structures to sustain continuous action potentials without accommodation and transmit the afferent message with high fidelity.

The dual mode of discharge patterns has several important implications for the network (population) behavior of neurons (Table I). First, the long lasting nature of AHP following burst discharges in individual neurons considerably facilitates the emergence of population synchrony (Buzsáki et al., 1988c; Traub et al., 1989). As hypothesized above, synchronous occurrence of AHP in large numbers of neurons results in summed extracellular currents and consequent slow delta waves in the EEG record. In contrast, blockade of the AHP by ACh and other monoamines of subcortical origin reduce the probability of population synchrony and result in desynchronized EEG (Buzsáki et al., 1988a). Population synchrony is largely a closed-loop phenomenon of the neuronal network (Traub et al., 1989), while the desynchronized (or "activated") state is dependent on external, arousing inputs both in thalamus and neocortex.

We suggest that the activation process implies a switching action between the two fundamental modes of operation of the central nervous system. In the activated state the brain is in continuous interaction with the environment. To date, no function has been assigned to the non-interactive mode of brain function. We have recently suggested, however, that population bursting, the characteristic pattern of the closed-loop state, is the most likely candidate for the induction of long-term plastic changes underlying memory formation (Buzsáki, 1989). From this perspective the arousal process is not simply a shift from the passive state to an active one, but is viewed as a fundamental change from the storage mode to the information processing mode of brain operation. As we have discussed in this chapter, the cholinergic basal forebrain plays a pivotal role in this important process.

CONCLUSIONS

The cholinergic NB plays an essential role in activation of the cerebral cortex via a dual mechanism. First, the cortical cholinergic projection from NB directly influences neocortical pyramidal cells mainly by blocking AHP and accommodation in these cells. Second, the cholinergic input from NB to RT suppresses the rhythmic oscillations of the "pacemaker" neurons of this thalamic nucleus. Thus, increased activity of NB neurons, e.g., during walking, will ensure neocortical activation by direct release of ACh in the neocortex and by dampening the oscillatory influences of the thalamus.

ACKNOWLEDGMENTS

The work reviewed here was supported by the Alzheimer's Disease and Related Disorders Association, The Sandoz Foundation for Gerontological Research and the Whitehall Foundation.

REFERENCES

Arendash, G., Millard, W.J., Dunn, A.J. and Meyer, E.M. (1987): Long-term neuropathological and neurochemical effects of nucleus basalis lesions in the rat. *Science* 238:952-956

Asanuma, C. (1989): Magnocellular basal nucleus projection to the thalamic reticular nucleus in rats: a structural substrate for the thalamic modulation of thalamic excitability by the basal forebrain. *Proc. Natl. Acad. Sci.* 86:4746-4750

Aston-Jones, G. and Bloom, F.E. (1981): Norepinephrine-containing locus coeruleus neurons in behaving rats exhibit pronounced responses to non-noxious stimuli. *J. Neurosci.* 1:887-900

Aston-Jones, G., Shaver, R. and Dinan, T.G. (1984): Cortically projecting nucleus basalis neurons in rat are physiologically heterogeneous. *Neurosci. Lett.* 46:19-24

Ball, G.J., Gloor, P. and Schaul, N. (1977): The cortical electromicrophysiology of cats. *Electroencephal. Clin. Neurophysiol.* 43:46-363

Belardetti, F., Borgia, R., and Mancia, M. (1977): Prosencephalic mechanisms of ECoG desynchronization in cerveau isole cats. *Electroencephal. Clin. Neurophysiol.* 42:213-225

Benardo, L.S. and Prince, D.A. (1982): Cholinergic excitation of mammalian hippocampal pyramidal cells. *Brain Res.* 249:315-331

Buzsáki, G. (1989): Two-stage model of memory trace formation: a role for "noisy" brain states. *Neurosci.* 31:551-570

Buzsáki, G., Bickford, T.G., Ponomareff, G., Thal, L.J., Mandel, R.J. and Gage, F.H. (1988a): Nucleus basalis and thalamic control of neocortical activity in the freely moving rat. *J. Neurosci.* 8:4007-4026

Buzsáki, G., Bickford, R.G., Armstrong, D.M., Ponomareff, G., Chen, K., Ruiz, R., Thal, L.J. and Gage, F.H. (1988b): EEG activity in the neocortex of freely moving young and aged rats. *Neurosci.* 26:735-744

Buzsáki, G., Ponomareff, G., Bayardo, F., Shaw, T. and Gage, F.H. (1988c): Suppression and induction of epileptic activity by neuronal grafts. *Proc. Natl. Acad. Sci.* 85:9327-9330

Buzsáki, G., Smith, A., Berger, S. Fisher, L.J. and Gage, F.H. (1990): Petit mal epilepsy and parkinsonian tremor: hypothesis of a common pacemaker. *Neurosci.* in press

Calvet, J. and Fourment, Michel, T. (1973): Electrical activity in neocortical projection and association areas during slow wave sleep. *Brain Res.* 5:173-187

Casamenti, F., Defenu, G., Abbamondi, A. L. and Pepeu, G. (1986): Changes in cortical acetylcholine output induced by modulation of the nucleus basalis. *Brain Res. Bull.* 16:689-695

Coben, L.A., Danzinger, W.L. and Starandt, M. (1985): A longitudinal study of mild senile dementia of Alzheimer type: changes at 1 year and 2.5 years. *Electroencephal Clin. Neurophysiol.* 61:101-112

Cole, A.E. and Nicoll, R.A. (1984): Characterization of a slow cholinergic postsynaptic potential recorded *in vitro* from rat hippocampal pyramidal cells. *J. Physiol.* (Lond) 352:173-188

Creutzfeldt, O., Watanabe, S. and Lux, H.D. (1966): Relations between EEG phenomena and potentials of single cortical cells. I. Evoked responses after thalamic and epicortical stimulation. *Electroencephal. Clin. Neurophysiol.* 20:1-18

DeLong, M. R. (1971): Activity of pallidal neurons during movement. *J. Neurophysiol.* 34:414-427

Detarí, L., Juhasz, G. and Kukorelli, T. (1984): Firing properties of cat basal forebrain neurons during sleep-wakefulness cycles. *Electroenceph. Clin. Neurophysiol.* 58:362-368

Detarí, L. and Vanderwolf, C.H. (1987): Activity of identified cortically projecting and other basal forebrain neurons during large slow waves and cortical activation in anesthetized rats. *Brain Res.* 437:1-10

Divac, I. (1975): Magnocellular nuclei of the basal forebrain project to neocortex, brain stem, and olfactory bulb. Review of some functional correlates. *Brain Res.* 93:385-398

Fibiger, H.C. (1982): The organization and some projections of cholinergic neurons of the mammalian forebrain. *Brain Res. Rev.* 4:327-388

Foote, S.L., Aston-Jones, G. and Bloom, F.E. (1980): Impulse activity of locus coeruleus neurons in awake rats and monkeys is a function of sensory stimulation and arousal. *Proc. Natl. Acad. Sci.* 77:3033-3037

Fox, K. and Armstrong-James, M. (1986): The role of the anterior intralaminar nuclei and N-methyl D-aspartate receptors in the generation of spontaneous bursts in rat neocortical neurones. *Exp. Brain Res.* 63:505-518

Funahashi, S. (1983): Responses of monkey prefrontal neurons during a visual tracking task reinforced by substantia innominata self-stimulation. *Brain Res.* 276:267-276

Griffith, W.H. and Matthews, R.T. (1986): Electrophysiology of AChE-positive neurons in basal forebrain slices. *Neurosci. Lett.* 71:171-174

Haas, H.L. and Konnerth, A. (1983): Histamine and noradrenaline decrease calcium-activated potassium conductance in hippocampal pyramidal cells. *Nature* (Lond.) 302:432-434

Hallanger, A. E., Levey, A. I., Lee, H. J., Rye, D. B. and Wainer, B. H. (1987): The origins of cholinergic and other subcortical afferents to the thalamus in the rat. *J. Comp. Neurol.* 262:105-124

Jahnsen, H. and Llinas, R. (1984): Electrophysiological properties of guinea-pig thalamic neurones: an *in vitro* study. *J. Physiol.* (Lond.) 349: 205-226

Jasper, H.H. (1949): Diffuse projection systems: the integrative action of the thalamic reticular system. *Electroenceph. Clin. Neurophysiol.* 1:405-420

Jones, E.G. (1985): *The Thalamus*. New York: Plenum Publishing Corp.

Jones, E.G., Burton, H., Saper, C.B. and Swanson, L.W. (1976): Midbrain, diencephalic and cortical relationships of the basal nucleus of Meynert and associated structures in primates. *J. Comp. Neurol.* 167:385-420

Klingberg, F. and Pickenhain, L. (1968): Das Aufreten von 'Spindelenthadinigen' bei der ratte in Beziehung zum Verhalten. *Acta Biol. Med. Germ.* 20:45-54

Krnjević, K., Pumain, R. and Renaud, L. (1971): The mechanism of excitation by acetylcholine in the cerebral cortex. *J. Physiol.* (Lond.) 215:247-268

Lamour, Y., Dutar, P., Rascol, O. and Joberts, A. (1986): Basal forebrain neurons projecting to the rat fronto-parietal cortex: electrophysiological and pharmacological properties. *Brain Res.* 362:122-131

Llinas, R.R. (1988): The intrinsic electrophysiological properties of mammalian neurons: insight into central nervous system. *Science* 242:1654-1664

Lo Conte, G., Casamenti, E., Bigl, V., Milaneschi, E. and Pepeu, G. (1982): Effect of magnocellular forebrain nuclei lesions on acetylcholine output from the cerebral cortex, electrocorticogram and behavior. *Arch. Ital. Biol.* 120:176-188

Longo, V.G. (1956): Effects of scopolamine and atropine on electro-encephalographic and behavioral reactions due to hypothalamic stimulation. *J. Pharmacol.* 116:198-208

Madison, D.V. and Nicoll, R.A. (1986): Actions of noradrenaline recorded intracellularly in rat hippocampal CA1 pyramidal neurons, *in vitro*. *J. Physiol.* (Lond.) 321:175-177

McCormick, D.A. and Prince, D.A. (1986): Mechanisms of action of acetylcholine in the guinea pig cerebral cortex *in vitro*. *J. Neurophysiol.* 375:169-194

McGinty, D.J. and Sterman, M.B. (1968): Sleep suppression after basal forebrain lesions in cat. *Science* 160:1253-1255

Mesulam, M.-M. and Van Hoesen, G.W. (1976): Acetylcholinesterase-rich projections from the basal forebrain of the rhesus monkey to neocortex. *Brain Res.* 109:152-157

Mesulam, M.-M., Mufson, E.J., Wainer, B.H. and Levey, A.I. (1983): Central cholinergic pathways in the rat: an overview based on an alternative nomenclature (Ch1-Ch6). *Neurosci.* 4:1185-1201

Mitchell, S.J., Richardson, R.T. and DeLong, M.R. (1987a): The primate globus pallidus: neuronal activity related to direction of movement. *Exp. Brain. Res.* 68:491-505

Mitchell, S.J., Richardson, R.T. and DeLong, M.R. (1987b): The primate nucleus basalis: neuronal activity related to behavior. *Exp. Brain Res.* 68:506-515

Moruzzi, G. and Magoun, H.W. (1949): Brainstem reticular formation and activation of the EEG. *Electroenceph. Clin. Neurophysiol.* 1:455-473

Nakajima, Y., Nakajima, S., Leonard, R.J. and Yamaluchi, K. (1986): Acetylcholine raises excitability by inhibiting the fast transient potassium current in cultured hippocampal neurons. *Proc. Natl. Acad. Sci.* 83:3022-3026

Nicoll, R.A. (1988): The coupling of neurotransmitter receptors to ion channels in the brain. *Science* 241:545-551

Papez, J.W. (1956): Central reticular path to intralaminar and reticular neurons of the thalamus for activating EEG related to consciousness. *Electroencephal. Clin. Neurophysiol.* 8:117-128

Pentilla, M., Partanen, J.V., Soinen, H. and Riekkinen, P. J. (1985): Quantitative analysis of occipital EEG in different stages of Alzheimer's disease. *Electroencephal. Clin. Neurophysiol.* 60:1-6

Phillis, J.W. (1980): Acetylcholine release from the cerebral cortex and its role in cortical arousal. *Brain Res.* 7:378-389

Rappelsberger, P., Pockberger, H. and Petsche, H. (1981): The contribution of the cortical layers to the generation of the EEG: field potential and current source density analyses in the rabbit's visual cortex. *Electroenceph. Clin. Neurophysiol.* 53:254-269

Reiner, P.B., Semba, K., Fibiger, H.C. and McGeer, E.G. (1987): Physiological evidence for subpopulations of cortically projecting basal forebrain neurons in the anesthetized rat. *Neurosci.* 20:629-636

Ribak, C.E. (1978): Aspinous and sparsely-spinous stellate neurons in the visual cortex of rats containing glutamic acid decarboxylase. *J. Neurocytol.* 7:461-478

Richardson, R.T. and DeLong, M.R. (1988): A reappraisal of the functions of the nucleus basalis of Meynert. *Trends Neurosci.* 11:264-267

Richardson, R.T., Mitchell, S.J., Baker, F.H. and DeLong, M.R. Responses of nucleus basalis of Meynert neurons in behaving monekys. In: *Cellular Mechanisms of Conditioning and Behavioral Plasticity*. C.D. Woody, D.L. Alkon and McGaugh, J.L., eds. New York: Plenus Publishing Corp. pp 161-173

Rigdon, G.C. and Pirch, J.H. (1986): Nucleus basalis involvement in conditioned neuronal responses in the rat frontal cortex. *J. Neurosci.* 6:2535-2542

Rolls, E.T., Sanghera, M.K. and Roper-Hall, A. (1979): The latency of activation of neurons in the lateral hypothalamus and substantia innominata during feeding in the monkey. *Brain Res.*164:121-135

Semba, K., Reiner, P.B., McGeer, E.G. and Fibiger, H.C. (1987): Morphology of cortically projecting basal forebrain neurons in the rat as revealed by intracellular iontophoresis of horseradish peroxydase. *Neurosci.* 20:637-351

Shute, C. D. and Lewis, P. R. (1967): The ascending cholinergic reticular systems: neocortical, olfactory and subcortical projections. *Brain* 90:497-520

Siegel, J., and Wang, R.Y. (1974): Electroencephalographic, behavioral and single-unit effects produced by stimulation of forebrain inhibitory structures in cats. *Exp. Neurol.* 42:28-50

Somogyi, P., Kisvarday, Z.F., Martin, K.A.C. and Whitteridge, D. (1983): Synaptic connections of morphologically identified and physiologically characterized large basket cells in the striate cortex of cat. *Neurosci.* 10:261-294

Steriade, M. (1970): Ascending control of thalamic and cortical responsiveness. *Int. Rev. Neurobiol.* 12:87-144

Steriade, M. and Buzsáki, G. (1989): Parallel activation of thalamic and cortical neurons by brainstem and forebrain cholinergic systems. In: *Brain Cholinergic Systems*. Steriade, M., Biesold, D., eds. Oxford: Oxford University Press

Steriade, M. and Deschenes, M. (1988): The thalamus as a neuronal oscillator. *Brain Res. Rev.* 8:1-63

Steriade, M. and Llinas, R. (1988): The functional states of the thalamus and the associated neuronal interplay. *Physiol. Rev.* 68:649-742

Steriade, M., Parent, A., Paré, D. and Smith, Y. (1987): Cholinergic and noncholinergic neurons of the cat basal forebrain project to reticular and mediodorsal thalamic nuclei. *Brain Res.* 408:372-376

Sterman, M.B. and Clemente, C.D. (1962): Forebrain inhibitory mechanisms: sleep patterns induced by forebrain stimulation in the behaving cat. *Exp. Neurol.* 6:103-117

Stern, W.C. and Pugh, W.W. (1984): Responses of frontal cortex single units to magnocellular basal forebrain stimulation. *Soc. Neurosci. Abstr.* 10:9.

Stewart, D.J., MacFabe, D.F. and Vanderwolf, C.H. (1984): Cholinergic activation of the electrocorticogram: role of substantia innominata and effects of atropine and quinuclidinyl benzylate. *Brain Res.* 322:219-232

Szymusiak, D. and McGinty, D. (1986): Sleep-related neuronal discharge in the basal forebrain of cats. *Brain Res.* 370:82-92

Traub, R.D., Miles, R. and Wong, R.K.S. (1989): Model of rhythmic population oscillation in the hippocampal slice. *Science* 243:1319-1325

Trulson, M.E. and Jacobs, B.L. (1979): Raphe unit activity in freely moving cats: correlation with level of behavioral arousal. *Brain Res.* 163:135-150

Vanderwolf, C.H. (1975): Neocortical and hippocampal activation in relation to behavior: effects of atropine, eserine, phenothiazines, and amphetamine. *J. Comp. Physiol. Psychol.* 88:300-323

Vanderwolf, C.H. (1988): Cerebral activity and behavior: control by central cholinergic and serotonergic systems. *Intl. Rev. Neurobiol.* 30:225-340

Vanderwolf, C.H. and Baker, G.B. (1986): Evidence that serotonin mediates non-cholinergic neocortical low voltage fast activity, non-cholinergic hippocampal rhythmical slow activity and contributes to intelligent behavior. *Brain Res.* 374:342-356

Vanderwolf, C.H. and Robinson, T.H. (1981): Reticulocortical activity and behavior: a critique of the arousal theory and a new synthesis. *Behav. Brain Sci.* 4:459-514

Vanderwolf, C.H. and Stewart, D.J. (1986): Joint cholinergic-serotonergic control of neocortical and hippocampal electrical activity in relation to behavior: effects of scopolamine, ditran, trifluoperazine and amphetamine. *Physiol. Behav.* 38:57-65

Vanderwolf, C.H. and Steward, D.J. (1988): Thalamic control of neocortical activation: a critical re-evaluation. *Brain Res. Bull.* 20:529-53

Wikler, A. (1952): Pharmacologic dissociation on behavior and EEG sleep patterns in dogs: morphine, N-allylnormorphine and atropine. *Proc. Soc. Exp. Biol.*, N.Y. 79:261-266

Functional Implications of Tonic and Phasic Activity Changes in Nucleus Basalis Neurons

Russell T. Richardson and Mahlon R. DeLong

INTRODUCTION

The basal forebrain cholinergic system (BFCS) has become a focus of research in many laboratories over the past decade. Current interest in this system began in the mid-1970s when a population of neurons in the basal forebrain was discovered to project to cerebral cortex (Divac, 1975; Kievit and Kuypers, 1975). It was later established that the neurotransmitter for the cortically projecting neurons was acetylcholine (ACh) (Mesulam et al., 1983; Rye et al., 1984) and that these neurons provided the major source of cholinergic input to cortex (Lehmann et al., 1980; Wenk et al., 1980; Johnston et al., 1981; Struble et al., 1986). Also in the mid-1970s, ACh became strongly implicated in Alzheimer's disease (AD) because cholinergic markers were found to be severely reduced in the brains of AD patients (Davies and Maloney, 1976; Perry et al., 1977; Spillane et al., 1977). By the early 1980s, the nucleus basalis, the largest component of the BFCS, was shown to have a substantial loss of neurons in patients with AD (Whitehouse et al., 1982). The depletion of nucleus basalis neurons was hypothesized to account for the decrease in cortical cholinergic markers which could possibly lead to the cognitive deterioration of AD (Bartus et al., 1982; Coyle et al., 1983). These findings stimulated a great deal of interest in the anatomical and physiological properties of the BFCS in an effort to understand its role in normal brain function and dementia.

Prior to recent studies of the cholinergic system, most of our understanding of the role of ACh in brain function came from studies of the effects of cholinergic drugs. Although the mechanisms or sites of action of cholinergic agents were unknown, the drugs had dramatic effects, suggesting certain processes in which ACh might be involved. One of the most profound effects was the influence of cholinergic agents on the cortical electroencephalogram (EEG). Cholinergic antagonists, such as atropine or scopolamine, produced a generally synchronized cortical EEG, whereas agonists, such as the acetylcholinesterase inhibitor physostigmine, produced a desynchronized EEG (Longo, 1955; Vanderwolf, 1975). Another prominent effect of cholinergic drugs was their ability to alter learning and memory processes. Cholinergic antagonists disrupted performance on memory tasks in several species from mice to humans, and cholinergic agonists sometimes improved performance on such tasks (Collerton, 1986; Smith, 1988). Thus, ACh was considered to play an important role in arousal and in learning and memory. Given the rapid increase in information regarding the BFCS, it is now possible to make hypotheses regarding the possible sites of action of ACh and mechanisms of its role in these processes.

This chapter approaches the question of the functions of the BFCS primarily from an electrophysiological point of view, and primarily from studies of the nucleus basalis in primates. Studies of the physiological properties of nucleus basalis neurons, combined with new information regarding the anatomical connections of these neurons, have provided insights into the possible functions of the cholinergic system, in particular its role in arousal and learning. In brief, much of the available evidence suggests that the cholinergic system may set the level of excitability of target neurons in cerebral cortex, amygdala, and hippocampus. An increase in excitability may contribute to the cortical activation component of arousal, and may also lead to a long-term facilitation of connections among selected cortical neurons, thereby contributing to the neuronal substrate of learning.

ANATOMICAL PROPERTIES

Details of the anatomical properties of the BFCS are discussed in other chapters in this book. Only the key anatomical features of the cholinergic system, particularly the nucleus basalis, are outlined here.

Perhaps the most important structural feature of the BFCS is that it projects to a substantial portion of the forebrain. Virtually all regions of cortex are innervated by the cholinergic system, although some regions receive a heavier input than others (Lehmann et al., 1984; Mesulam et al., 1986). The cholinergic system also projects to the hippocampal formation, the amygdaloid complex, and the olfactory bulb. Interestingly, one of the few regions of the thalamus to which the BFCS projects is the reticular thalamic nucleus (Levey et al., 1987; Parent et al., 1988), which influences most of the thalamus, which, in turn, influences most of the cerebral cortex. Thus, the cholinergic system can directly and indirectly influence a remarkably large region of the forebrain.

Although the cholinergic system as a whole projects to a widespread region of the forebrain, individual neurons of the cholinergic system project to fairly restricted areas. Single neurons from the nucleus basalis do not appear to have long collateral branches that could innervate disparate cortical areas (Bigl et al., 1982; Walker et al., 1985; Koliatsos et al., 1988). The terminal field of a single basalis neuron has been estimated to be approximately 1.5 mm in diameter in rodents (Price and Stern, 1983). Given that there are approximately 400,000 neurons in the human nucleus basalis (Arendt et al., 1985) and that the human neocortical surface is approximately 227,500 mm^2 (Elias and Schwartz, 1969), the average size of non-overlapping terminal fields of cortically projecting basalis neurons would be slightly more than 0.5 mm^2. Based on anterograde tracing studies using *Phaseolus* lectin (Luiten et al., 1987), cholinergic neurons may have extensive collateral branching within their terminal fields, but they do not appear to innervate large or discontiguous cortical areas.

Cortically projecting cholinergic neurons are not the only neurons that exist in the basal forebrain. The nucleus basalis itself is identified by its large, hyperchromic neurons, and if a basalis neuron projects to cortex, there is an approximately 90% chance that it contains choline-acetyltransferase (ChAT), the synthetic enzyme for ACh (Mesulam et al., 1983; Rye et al., 1984). Therefore, only a small proportion of nucleus basalis neurons that project to cortex are non-cholinergic. On the other hand, if a basalis neuron contains ChAT, it is not known what the chances are that it projects to distal targets or terminates within the BFCS.

There are a number of smaller non-cholinergic neurons intermixed with the larger neurons of the nucleus basalis (Walker et al., 1989a; 1989b). Moreover, in most mammalian species, basalis neurons are dispersed throughout the ventral part of the globus pallidus and are therefore intermixed with pallidal neurons (Parent et al., 1981). In primates, however, basalis neurons are mostly segregated from pallidal neurons, but numerous cortically projecting cholinergic neurons lie within the medullary laminae along the lateral borders of the pallidal segments (Mesulam et al., 1983). Thus, there are "non-basalis" neurons intermixed with basalis neurons within the main body of the nucleus basalis, and there are basalis neurons intermixed with other neurons outside the main body of the nucleus basalis.

In summary, the nucleus basalis is a loose aggregate of large, hyperchromic neurons in the basal forebrain. Most basalis neurons contain ChAT, the synthetic enzyme for ACh, and are intermixed with smaller non-cholinergic neurons. The nucleus basalis as a whole projects to widespread regions of cerebral cortex, but individual basalis neurons appear to project to single target areas on the order of 1 mm^2 in cortex.

CORTICAL ACTIVATION

There is now considerable evidence that the nucleus basalis is involved in the process of arousal. More specifically, it appears to be related to cortical activation in that increased discharge rates of basalis neurons may initiate or maintain EEG desynchronization. A desynchronized EEG is usually characteristic of increased levels of arousal, whereas synchronized EEG is generally indicative of drowsiness or slow wave sleep. However, desynchronized EEG is not synonymous with behavioral arousal because the two can be dissociated under certain conditions. For example, during REM sleep, an animal is clearly not in a behaviorally aroused state, but the EEG is desynchronized. In addition, animals given cholinergic blockers, such as scopolamine, can be awake and moving about while their EEG is highly synchronized. The key distinction is that EEG desynchronization is a *component* of arousal, just as directed movements, orientation to stimuli, and increased muscle tone are components of arousal. Hence, the nucleus basalis appears to be involved with a specific component of arousal, namely EEG desynchronization.

Desynchronized EEG activity is indicative of cortical activation, which has been defined as "a tonic state of response readiness in neuronal networks of the cerebrum" (Steriade, 1984). During cortical activation, there is a high fidelity transfer of information through the thalamus to cerebral cortex. In contrast, during periods of drowsiness or slow wave sleep, characterized by EEG synchronization, thalamic and cortical projection neurons do not respond reliably to external stimuli, but tend to fire in a repetitive, cyclical fashion.

During cortical activation, there is an increased excitability of cortical and thalamic projection neurons in that they are more likely to respond to excitatory stimulation (Steriade, 1984). Cortical neurons also have increased responsiveness during cortical activation in that they discharge more spikes in response to excitatory afferent stimulation (Singer et al., 1976; Livingstone and Hubel, 1981). Recent findings suggest that the cholinergic projection from the nucleus basalis may enhance both the excitability and responsiveness of cortical neurons during cortical activation.

Tonic Discharge Rates of Basalis Neurons

In an awake animal, nucleus basalis neurons have a characteristic steady firing pattern of approximately 20 spikes/second with little variability in the time between cell discharges (DeLong, 1971; Lamour et al., 1986; Richardson and DeLong, 1987). However, as the animal becomes drowsy or falls asleep, basalis neurons begin to fire more slowly and sporadically. When the animal becomes alert again, basalis neurons resume their steady firing. Accordingly, there is a tight coupling of the discharge rates of basalis neurons with cortical EEG desynchronization (Detarí and Vanderwolf, 1987; Szymusiak and McGinty, 1989), as shown in Fig. 1. Higher discharge rates in basalis neurons are consistently associated with EEG desynchronization, and lower discharge rates are associated with cortical synchronization. Cortical EEG desynchronization is also associated with an increased release of ACh in cortex. In general, there is a robust increase in the amount of ACh that can be collected from cerebral cortex during periods of cortical EEG desynchronization due to reticular formation stimulation or normal waking (Celesia and Jasper, 1966; Pepeu, 1974). Direct electrical stimulation of the nucleus basalis also increases the amount of ACh released in cortex (Casamenti et al., 1986; Kurosawa et al., 1989). Thus, the increase in ACh release in cerebral cortex during periods of EEG desynchronization appears to result directly from the increased firing rates of basalis neurons.

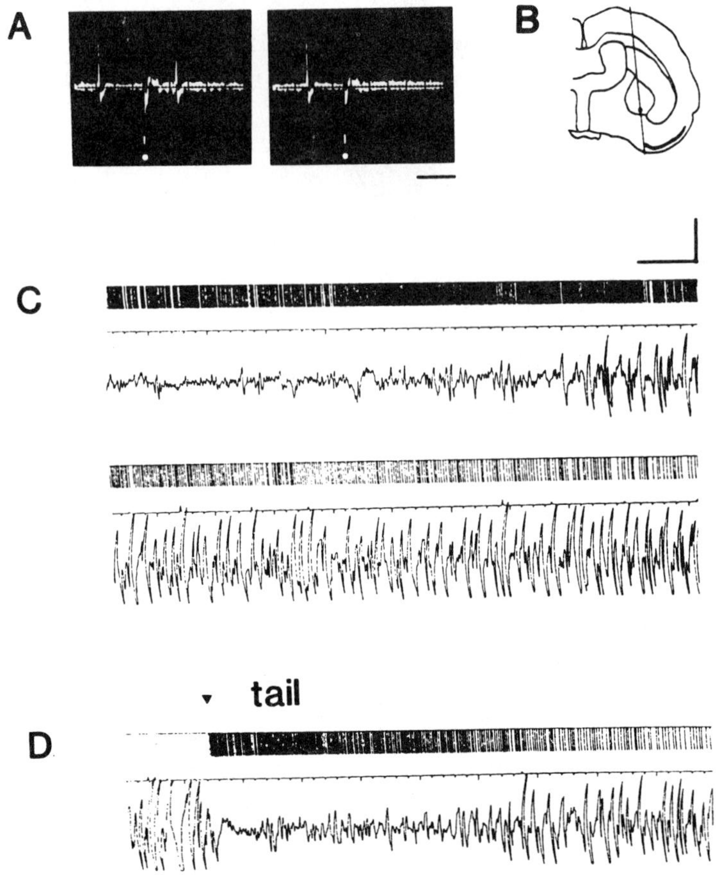

Figure 1. Discharge rate of a cortically projecting basalis neuron corresponds to EEG desynchronization in rat. A. Collision test. The neuron is antidromically activated from stimulation sites in cortex when the stimulation occurs 11 msec after the cell discharges spontaneously, but not at 9 msec. Horizontal bar is 10 msec. B. Location of the recorded neuron in the ventral globus pallidus. C. Continuous recording over 100 sec, displayed as two traces. In each trace, the top row represents discharges of the neuron, the bottom trace shows the concurrent EEG, and the middle trace shows timing marks. Calibration bars are 0.25 mV for the EEG record and 5 sec. Note that as large synchronized waves appear in the EEG, the discharge rate of the neuron slows markedly. D. After approximately 70 sec of synchronized EEG, the neuron is silent, but a tail pinch (at the arrow) elicits rapid firing in the neuron and transient EEG desynchronization. As the EEG becomes synchronized, the discharge rate of the basalis neuron again decreases. Reproduced with permission of Elsevier Science Publishers, B.V. from Detarí and Vanderwolf, (1987): Activity of identified cortically projecting and other basal forebrain neurones during large waves and cortical activation in anesthetized rats. *Brain Res.* 437:1-8.

Modulatory Effects of ACh on Cortical Neurons

The net effect of the increased release of ACh during cortical activation is likely to be an enhancement of the response properties of cortical neurons. ACh applied directly to cortical neurons increases the discharge rate in 11 to 38% of all cortical neurons tested (Krnjević and Phillis, 1963; Sillito and Kemp, 1983; Metherate et al., 1987; Lamour et al., 1988; McKenna et al., 1988). Less often, ACh decreases discharge rates of cortical neurons (Jordan and Phillis, 1972) which may be due to a rapid excitation of GABAergic interneurons (McCormick and Prince, 1985). The most profound effect of ACh, however, is its ability to alter the responses of cortical neurons to other stimuli. In some studies, over 90% of all cortical neurons have shown altered response properties after ACh application (Sillito and Kemp, 1983; Sato et al., 1987a).

Most neurons affected by ACh show facilitated response properties in that they have an increased magnitude of response (i.e., number of spikes) to a particular stimulus. Some cortical neurons have diminished responses following ACh application, but they are far less common than those with enhanced responses. Furthermore, Sato et al. (1987b) have found that, in cats, lesions of the nucleus basalis that destroy much of the cholinergic input to visual cortex strongly reduce the responses of cortical neurons to visual stimuli. Somewhat normal responses can then be restored by local application of ACh. Hence, the cholinergic projection from the nucleus basalis appears to have a modulatory effect on cortical neurons in that it generally enhances their responses to other afferent inputs.

ACh Effects on Ion Channels

The enhanced excitability of cortical neurons appears to result from the effect of ACh on a number of ion currents. ACh blocks the M-current, which is a K^+ current that resists depolarization of the resting membrane potential (Halliwell and Adams, 1982; Brown, 1983). Hence, an ACh induced decrease in the M-current would make a neuron more likely to discharge in response to a depolarizing input. As mentioned earlier, one of the characteristics of cortical activation is an enhanced excitability of cortical neurons.

Another consistent effect of ACh is an increase in the input resistance of cortical and hippocampal neurons (Krnjević et al., 1971; Woody et al., 1978; Benardo and Prince, 1982). The input resistance appears to be enhanced primarily by ACh blocking a slow K^+ leak current (Madison et al., 1987; Benson et al., 1988). Decreasing the K^+ leak current can also slightly depolarize the neuron. Both the depolarization and increased input resistance could increase a neuron's excitability during cortical activation.

Another feature of cortical activation is a decrease in the long duration afterhyperpolarization in cortical neurons (Steriade, 1984) which may be due to a Ca^{++} activated K^+ current ($I_{K/Ca}$). ACh strongly inhibits a $I_{K/Ca}$ in cortical and hippocampal neurons, and the decreased afterhyperpolarization enhances neuronal responsiveness by allowing the cells to discharge repeatedly in response to an excitatory input (Cole and Nicoll, 1984; McCormick and Prince, 1985). Thus, by altering specific ion currents, increased ACh release can increase both the excitability of a neuron (the probability that it will discharge) and the responsiveness of a neuron (the number of discharges.)

There is some debate about whether the facilitory effect of ACh actually increases response specificity in cortical neurons. For example, ACh can enhance neuronal responses to a particular stimulus, but ACh may also increase the background firing rate of the neuron, thereby reducing the signal-to-noise ratio of the neuronal response. In some studies of visual cortex, ACh appears to enhance a neuron's responses only to a preferred stimulus, thereby increasing the neuron's selectivity (Sillito and Kemp, 1983), but in other studies, response selectivity may be unchanged or worsened by ACh (Sato et al., 1987a). In somatosensory cortex, ACh may reveal a receptive field that would otherwise not be detected for a neuron, thereby improving the cell's selectivity, but it may also enlarge a neuron's pre-existing receptive field, thereby decreasing the cell's selectivity (Lamour et al., 1988). Although ACh generally enhances the overall magnitude of a cortical neuron's responses to stimuli, it is not clear under what circumstances the selectivity of the neuron's responses would also be enhanced.

Structures Affecting Cortical EEG

It appears that one of the primary functions of the nucleus basalis is to maintain generalized cortical activation during wakefulness and paradoxical sleep. An increase in the discharge rates of nucleus basalis neurons is hypothesized to produce an increase in ACh release in cerebral cortex, which enhances the excitability and responsiveness of cortical neurons by altering specific ion currents. The changes in the membrane properties of cortical neurons may form the neuronal substrate of cortical activation, or at least contribute to it.

Of course, the nucleus basalis is not the only structure that plays a role in cortical activation. There is evidence that cortical activation can occur without an increase in ACh release in cortex (Casamenti et al., 1986), which suggests that other projection systems may be able to maintain cortical activation. Other structures that may promote cortical activation include the locus coeruleus, raphe nuclei, and intralaminar thalamic nuclei.

Nevertheless, there are numerous suggestions that the cholinergic system may have the most prominent influence on cortical activation. Lesions in the basal forebrain that damage the cholinergic projection to cortex also affect the EEG. In general, such lesions diminish the high frequency components or enhance the low frequency components of the EEG (LoConte et al., 1982; Stewart et al., 1984; Buzsáki et al., 1988), resulting in a shift from desynchronized to synchronized EEG activity. Comparable changes in EEG can be produced by blocking cholinergic receptors with atropine or scopolamine (Longo, 1955; Vanderwolf, 1975).

In contrast to basal forebrain lesions, extensive lesions of the reticular or intralaminar thalamic nuclei have little effect on cortical EEG desynchronization, although they clearly diminish various forms of synchronized EEG activity (Stewart et al., 1984; Buzsáki et al., 1988). Thus, these thalamic nuclei may not be critical for cortical activation. Nor, in addition, may the the locus coeruleus and raphe nuclei be essential for cortical activation. If the ascending afferents from these structures are effectively disconnected from cortex by cryogenic blockade at the mesencephalon, animals can still show desynchronized EEG in frontal cortex (Skinner, 1970). If the mesencephalon is disconnected from cortex by complete transection, desynchronized EEG patterns return after several days (Batsel, 1960; Villablanca, 1962). Such manipulations remove the noradrenergic and serotonergic projections to cortex but do not disrupt the cholinergic projection.

Cortical activation that occurs during REM sleep is also probably not contingent on the locus coeruleus or raphe because the discharge rates of neurons in these structures are strongly suppressed during REM sleep (Trulson and Jacobs, 1979; Aston-Jones and Bloom, 1981; Rasmussen et al., 1986). In contrast, neurons in the nucleus basalis that have increased firing rates during wakefulness also have increased firing rates during REM sleep (Szymusiak and McGinty, 1986, 1989). Hence, the nucleus basalis may be the primary subcortical structure involved in cortical activation during REM sleep as well as wakefulness.

Afferent Control of Nucleus Basalis Activity

If increased activity in the nucleus basalis promotes cortical activation, it then becomes important to know what triggers or maintains the increased discharge rates of basalis neurons. Considering the anatomical properties of the nucleus basalis, two main categories of inputs appear to be most likely: (1) "ascending" inputs from the brainstem and hypothalamus, and (2) "descending" inputs from the amygdaloid complex and specific regions of cerebral cortex.

Ascending inputs have been identified from the peripeduncular nucleus, parabrachial nucleus, locus coeruleus, dorsal and median raphe nuclei, ventral tegmental area, and posterior and lateral hypothalamus (Russchen et al., 1985; Irle and Markowitsch, 1986). Each of these areas could be involved in either inducing or maintaining the increased firing rates of basalis neurons, which would be consistent with the concept of a unified system of ascending cortical afferents (Saper, 1987).

Another interesting possibility is that increased firing rates of basalis neurons may be induced by cortical neurons which are themselves influenced by basalis neurons. The nucleus basalis receives a heavy input from the amygdaloid complex and the entorhinal, prepiriform, posterior orbitofrontal, anterior insular, and polar temporal cortical areas (Mesulam and Mufson, 1984; Russchen et al., 1985; Irle and Markowitsch, 1986). In turn, the nucleus basalis has heavy projections back to each of these areas (Lehmann et al., 1984; Mesulam et al., 1986). Each of these cortical areas receives highly processed sensory information since they are several synapses away from primary sensory areas. One or more of the cortical or amygdaloid regions may influence the firing rates of basalis neurons, which could then alter the activation of the entire cerebral cortex. The nucleus basalis may thereby provide a mechanism by which small regions of cortex (perhaps those regions with access to the most highly processed information) may control the general level of activation of the rest of the cortex.

Another possibility is that the firing patterns of basalis neurons may not be influenced primarily by a single set of afferents, but they may be indirectly influenced by structures whose fibers pass through the basal forebrain on their way to other target areas. Basalis neurons are usually found in or along fiber pathways (such as the anterior commissure, ansa lenticularis, and the medullary laminae), and the dendrites of basalis neurons often extend into fiber pathways (Das and Kreutzberg, 1968). It is possible that basalis neurons receive collateral inputs from passing axons and are therefore influenced by numerous structures that project through the basal forebrain.

Another mechanism by which the nucleus basalis may influence cortical activation is through the reticular nucleus of the thalamus (Re). Whereas most of the thalamic nuclei receive cholinergic innervation from the pedunculopontine and laterodorsal tegmental nuclei (Mesulam et al., 1983; Sofroniew et al., 1985), the Re receives a substantial part of its cholinergic input from the nucleus basalis (Levey et al., 1987; Parent et al., 1988). The basalis input to Re appears to be inhibitory since direct application of ACh inhibits Re neurons (McCormick and Prince, 1986; Francesconi et al., 1988). The Re is involved in the generation of thalamocortical spindles and EEG synchronization during periods of decreased arousal (Steriade, 1984). If increased firing of the cholinergic basalis neurons that project to Re produce a sustained inhibition of Re neurons, the processes that induce EEG synchronization may be inoperable, which would indirectly promote EEG desynchronization. The primary problem with this idea is that Re neurons discharge most rapidly at the same times as basalis neurons: during wakefulness and REM sleep (Mukhametov et al., 1970; Hirsch et al., 1982). Therefore, either Re neurons are not normally inhibited by ACh or they may not be strongly influenced by the relatively small projection from the nucleus basalis.

LEARNING

As suggested in the preceding section, increases in the baseline discharge rates of basalis neurons may enhance the response properties of cortical neurons during periods of cortical activation. Under certain circumstances, however, the changes in cortical neurons may persist indefinitely. Such long lasting changes may result from brief increases in firing in basalis neurons in the awake animal. We have hypothesized that the resulting long-term changes in the effective synaptic strengths among certain cortical neurons may contribute to the neuronal substrate of learning (Richardson and DeLong, 1988; Richardson et al., 1988).

Persistent Cholinergic Facilitation

As discussed earlier, the most common effect of ACh applied directly to a cortical neuron appears to be an enhancement of the neuron's responses to other afferent inputs. ACh typically has a transient effect in that the response properties of cortical neurons return to normal soon after the end of ACh application. However, ACh can also have a persistent modulatory effect lasting an hour or longer when it is applied directly to a cortical neuron that has been induced to discharge rapidly. Such long-term changes have been reported in motor (Woody et al., 1978), somatosensory (Metherate et al., 1987; Lamour et al., 1988), and visual (Sillito and Kemp, 1983) cortical areas. Increased discharge rates in cortical neurons have been produced by intracellular current injection, glutamate application, thalamic afferent stimulation, and receptive field stimulation. If the neuron is induced to fire rapidly but no ACh is applied, the persistent change in responsiveness does not occur (Woody et al., 1978). Likewise, if ACh is applied to the neuron, but the cell fires at its normal rate, there is no long-lasting change in responsiveness. Hence, persistent cholinergic facilitation has two critical requirements: (1) ACh must be applied to the neuron, and (2) the neuron must be stimulated to fire rapidly.

Although ACh can produce a persistent facilitation of the responses of cortical neurons, only 20 to 50% of cortical neurons studied thus far have shown such long-term changes after ACh application (Woody et al., 1978; Lamour et al., 1988). Also, a small percentage of neurons have a persistent decrease in responsiveness following combined ACh application and stimulation (Metherate et al., 1987). However, as with short term modulation by ACh, the most common persistent effect by far has been an enhancement of neuronal responsiveness.

There are several important aspects of persistent cholinergic facilitation that are unknown. For example, it is not clear whether the application of ACh and stimulation of the neuron must coincide, or whether they could be slightly separated in time. It is also not known whether the affected cortical neuron is more responsive to all of its inputs, or whether the facilitation is specific for a subset of connections to the neuron. Pairing ACh application with intracellular stimulation produces an increased input resistance in the neuron which would make it more responsive to all afferent inputs (Woody et al., 1978). On the other hand, ACh application paired with receptive field stimulation appears to produce a more selective enhancement that could be due to facilitation of a select subset of inputs (Metherate and Weinberger, 1989). These differing findings suggest that cholinergic facilitation occurring under experimental conditions may affect the entire neuron to make it more responsive to all inputs, whereas naturally occurring cholinergic facilitation may produce a more selective enhancement, possibly by being restricted to small sections of the dendrites.

If cholinergic facilitation does occur naturally, there must be a mechanism to increase the release of ACh onto cortical neurons at specific times. Such an increase in ACh release would presumably result from increased firing of neurons in the nucleus basalis. Basalis neurons have increased tonic discharge rates during waking and REM sleep, which, as discussed above, appears to set the general level of activity of cortical neurons. Basalis neurons also have brief, phasic changes in firing when certain stimuli are presented to the animal, and the resulting increases in ACh output may facilitate the responses of certain cortical neurons. Hence, knowing when basalis neurons increase their firing may indicate when persistent cholinergic facilitation could occur, and such information may help to identify the processes in which the nucleus basalis is involved.

Phasic Activity in Basalis Neurons During Behavior

Neuronal activity in the nucleus basalis has been studied most extensively in monkeys engaged in various behavioral tasks. The most common finding has been that basalis neurons respond to rewards and events associated with rewards (Richardson et al., 1988). Many basalis neurons respond to the delivery of a reward with a clear increase or decrease in firing, as shown in Fig. 2. In most studies, the reward has consisted of a small volume of water delivered at the end of a correctly executed trial in a behavioral task. In a series of three behavioral tasks, 41% of all sampled basalis neurons had detectable changes in firing after water delivery (Richardson et al., 1988; Richardson and DeLong, 1990a). In water-restricted monkeys that had not been trained to perform a behavioral task, approximately 50% of all basalis neurons were responsive to the delivery of water. The responses to a reward are therefore probably not a result of training but are an inherent property of basalis neurons.

In trained monkeys, approximately half of the basalis neurons responding to the water reward had increases in firing, whereas in untrained monkeys, approximately 60% had increases (Richardson and DeLong, 1990a). In both trained and untrained animals, neurons responding to water were distributed throughout the nucleus basalis. Thus, water appears to be a salient stimulus for basalis neurons in thirsty animals, and it may lead to a transient increase in ACh release throughout cortex.

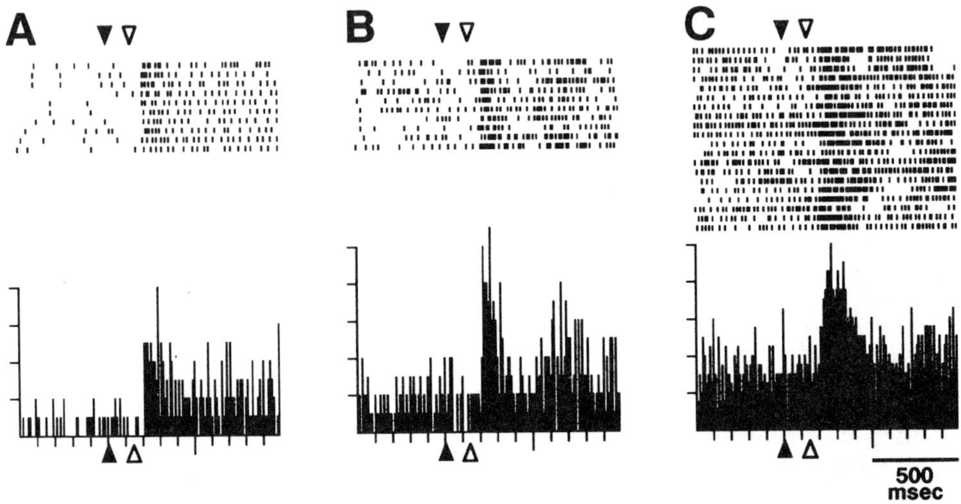

Figure 2. Responses of three basalis neurons to water delivery. Each dot in the raster represents one discharge of the neuron, and each line of dots is from a single trial. The histograms are generated by collapsing the rasters across trials into 10 msec bins. Each raster and histogram is aligned on solid triangles, representing the opening of a solenoid valve inside a sound-proof container. The open triangles represent the approximate time at which the water actually arrives at the monkey's mouth 135 msec after the valve opens. Each mark on the horizontal axis is 100 msec, and each vertical mark represents a discharge rate of 20 spikes/sec. All three basalis neurons have a sharp increase in firing, beginning at approximately 75 msec following the water arrival. In A and B, the monkey was untrained. In C, the monkey had learned that a torque to the right always preceded the water, but no torques were given on the series of trials shown here. The neuron in C is the same as in Fig. 5 A and B.

A Model of the Role of the Nucleus Basalis in Learning

Given the observation that basalis neurons generally respond to water delivery with an increase in firing, the following model is proposed for the role of the nucleus basalis in simple classical conditioning paradigms. In such paradigms, an animal learns to associate a conditioned stimulus (CS) with an unconditioned stimulus (US). The CS is typically an auditory or visual stimulus which produces no apparent change in the animal's behavior, whereas the US is an appetitive or aversive stimulus (such as water delivery or air puff, respectively) which elicits an overt behavioral response. Training the animal to associate the CS with the US comes about by consistently presenting the CS just prior to the US. Over the course of conditioning, the animal begins to show behavioral responses following the CS that are similar to the responses to the US. The development of the behavioral response to the CS indicates that an association has been made between the CS and the US.

The search for the neural substrate of a learned association has been the topic of intense research for many years. The brain regions that have been studied most extensively in this regard are the cerebral cortex, hippocampus, amygdala, and cerebellum (Thompson, 1986), the first three of which are innervated by the basal forebrain cholinergic system. Some of the current evidence for the cerebral cortex being a site of CS-US association is presented in the chapters by Gorman and Woody, and Ashe and Weinberger in this book.

Our model of the nucleus basalis role in conditioning assumes that the presentation of a stimulus activates a specific set of cortical neurons which constitutes the neural representation of that stimulus. It also assumes that some of the cortical neurons that represent the CS have weak excitatory projections to some of the cortical neurons that represent the US. These assumptions are diagrammed in Fig. 3 which shows sensory input from a CS and a US to two different sets of neurons. Before training, when there is no association between the CS and US, activation of the CS representation would have little effect on the US representation, but the process of conditioning would eventually strengthen the excitatory connections from the CS representation to the US representation. Hence, the neural basis of the learned association would be the strengthening of connections from neurons representing the CS to neurons representing the US.

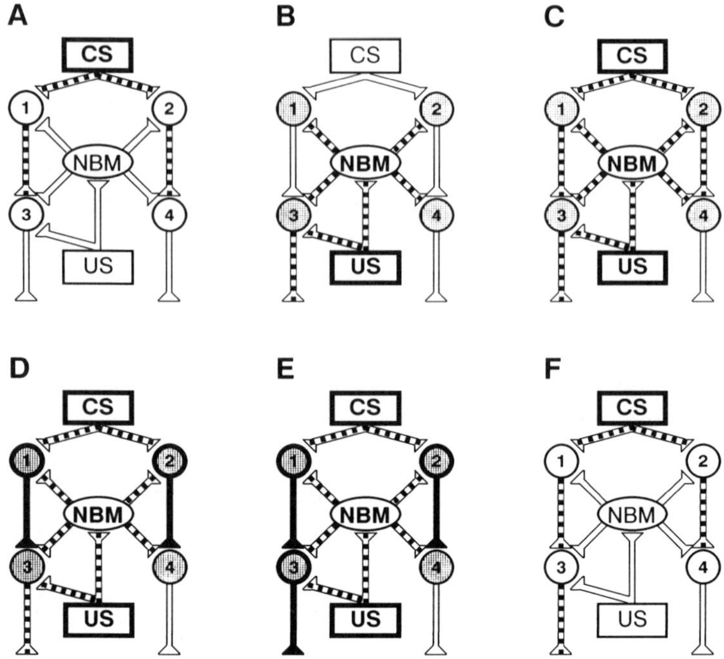

Figure 3. A model of the nucleus basalis role in classical conditioning. Neurons 1 and 2 are part of the CS representation, neuron 3 is part of the US representation, and neuron 4 is not part of either representation. Only neuron 1 in the CS representation projects to neurons in the US representation, namely neuron 3. Open axons indicate normal levels of activity; dashed axons indicate increased discharge rates; and solid axons indicate persistent cholinergic facilitation (PCF). Shaded neurons indicate increased exposure to ACh from nucleus basalis of Meynert (NBM) projections. A. CS presentation before training. Only neurons 1 and 2 have increased firing rates. B. US presentation before training. The US increases firing in neuron 3 and NBM neurons. Increased firing of NBM neurons increases the release of ACh to neurons 1 - 4. Some PCF may occur in neuron 3, which would be further increased during conditioning (see E below). C. Initial phase of training. Because the US occurs soon after the CS, neurons 1 and 2 are exposed to enhanced levels of ACh while they are firing at a higher than normal rate. D. Facilitation of CS representation. The combination of increased discharge rates and increased exposure to ACh leads to PCF in the CS representation neurons, which in turn increases the excitatory drive onto neurons 3 and 4. E. Facilitation of US representation. The increased excitatory input from neuron 1 leads to further PCF of neuron 3. Despite the increased input to neuron 4, it is not activated sufficiently to induce PCF. F. Fully conditioned. Since neurons 1, 2, and 3 (but not 4) are facilitated, the CS activates both the CS representation and part of the US representation (neuron 3). Hence, the CS is now associated with the US.

In our model, the connections between the CS and US representations would be facilitated by ACh released from nucleus basalis neurons. As described above, there appears to be a general increase in the firing of basalis neurons in response to water, an appetitive stimulus. The increase in activity in the nucleus basalis would briefly increase ACh levels throughout cortex, and cortical neurons that are activated (i.e., firing more rapidly) at the time of the increased release of ACh would develop an increased responsiveness due to persistent cholinergic facilitation. In a simple conditioning paradigm, the cortical neurons that would most likely be activated at the time of the increased ACh release would be those responding to the US and those having long duration responses to the preceding CS.

Before training, presentation of the CS alone would activate only the CS representation neurons, depicted as neurons 1 and 2 in Fig. 3A. Presentation of the US (Fig. 3B) would activate the US representation neurons and the nucleus basalis, thereby increasing the release of ACh onto all cortical neurons. The increase in ACh release would facilitate neurons responding to the US to a degree regardless of whether the US was preceded by a CS. Therefore, early in training (Fig. 3C), when the CS is initially paired with the US, no additional facilitation would be induced in neurons representing the US. Neurons representing the CS, however, would be facilitated by the increase in ACh levels, and would then have stronger responses, (i.e., more rapid firing), to subsequent presentations of the CS, as illustrated in Fig. 3D. The increased firing might produce further cholinergic facilitation of the same neurons on subsequent trials.

In this model, the facilitated neurons that respond to the CS (neurons 1 and 2 in Fig. 3) have excitatory connections to other cortical neurons, some of which represent the US (neuron 3) and some of which represent other stimuli (neuron 4). Each of these target neurons would receive an increased excitatory input from the facilitated neurons that responded to the CS, but the greatest net excitatory effect would be on those neurons that are also excited by the subsequent presentation of the US. As depicted in Fig. 3E, the neurons that are activated by both the US and the increased excitatory input from CS representation neurons would be further facilitated by the release of ACh. Neurons that only receive an enhanced input from CS representation neurons would not be activated sufficiently to be facilitated. As a result of training, the neurons facilitated the most would be (1) those that respond to the CS and (2) those that respond to the US and also receive excitatory inputs from facilitated neurons representing the CS. The net effect (Fig. 3F) is that activation of the neuronal representation of the CS is now more likely to activate neurons in the neuronal representation of the US, thus indicating that the CS has become associated with the US.

There are numerous aspects of this model that could be modified to make it more sophisticated and complex. For example, the direct connections among neurons representing the CS and US could be replaced with multisynaptic pathways. Also, rather than whole neurons becoming more responsive, restricted parts of the dendrites could develop increased excitability. Another possibility is that ACh may not act directly on a neuron to produce long-term changes in its excitability, but it may enhance the responses of a neuron enough to allow other long-term changes, such as cortical long-term potentiation (Artola and Singer, 1987; Baranyi and Szente, 1987; Iriki et al., 1989) to take place. Regardless of such modifications, the principle of the model remains unchanged in that the cholinergic system is suggested to promote learning by selectively enhancing the excitability of neurons that respond to the conditioned or unconditioned stimuli.

This model of cholinergic involvement in simple conditioning is an example of how the cholinergic system could effectively induce changes in the strengths of synaptic connections among cortical neurons. Since more complicated learning paradigms can also be interpreted as changes in synaptic efficacy among cortical neurons, the above model could easily be expanded to explain how the cholinergic system might be involved in those learning situations as well. The idea that the cholinergic system has such a fundamental role in cortical plasticity is consistent with the numerous studies that have found learning and memory deficits following lesions of the basal forebrain in rodents and primates (Collerton, 1986; Smith, 1988). Damage to the cholinergic system in Alzheimer's disease and other dementing illnesses may also contribute to the learning and memory deficits in those disorders. If the cholinergic system has such an extensive involvement in learning and memory, nucleus basalis neurons might be expected to be responsive to more than simple appetitive stimuli. Indeed, there are numerous examples of other situations in which basalis neurons show phasic changes in activity which could potentially lead to changes in synaptic connections among cortical neurons. In particular, there is evidence that basalis neurons are responsive to aversive stimuli and to conditioned stimuli that precede appetitive stimuli.

Aversive Stimuli

Neuronal activity in the nucleus basalis has been associated most often with appetitive stimuli, but there is now clear evidence that many basalis neurons also respond to aversive stimuli. Earlier studies found that basal forebrain neurons that responded selectively to the sight of food objects did not show sustained changes in firing following an air puff to the monkey's face (Rolls et al., 1976). However, over half of a sample of 39 basalis neurons had a brief change in firing in the 500 msec period following a similar air puff (Richardson and DeLong, 1990a). Over half of the basalis neurons responding to the air puff had qualitatively similar responses to the delivery of water. Similar to the responses of basalis neurons to water, a high percentage (81%) of the responses to the air puff consisted of increases in firing. Examples of basalis neurons responding to an air puff are shown in Fig. 4.

One caveat in the use of an air puff as an aversive stimulus is that it created a very loud hiss. It is possible that basalis neurons could have been responsive to the sound of the air puff rather than to its aversive quality. To test this possibility, the air puff nozzle was sometimes aimed away from the monkey's snout rather than toward it, so that the auditory component remained but the tactile component was removed. Most of the basalis neurons had responses to the sound of the air puff that were slightly reduced in magnitude compared to responses to the air puff itself, as demonstrated in Fig. 4. However, the monkey usually flinched if the air puff was directed at his snout, but he consistently blinked when it was turned away from his snout. Hence, the sound of the air puff apparently startled the animal and may have therefore been aversive by itself.

The air puff was clearly not an appetitive stimulus, yet a substantial proportion of basalis neurons had robust changes in firing in response to it. Therefore, basalis neurons do not appear to be exclusively responsive to appetitive stimuli, such as a water reward. However, a feature that aversive and appetitive stimuli have in common is that they are both arousing to the animal. Basalis neurons may, in general, be responsive to any arousing stimulus, which would explain why a large number of them responded to both the water and the air puff. Unfortunately, this interpretation cannot easily be applied to neurons that responded to only the air puff or the water but not both.

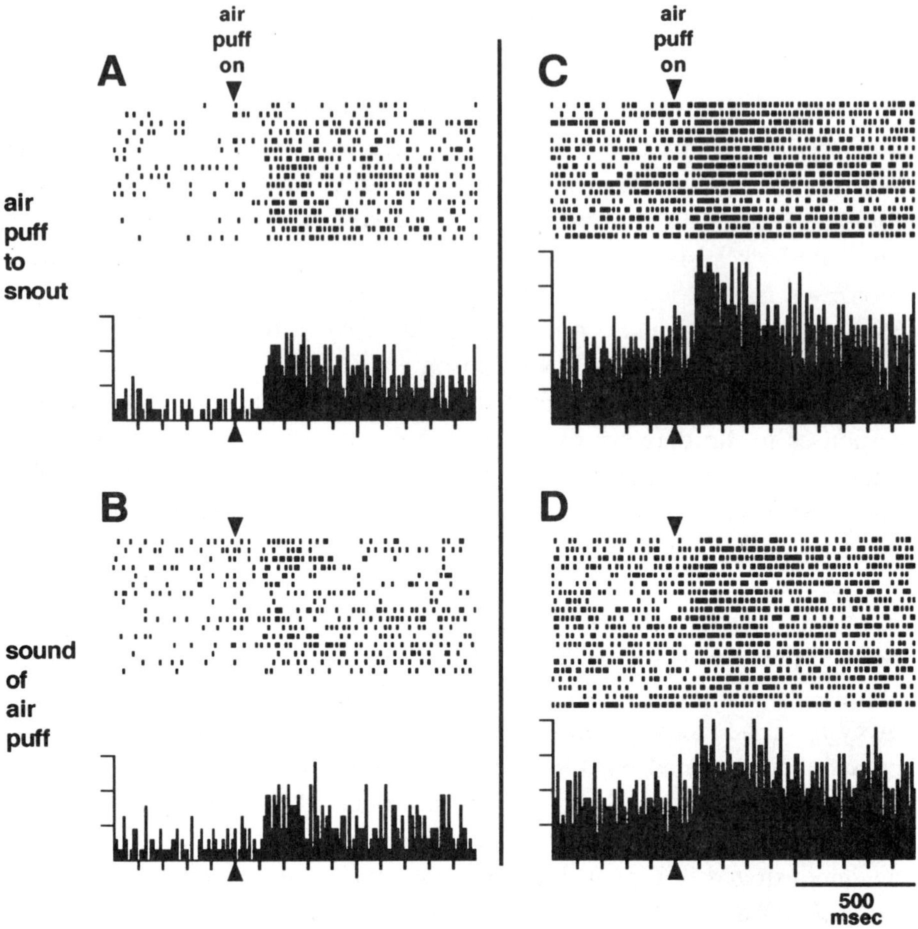

Figure 4. Responses of two basalis neurons to an air puff. Conventions are the same as in Fig. 2. In A and C, the air puff was directed at the monkey's snout, and both neurons had a brisk increase in firing at a latency of approximately 110 msec. Slightly diminished responses occurred in B and D when the air puff was directed away from the monkey. As explained in the text, the sound of the air puff may have startled the animal.

Conditioned Stimuli

Several studies have demonstrated that basalis neurons are particularly responsive to conditioned stimuli that precede rewards. Rolls and associates studied a population of neurons in the region of the nucleus basalis in monkeys that responded selectively to the sight of food or to stimuli that the animal had learned to associate with food (Rolls et al., 1976; 1979). The neuronal responses to a stimulus developed as the animal learned that the stimulus always preceded a food or juice reward (Mora et al., 1976), and diminished as the animal became satiated and rejected the food (Burton et al., 1976).

Our studies in monkeys have demonstrated that approximately 75% of all basalis neurons respond to events occurring in behavioral tasks, and up to 70% of those neurons respond in the part of the task that immediately precedes the delivery of a water reward (Richardson et al., 1988). The responses of basalis neurons are not dependent on movements made by the animal to obtain the water reward nor to specific visual stimuli per se, but they appear to reflect the meaning or significance of the stimuli (Mitchell et al., 1987; Richardson and DeLong, 1990b). In other words, basalis neurons rarely respond to a stimulus when it does not signify that a water reward is imminent, but they often respond to the same stimulus when it does signify that a reward will soon be delivered. Thus, the responses of basalis neurons to a sensory stimulus appear to be strongly influenced by the significance of the stimulus.

In an ongoing study using classical conditioning procedures, we have found that many basalis neurons respond more vigorously to a stimulus that precedes a water reward than to a similar stimulus that does not. As in the more complicated behavioral tasks used in earlier studies, approximately 75% of all basalis neurons were responsive in the conditioning task, and the vast majority responded to a brief arm perturbation that immediately preceded a water reward. More than half of the responsive neurons had substantially smaller changes in firing following an arm perturbation in the opposite direction which did not precede a water reward. Examples of basalis neurons with such differential responses are shown in Fig. 5.

Similarities in Tonic and Phasic Activity

It appears likely that the key feature of a stimulus that elicits responses in basalis neurons is its arousal value. Basalis neurons may be more responsive to a stimulus that predicts a reward because it is more arousing than a stimulus that signifies nothing of importance to the animal. They

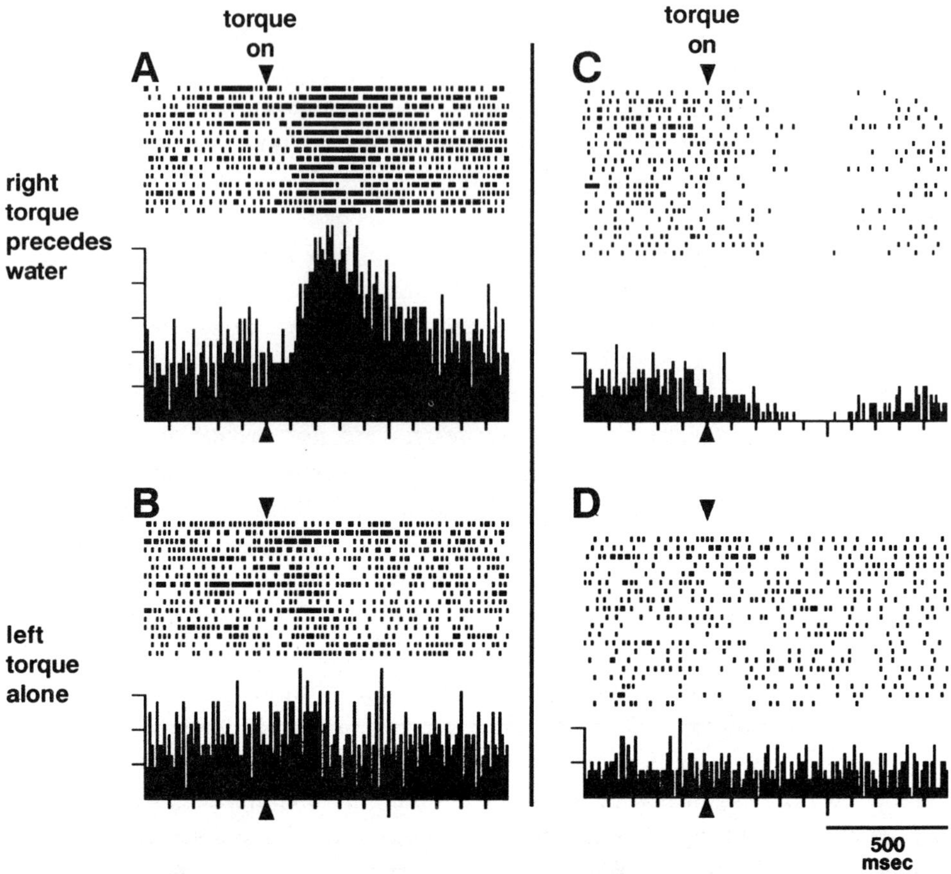

Figure 5. Differential responses of two basalis neurons to conditioned stimuli. Conventions are the same as in Fig. 2. In A and C, a brief torque that moved the monkey's arm to the right was consistently followed 1 to 1.5 sec later by a drop of water. In B and D, a torque of equal magnitude to the left did not precede water or any other unconditioned stimulus. In A and B, the basalis neuron had a strong increase in firing after the right torque, but no consistent change after the left torque. This same neuron had a similar increase in firing when water was delivered without the preceding torque, as shown in Fig. 2 C. In C and D, the basalis neuron had a sharp pause in firing after the right torque, but no change in activity after the left torque.

may also be particularly responsive to appetitive and aversive stimuli because such stimuli are arousing to the animal. Hence, phasic changes in the activity of basalis neurons may be related to arousing events, just as tonic changes in the background firing rates of basalis neurons appear to be related to the animal's state of arousal.

Different states of arousal are usually considered to persist over prolonged periods of time, certainly longer than fractions of a second. Periods of wakefulness generally last for hours, and, as mentioned above, cortical activation which accompanies wakefulness may result from increased tonic firing rates in nucleus basalis neurons. Phasic increases in the firing rates of basalis neurons may therefore be related to brief increases in cortical activation lasting only seconds. However, it is debatable whether a brief change in cortical activation would constitute a change in the animal's overall level of arousal. Cortical activation is only one component of arousal, and the other components of arousal would not necessarily be affected by basalis neurons. Therefore, to hypothesize that basalis neurons respond to "arousing" stimuli is not to imply that there is a state change in the animal, but rather that there may be a brief increase in cortical activation.

Both the tonic and phasic changes in the firing rates of basalis neurons may also be related to learning. As outlined above, phasic increases in the activity of basalis neurons may induce changes in the synaptic efficacy of cortical neurons that form the neuronal substrate of learning. The tonic discharge rates of basalis neurons may be indirectly related to learning since, according to the Yerkes-Dodson law (Broadhurst, 1959), learning is most efficient at particular levels of arousal. Cortical activation may be the specific component of arousal affecting the efficiency of learning because cortical neurons are then more excitable and more responsive. Cortical neurons may only be able to develop long-lasting physiological changes when sufficient levels of ACh are present, which would depend on the tonic discharge rates of basalis neurons.

Spatial Limits of the Basalis Influence on Cortex

Our hypotheses regarding the functional role of the nucleus basalis have not emphasized the potential specificity of the effects of single neurons or groups of neurons on subregions of cortex. As mentioned earlier, the nucleus basalis as a whole projects to widespread cortical areas, but each individual neuron projects to only a small area of cortex of approximately 1 mm^2. Moreover, there is a rough topography in the basalis projection to cortex, which would make it possible for a subregion of the nucleus basalis to selectively influence a subregion of cortex.

This unique structure gives the nucleus basalis the potential ability to control which areas of cortex undergo changes related to learning and which areas have enhanced neuronal responses, such as those that occur with increased arousal levels. It is conceivable that the enhanced responses of neurons in restricted zones of cortex may constitute the neuronal basis of selective attention. For example, increased tonic firing in only those basalis neurons that project to auditory cortical areas may enhance the animal's attention to auditory stimuli. Thus, the restricted projection areas of basalis neurons may give them the capacity to have a finer control over the changes in cortical neuronal activity related to learning, arousal, and possibly attention.

Despite the capacity of the nucleus basalis to selectively influence subregions of cortex, there has been little physiological evidence to support this idea. A selective effect would be suggested by the finding that certain areas of the nucleus basalis contain neurons that respond differently from neurons in other areas. In general, however, the neuronal responses found in one subregion of the nucleus basalis are found in all other subregions (Richardson and DeLong, 1986; 1990a,b). There appears to be an anterior to posterior gradient of increasing baseline firing rates of basalis neurons (Richardson and DeLong, 1990b), and there have been slight differences in the distribution of neurons showing certain response types (Richardson and DeLong, 1990a). Otherwise, each subregion of the nucleus basalis appears to have roughly the same proportion of cells that respond with an increase or decrease in firing in each part of a behavioral task. Given the lack of evidence for selective influences, the ideas discussed in this chapter have been based on the assumption that all cortical areas receive a similar input from the nucleus basalis. The hypotheses presented here could be modified, however, if future studies provide evidence for a more selective effect of the nucleus basalis on restricted cortical areas.

SUMMARY

The basal forebrain cholinergic system has the potential to influence a broad range of brain functions since it is the primary source of cholinergic input to the hippocampal formation, the amygdaloid complex, and all areas of cerebral cortex. Recent physiological studies have suggested how nucleus basalis neurons and ACh may be directly involved in cortical activation and learning. ACh appears to act primarily as a neuromodulator to enhance the responsiveness of cortical neurons to other inputs. This enhancement effect may be transient, lasting only a few seconds, or it may be persistent, lasting an hour or more. Transient and persistent facilitation by ACh may correspond, respectively, to tonic and phasic changes in the discharge rates of nucleus basalis neurons that project to cerebral cortex.

The tonic discharge rates of basalis neurons are generally increased when cortical EEG is desynchronized during wakefulness and REM sleep, and decreased when the EEG is synchronized during drowsiness and slow wave sleep. EEG desynchronization is indicative of cortical activation in which cortical neurons are more excitable and responsive. The altered response properties of cortical neurons are hypothesized to be due in part to changes in specific ion currents that are affected by ACh released from nucleus basalis neurons projecting to cortex. Thus, the tonic increase in discharge rates of basalis neurons during cortical activation appears to set the level of excitability and responsiveness of cortical neurons.

In addition to the tonic increases in discharge rates of basalis neurons during wakefulness, phasic changes in firing occur in response to certain stimuli. Basalis neurons are particularly responsive to events that are of significance to the animal, such as appetitive or aversive stimuli. Phasic increases in the firing of basalis neurons may produce a persistent cholinergic facilitation in cortical neurons that are stimulated by other inputs simultaneously with the enhanced release of ACh. According to our proposed model of associative conditioning, the persistent facilitation of selected cortical neurons may contribute to the neuronal substrate of learning. Thus, the role of the nucleus basalis in learning and memory may be related to its ability to induce long-term changes in the response properties of selected cortical neurons.

In conclusion, if the properties of nucleus basalis neurons are applicable to the entire BFCS, then the cholinergic system may be able to modulate the responses of neurons throughout the forebrain. Increases in the tonic discharge rates of cholinergic neurons may transiently enhance the response properties of all target neurons, and this effect may be a component of arousal. Phasic increases in firing in cholinergic neurons may induce a long-term enhancement of responses properties only in selected target neurons, and this effect may contribute to the neuronal substrate of learning.

REFERENCES

Arendt, T., Bigl, V., Tennstedt, A. and Arendt, A. (1985): Neuronal loss in different parts of the nucleus basalis is related to neuritic plaque formation in cortical target areas in Alzheimer's Disease. *Neurosci.* 14:1-14

Artola, A. and Singer, W. (1987): Long-term potentiation and NMDA receptors in rat visual cortex. *Nature* 330:649-652

Aston-Jones, G. and Bloom, F.E. (1981): Activity of norepinephrine-containing locus coeruleus neurons in behaving rats anticipates fluctuations in the sleep-waking cycle. *J. Neurosci.* 1:876-886

Baranyi, A. and Szente, M.B. (1987): Long-lasting potentiation of synaptic transmission requires postsynaptic modifications in the neocortex. *Brain Res.* 423: 378-384

Bartus, R.T., Dean III, R.L., Beer, B. and Lippa, A.S. (1982): The cholinergic hypothesis of geriatric memory dysfunction. *Science* 217:408-417

Batsel, H.L. (1960): Electroencephalographic synchronization and desynchronization in the chronic 'cerveau isole' of the dog. *Electroenceph. Clin. Neurophysiol.* 12:421-430

Benardo, L.S. and Prince, D.A. (1982): Ionic mechanisms of cholinergic excitation in mammalian hippocampal pyramidal cells. *Brain Res.* 249:333-344

Benson, D.M., Blitzer, R.D. and Landau, E.M. (1988): An analysis of the depolarization produced in guinea-pig hippocampus by cholinergic receptor stimulation. *J. Physiol.* 404:479-496

Bigl, V., Woolf, N.J. and Butcher, L.L. (1982): Cholinergic projections from the basal forebrain to frontal, parietal, temporal, occipital, and cingulate cortices: a combined fluorescent tracer and acetylcholinesterase analysis. *Brain Res. Bull.* 8:727-749

Broadhurst, P.L. (1959): The interaction of task difficulty and motivation: the Yerkes-Dodson Law revived. *Acta Psychologica* 16:321-338

Brown, D.A. (1983): Slow cholinergic excitation – a mechanism for increasing neuronal excitability. *Trends Neurosci.* 6:302-307

Burton, M.J., Rolls, E.T. and Mora, F. (1976): Effects of hunger on the responses of neurons in the lateral hypothalamus to the sight and taste of food. *Exp. Neurol.* 51:668-677

Buzsáki, G., Bickford, R.G., Ponomareff, G., Thal, L.J., Mandel, R. and Gage, F. (1988): Nucleus basalis and thalamic control of neocortical activity in the freely moving rat. *J. Neurosci.* 8:4007-4026

Casamenti, F., Deffneu, G., Abbamondi, A.L. and Pepeu, G. (1986): Changes in cortical acetylcholine output induced by modulation of the nucleus basalis. *Brain Res. Bull.* 16:689-695

Celesia, G.G. and Jasper, H.H. (1966): Acetylcholine released from cerebral cortex in relation to state of activation. *Neurol.* 16:1053-1063

Cole, A.E. and Nicoll, R.A. (1984): Characterization of a slow cholinergic post-synaptic potential recorded in vitro from rat hippocampal pyramidal cells. *J. Physiol.* 352:173-188

Collerton, D. (1986): Cholinergic function and intellectual decline in Alzheimer's disease. *Neurosci.* 19:1-28

Coyle, J.T., Price, D.L. and DeLong, M.R. (1983): Alzheimer's Disease: a disorder of cortical cholinergic innervation. *Science* 219:1184-1190

Das, G.D. and Kreutzberg, G.W. (1968): Evaluation of interstitial nerve cells in the central nervous system: a correlative study using acetylcholinesterase and Golgi techniques. *Ergeb. Anat. Entwickl. Gesch.* 41:1-58

Davies, P. and Maloney, A.J.F. (1976): Selective loss of central cholinergic neurons in Alzheimer's Disease. *Lancet* 2:1403

DeLong, M.R. (1971): Activity of pallidal neurons during movement. *J. Neurophysiol.* 34:414-427

Detarí, L. and Vanderwolf, C.H. (1987): Activity of identified cortically projecting and other basal forebrain neurones during large slow waves and cortical activation in anaesthetized rats. *Brain Res.* 437:1-8

Divac, I. (1975): Magnocellular nuclei of the basal forebrain project to neocortex, brain stem, and olfactory bulb. Review of some functional correlates. *Brain Res.* 93:385-398

Elias, H. and Schwartz, D. (1969): Surface areas of cerebral cortex of mammals determined by stereological methods. *Science* 166:111-113

Francesconi, W., Muller, C.M. and Singer, W. (1988): Cholinergic mechanisms in the reticular control of transmission in the cat lateral geniculate nucleus. *J. Neurophysiol.* 59:1690-1718

Halliwell, J.V. and Adams, P.R. (1982): Voltage-clamp analysis of muscarinic excitation in hippocampal neurons. *Brain Res.* 250:71-92

Hirsch, J.C., Fourment, A. and Marc, M.E. (1982): Electrophysiological study of the perigeniculate region during natural sleep in the cat. *Exp. Neurol.* 77:436-454

Iriki, A., Pavlides, C., Keller, A. and Asanuma, H. (1989): Long-term potentiation in the motor cortex. *Science* 245:1385-1387

Irle, E. and Markowitsch, H.J. (1986): Afferent connections of the substantia innominata/basal nucleus of Meynert in carnivores and primates. *J. Hirnforsch.* 27:343-367

Johnston, M.V., McKinney, M. and Coyle, J.T. (1981): Neocortical cholinergic innervation: a description of extrinsic and intrinsic components in the rat. *Exp. Brain Res.* 43:159-172

Jordan, L.M. and Phillis, J.W. (1972): Acetylcholine inhibition in the intact and chronically isolated cerebral cortex. *Br. J. Pharmacol.* 45:584-595

Kievit, J. and Kuypers, H.G.J.M. (1975): Basal forebrain and hypothalmic connections to the frontal and parietal cortex in the rhesus monkey. *Science* 187:600-662

Koliatsos, V.E., Martin, L.J., Walker, L.C., Richardson, R.T., DeLong, M.R. and Price, D.L. (1988): Topographic, non-collateralized basal forebrain projections to amygdala, hippocampus, and anterior cingulate cortex in the rhesus monkey. *Brain Res.* 463:133-139

Krnjević, K. and Phillis, J.W. (1963): Acetylcholine-sensitive cells in the cerebral cortex. *J. Physiol.* 166:296-327

Krnjević, K., Pumain, R. and Renaud, L. (1971): The mechanism of excitation by acetylcholine in the cerebral cortex. *J. Physiol.* 215:247-268

Kurosawa, M., Sato, A. and Sato, Y. (1989): Stimulation of the nucleus basalis of Meynert increases acetylcholine release in the cerebral cortex in rats. *Neurosci. Lett.* 98:45-50

Lamour, Y., Dutar, P., Rascol, O. and Jobert, A. (1986): Basal forebrain neurons projecting to the rat frontoparietal cortex: electrophysiological and pharmacological properties. *Brain Res.* 362:122-131

Lamour, Y., Dutar, P., Jobert, A. and Dykes, R.W. (1988): An iontophoretic study of single somatosensory neurons in rat granular cortex serving the limbs: a laminar analysis of glutamate and acetylcholine effects on receptive-field properties. *J. Neurophysiol.* 60:725-750

Lehmann, J., Nagy, J.I., Armadja, S. and Fibiger, H.C. (1980): The nucleus basalis magnocellularis: the origin of a cholinergic projection to the neocortex of the rat. *Neurosci.* 5:1161-1174

Lehmann, J., Struble, R.G., Antuono, P.G., Coyle, J.T., Cork, L.C. and Price, D.L. (1984): Regional heterogeneity of choline acetyltransferase activity in primate neocortex. *Brain Res.* 322:361-364

Levey, A.I., Hallanger, A.E. and Wainer, B.H. (1987): Cholinergic nucleus basalis neurons may influence the cortex via the thalamus. *Neurosci. Lett.* 74:7-13

Livingstone, M.S. and Hubel, D.H. (1981): Effects of sleep and arousal on the processing of visual information in the cat. *Nature* 291:554-561

LoConte, G., Casamenti, F., Bigl, V., Milaneschi, E. and Pepeu, G. (1982): Effect of magnocellular forebrain nuclei lesions on acetycholine output from the cerebral cortex, electrocorticogram and behaviour. *Arch. Ital. Biol.* 120:176-188

Longo, V.G. (1955): Effects of scopolamine and atropine on electroencephalographic and behavioral reactions due to hypothalamic stimulation. *J. Pharmacol.* 116:198-208

Luiten, P.G.M., Gaykema, R.P.A., Traber, J. and Spencer Jr, D.G. (1987): Cortical projection patterns of magnocellular basal nucleus subdivisions as revealed by anterogradely transported phaseolus vulgaris leucoagglutin. *Brain Res.* 413:229-250

Madison, D.V., Lancaster, B. and Nicoll, R.A. (1987): Voltage clamp analysis of cholinergic action in the hippocampus. *J. Neurosci.* 7:733-741

McCormick, D.A. and Prince, D.A. (1985): Mechanisms of action of acetylcholine in the guinea-pig cerebral cortex *in vitro*. *J. Physiol.* 169-194

McCormick, D.A. and Prince, D.A. (1986): Acetylcholine induces burst firing in thalamic reticular neurons by activating a potassium conductance. *Nature* 319:402-405

McKenna, T.M., Ashe, J.H., Hui, G.K. and Weinberger, N.M. (1988): Muscarinic agents modulate spontaneous and evoked unit discharge in auditory cortex of cat. *Synapse* 2:54-68

Mesulam, M.-M., Mufson, E.J., Levey, A.I. and Wainer, B.H. (1983): Cholinergic innervation of cortex by the basal forebrain: cytochemistry and cortical connections of the septal area, diagonal band nuclei, nucleus basalis (substantia innominata), and hypothalamus in the rhesus monkey. *J. Comp. Neurol.* 214:170-197

Mesulam, M.-M., Mufson, E.J., Wainer, B.H. and Levey, A.I. (1983): Central cholinergic pathways in the rat: an overview based on an alternative nomenclature (Ch1-Ch6). *Neurosci.* 10:1185-1201

Mesulam, M.-M. and Mufson, E.J. (1984): Neural inputs into the nucleus basalis of the substantia innominata (Ch4) in the rhesus monkey. *Brain* 107:253-274

Mesulam, M.-M., Volicer, L., Marquis, J.K., Mufson, E.J. and Green, R.C. (1986): Systematic regional differences in the cholinergic innervation of the primate cerebral cortex: distribution of enzyme activities and some behavioral implications. *Ann. Neurol.* 19:144-151

Metherate, R., Tremblay, N. and Dykes, R.W. (1987): Acetylcholine permits long-term enhancement of neuronal responsiveness in cat primary somatosensory cortex. *Neurosci.* 22:75-81

Metherate, R. and Weinberger, N.M. (1989): Acetylcholine produces stimulus-specific receptive field alterations in cat auditory cortex. *Brain Res.* 480:372-377

Mitchell, S.J., Richardson, R.T., Baker, F.H. and DeLong, M.R. (1987): The primate nucleus basalis of Meynert: neuronal activity related to a visuomotor tracking task. *Exp. Brain Res.* 68:506-515

Mora, F., Rolls, E.T. and Burton, M.J. (1976): Modulation during learning of the responses of neurons in the lateral hypothalamus to the sight of food. *Exp. Neurol.* 53:508-519

Mukhametov, L.M., Rizzolatti, G. and Tratardi, V. (1970): Spontaneous activity of neurons of nucleus reticularis thalami in freely moving cats. *J. Physiol.* 210:651-667

Parent, A., Gravel, S. and Boucher, R. (1981): The origin of forebrain afferents to the habenula in rat, cat and monkey. *Brain Res. Bull.* 6:23-38

Parent, A., Pare, D., Smith, Y. and Steriade, M. (1988): Basal forebrain cholingeric and noncholinergic projections to the thalamus and brainstem in cats and monkeys. *J. Comp. Neurol.* 277:281-301

Pepeu, G. (1974): The release of acetylcholine from the brain: an approach to the study of the central cholinergic mechanisms. *Prog. Neurobiol.* 2:257-288

Perry, E., Perry, R., Blessed, G. and Tomlinson, B. (1977): Necropsy evidence of central cholinergic deficits in senile dementia. *Lancet* 1:189

Price, J.L. and Stern, R. (1983): Individual cells in the nucleus basalis-diagonal band complex have restricted axonal projections to the cerebral cortex in the rat. *Brain Res.* 269:352-356

Rasmussen, K., Morilak, D.A. and Jacobs, B.L. (1986): Single unit activity of locus coeruleus neurons in the freely moving cat. I. During naturalistic behaviors and in response to simple and complex stimuli. *Brain Res.* 371:324-334

Richardson, R.T. and DeLong, M.R. (1986): Nucleus basalis of Meynert neuronal activity during a delayed response task in monkey. *Brain Res.* 399:364-368

Richardson, R.T. and DeLong, M.R. (1987): Tonically active nucleus basalis neurons in the awake monkey project to cerebral cortex. *Soc. Neurosci. Abstr.* 13:1027

Richardson, R.T. and DeLong, M.R. (1988): A reappraisal of the functions of the nucleus basalis of Meynert. *Trends Neurosci.* 11:264-267

Richardson, R.T. and DeLong, M.R. (1990a): Responses of primate nucleus basalis neurons to water rewards and related stimuli. In: *Brain Cholinergic Systems.* Steriade, M., and Biesold, D., eds. Oxford: Oxford University Press, in press

Richardson, R.T. and DeLong, M.R. (1990b): Context dependent responses of primate nucleus basalis neurons in a go/no-go task. J *Neurosci.*, in press

Richardson, R.T., Mitchell, S.J., Baker, F.H. and DeLong, M.R. (1988): Responses of nucleus basalis of Meynert neurons in behaving monkeys. In: *Cellular mechanisms of conditioning and behavioral plasticity.* Woody, C.D., Alkon, D.L., and McGaugh, J.L., eds. New York: Plenum Publishing Corp, pp. 161-173

Rolls, E.T., Burton, M.J. and Mora, F. (1976): Hypothalamic neuronal responses associated with the sight of food. *Brain Res.* 111:53-66

Rolls, E.T., Sanghera, M.K. and Roper-Hall, A. (1979): The latency of activation of neurons in the lateral hypothalamus and substantia innominata during feeding in the monkey. *Brain Res.* 164:121-135

Russchen, F.T., Amaral, D.G. and Price, J.L. (1985): The afferent connections of the substantia innominata in the monkey, Macaca fascicularis. *J. Comp. Neurol.* 242:1-27

Rye, D.B., Wainer, B.H., Mesulam, M.M., Mufson, E.J. and Saper, C.B. (1984): Cortical projections arising from the basal forebrain: a study of cholinergic and noncholinergic components employing combined retrograde tracing and immunohistochemical localization of choline acetyltransferase. *Neurosci.* 13:627-643

Saper, C.B. (1987): Diffuse cortical projection systems: anatomical organization and role in cortical function. In: *Handbook of Physiology. The Nervous System. Higher Functions of the Brain.* Mountcastle, V.B., and Plum, F., eds. Bethesda: American Physiological Society, pp. 169-209

Sato, H., Hata, Y., Masui, H. and Tsumoto, T. (1987a): A functional role of cholinergic innervation to neurons in the cat visual cortex. *J. Neurophysiol.* 58:765-780

Sato, H., Hata, Y., Hagihara, K. and Tsumoto, T. (1987b): Effects of cholinergic depletion on neuron activities in the cat visual cortex. *J. Neurophysiol.* 58:781-794

Sillito, A.M. and Kemp, J.A. (1983): Cholinergic modulation of the functional organization of the cat visual cortex. *Brain Res.* 289:143-155

Singer, W., Tretter, F. and Cynader, M. (1976): The effect of reticular stimulation on spontaneous and evoked activity in the cat visual cortex. *Brain Res.* 102:71-90

Skinner, J.E. (1970): Electrocortical desynchronization during functional blockade of the mesencephalic reticular formation. *Brain Res.* 22:254-258

Smith, G. (1988): Animal models of Alzheimer's disease: experimental cholinergic denervation. *Brain Res. Rev.* 13:103-116

Sofroniew, M.V., Priestley, J.V., Consolazione, A., Eckenstein, F. and Cuello, A.C. (1985): Cholinergic projections from the midbrain and pons to the thalamus in the rat, identified by combined retrograde tracing and choline acetyltransferase immunohistochemistry. *Brain Res.* 329:213-223

Spillane, J.A., White, P., Goodhardt, M.J., Flack, R.H.A., Bowen, D.M. and Davison, A.N. (1977): Selective vulnerability of neurons in organic dementia. *Nature* 266:558-559

Steriade, M.(1984): The excitatory-inhibitory response sequence in thalamic and neocortical cells: state-related changes and regulatory systems. In: *Dynamic Aspects of Neocortical Function.* Edelman, G.M., Gall, W.E., and Cowan, W.M,. eds. New York: John Wiley & Sons, pp. 107-157

Stewart, D.J., Macfabe, D.F. and Vanderwolf, C.H. (1984): Cholinergic activation of the electrocorticogram: role of the substantia innominata and effects of atropine and quinuclidinyl benzilate. *Brain Res.* 322:219-232

Struble, R.G., Lehmann, J.L., Mitchell, S.J., McKinney, M., Price, D.L., Coyle, J.T. and DeLong, M.R. (1986): Basal forebrain neurons provide major cholinergic innervation of primate neocortex. *Neurosci. Lett.* 66:215-220

Szymusiak, R. and McGinty, D. (1986): Sleep-related neuronal discharge in the basal forebrain of cats. *Brain Res.* 370:82-92

Szymusiak, R. and McGinty, D. (1989): Sleep-waking discharge of basal forebrain projection neurons in cats. *Brain Res. Bull.* 22:423-430

Thompson, R.F. (1986): The neurobiology of learning and memory. *Science* 233: 941-947

Trulson, M.E. and Jacobs, B.L. (1979): Raphe unit activity in freely moving cats: correlation with level of behavioral arousal. *Brain Res.* 16:135-150

Vanderwolf, C.H. (1975): Neocortical and hippocampal activation in relation to behavior: effects of atropine, eserine, phenothiazines, and amphetamine. *J. Comp. Physiol.* 88:300-323

Villablanca, J. (1962): Electroencephalogram in the permanently isolated forebrain of the cat. *Science* 138:44-46

Walker, L., Kitt, C.A., DeLong, M.R. and Price, D.L. (1985): Noncollateral projections of basal forebrain neurons to frontal and parietal neocortex in primates. *Brain Res. Bull.* 15:307-314

Walker, L.C., Koliatsos, V.E., Kitt, C.A., Richardson, R.T., Rokaeus, A. and Price, D.L. (1989a): Peptidergic neurons in the basal forebrain magnocellular complex of the rhesus monkey. *J. Comp. Neurol.* 280:272-282

Walker, L.C., Price, D.L. and Young, W.S. (1989b): Gabaergic neurons in the primate basal forebrain magnocellular complex. *Brain Res.* 499:188-192

Wenk, H., Bigl, V. and Meyer, U. (1980): Cholinergic projections from magnocellular nuclei of the basal forebrain to cortical areas in rats. *Brain Res. Rev.* 2:295-316

Whitehouse, P.J., Price, D.L., Struble, R.G., Clark, A.W., Coyle, J.T. and DeLong, M.R. (1982): Alzheimer's disease and senile dementia: loss of neurons in the basal forebrain. *Science* 215:1237-1239

Woody, C.D., Swartz, B.E. and Gruen, E. (1978): Effects of acetylcholine and cyclic GMP on input resistance of cortical neurons in awake cats. *Brain Res.* 158:373-395

Actions of Acetylcholine on Cortical Neurons: Pieces in the Puzzle About Mechanisms Underlying Learning

Linda K. Gorman and Charles D. Woody

INTRODUCTION

Evidence from earlier investigations suggests that acetylcholine (ACh) plays a significant role in cortical mechanisms underlying learning, but understanding this role is much like solving a jigsaw puzzle. Many pieces are visible; the challenge is to solve their relationships. There is also the possibility that one or two key pieces are missing.

This chapter will focus on pieces of the puzzle concerning ACh, and will also consider relevant pieces concerning glutamate (Glut) including its contribution to long term potentiation (LTP) and the acceleration of conditioning.

IMPLICATIONS OF ACh IN LEARNING

The earliest evidence for a role for the central cholinergic system in learning and memory processes arose from the use of anticholinergic drugs such as atropine and scopolamine. Clinically, the effects of scopolamine are well known (Weiner, 1980). Scopolamine, used in conjunction with morphine, produces a condition of amnesia and partial analgesia known as "twilight sleep." Scopolamine apparently causes the impairment of recollection for events occurring while the drug is effective.

Studies using various anticholinergic drugs have found deficits in most aspects of learning and memory processes tested, including impairment of performance of a broad variety of behavioral tasks and interference with the acquisition of conditioned behavior (Deutsch, 1971; Woody, 1982b; Collerton, 1986). Because of the widespread effects of these drugs, it is difficult to separate primary deficits from secondary or indirectly-produced deficits. Thus, although a number of different theories have been proposed (Deutsch, 1971; Drachman and Leavitt, 1974; Divac, 1975; Bartus et al., 1985; Dunnet, 1985; Hepler et al., 1985), the precise role of the central cholinergic system in learning and memory remains unclear.

Anticholinergic drugs, such as scopolamine or atropine, lead to a decrease in the ACh content of the brain (Campbell et al., 1970; Cooper et al., 1986). This reduction seems to be confined largely to the cerebral cortex. It has been shown, however, that these antimuscarinic agents can also produce a releasing effect of ACh, and an increase in ACh turnover with scopolamine has also been reported (Csaky, 1979). Although the exact mechanism by which these agents lower ACh content or stimulate release is not known, it has been suggested that the decreased ACh content may be a reflection of blocked presynaptic muscarinic receptors. If these receptors are blocked, the cells may not accurately sense the amount of ACh in the synapse. This could cause an alteration in the synthesis and release of ACh.

While muscarinic receptors (m_1 and m_2) have been shown to be moderately decreased in diseases affecting mnemonic processes, nicotinic receptors are also decreased (Perry et al.,1986), and the role that those receptors play in learning and memory processes is unknown.

Cholinergic *agonist* drugs sometimes facilitate performance of learned behavior, but can also impair performance or have no effect. Since cholinergic neurons innervate most of the brain in discrete pathways, each may have a different function. Stimulating the entire system by systemic administration of a cholinergic drug would be unlikely to produce specific changes in a single function. Acetylcholinesterase (AChE) inhibitors such as physostigmine, the most commonly used cholinergic agonist, inactivate acetylcholinesterase and slow down the destruction of ACh. These drugs thus tend to elevate total brain levels of ACh (Campbell et al., 1970). The difficulty in getting cholinergic agonists to act on the nervous system at the precise time necessary to affect performance of a previously learned behavioral task may explain some of the variability observed when using these pharmacologic agents, as may ancillary effects of some agonists on nicotinic receptors and other peripheral or systemic actions of many agonists beyond their primary actions within the CNS.

There are thus several confounding factors to consider when using drugs to dissect the role of the cholinergic system in memory and cognition. Davies (1985) also points to the regional distribution of drugs in the brain, regional variations in receptor concentrations and/or the affinity for the drug, and regional variations in the baseline activity of the system. The administrative route as well as dosage have consequences that also need to be considered.

Secondary effects of cholinergic and anticholinergic drugs can easily interfere with the assessment of learned behavior. It is well known that scopolamine suppresses arousal (Woody, 1982b) and causes drying of the mouth, motor incoordination, nausea, drowsiness, and dilation of the pupils, which may lead to a loss of accommodation and blurred vision (Martindale, 1982). These effects could themselves lead to performance deficits. Cholinergic drugs cause salivation, constriction of the pupils and hyperarousal (Martindale, 1982). The facilitation of performance of behavioral tasks by cholinergic agonists could, therefore, be secondary to arousal.

A final problem, elucidated by Collerton (1986), is the potential hindrance in defining the behavioral role of cholinergic function in terms of statistical power, the measure of probability that a given test will detect a given change in a parameter at a given level of statistical significance. The assessment of the effects of cholinergic drugs with tasks of different sensitivities is bound to produce apparent differential deficits regardless of the actual changes being produced in behavior.

ACh, THE FRONTAL CORTEX, AND MEMORY

The deficits produced by muscarinic cholinergic blocking agents resemble those of frontal cortical destruction. Deficits produced by frontal cortical destruction include forgetfulness, absent-mindedness, perseveration, inattention, defects in recent and long term memory, impaired associative power, and loss of recently acquired habits (Woody, 1982b).

Destruction of the frontal cortex has long been known to result in the impairment of learned behavior and memory loss associated with senility and Alzheimer's disease. Both Alzheimer's disease and senility have been linked to neocortical cell loss and degeneration with accompanying placques, neurofibrillary tangles and, more recently, reduction of choline acetyltransferase (ChAT) immunohistochemically.

Anatomical evidence suggests that both frontal cortex and hippocampus receive cholinergic input from the same region of the basal forebrain system, the vertical limb of the diagonal band (Divac, 1981). The prefrontal cortex may be the only neocortical area that receives projections from the portion of the magnocellular basal forebrain that also goes to the entorhinal cortex and the hippocampus.

Destruction of the hippocampus has also been linked to learning and memory deficits. Careful examination of symptomatology associated with hippocampal lesions suggests an effect such as might be seen with destruction of a retrieval system, as opposed to the primary system for induction of the physical changes supporting learning directly (Woody, 1982b). This is not surprising if one thinks of learning as a cellular process involving changes in conductance across nerve membranes and if one notes the vastly greater volume of brain tissue comprised of neocortex than archicortex in most mammals.

BASAL FOREBRAIN CHOLINERGIC SYSTEMS TO CORTEX

One might thus ask: what neurons and synaptic boutons supply cholinergic projections to the cortex and what areas of cortex receive these projections? In 1963, Hebb et al. used cortical undercutting and an assay for ChAT, the enzyme that synthesizes ACh, to determine that subcortical cholinergic neurons projected to the cortex. Horseradish peroxidase (HRP) studies by Divac (1975) and also by Kievit and Kuypers (1975) described magnocellular nuclei in the basal forebrain that projected to cortex. According to Lehmann et al. (1980) this projection was first described by Kodama in 1929. Krnjević and Phillis (1963) found cells excited by iontophoretically applied ACh in most areas of the cerebral cortex, and especially cells near the primary sensory areas.

The likelihood that cortical cholinergic transmission plays an integral role in learning, memory and higher cognitive function has led to more detailed anatomical studies of the cholinergic projections from the magnocellular neurons of the basal forebrain. Using radiofrequency lesions and histochemistry for the degradative enzyme, acetylcholinesterase (AChE), Shute and Lewis (1967; cf. Lewis and Shute 1967) have described an *ascending cholinergic reticular system* and a *cholinergic limbic system.*

The *ascending cholinergic reticular system* has two components, a dorsal tegmental pathway and a ventral tegmental pathway. These components were originally thought to mediate electrocortical arousal via corticopetal radiations. Later, the ventral tegmental pathway was found to be dopaminergic. The *cholinergic limbic system* had two groups of cells, one which projected to the hippocampus, and one which received input from the hippocampus and projected to the medial cortex, cerebellum and ascending cholinergic reticular system. Altogether this central cholinergic system was thought to play a role in learning and memory processes and to support arousal and attentional processes.

As methodologies became more precise and the mapping of the central cholinergic system continued, McGeer et al. (1971) measured AChE and ChAT activity in the neostriatum. Hoover et al. (1978) used micropunches of discrete brain areas and a radioenzymatic assay to map ACh content in the brains of rats. In 1979, Johnston et al., using kainate acid and electrocoagulation lesions, found direct projections of the basal forebrain, medial globus pallidus and substantia innominata to frontal and parietal cortex.

Further advances brought the advent of immunohistochemical procedures for identifying neurons containing ChAT. Because AChE has been localized in other transmitter systems (Lewis and Schon, 1975; Lehmann and Fibiger, 1978), ChAT is thought to be the more definitive marker for cholinergic neurons. A ChAT antibody was used by McGeer et al. (1974) to identify cholinergic neurons in the cerebral cortex of the rat, but the possibility was raised that the antibody might not be completely specific (Rossier, 1981). Since then, numerous investigators (Kimura et al., 1980; Wenk et al., 1980; Armstrong et al., 1983; Eckenstein and Sofroniew, 1983; Eckenstein and Thoenen, 1983; Houser et al., 1983; Levey et al., 1983; Mesulam et al., 1983a,b; Saper, 1984) have used ChAT immunohistochemical techniques to map the cholinergic neurons and their projections.

A useful nomenclature, across species, of the basal forebrain system comes from Mesulam et al. (1983b). He describes four nuclei or regions with neurons that project to the cortex. Ch1 corresponds to the medial septal nucleus. In primate, 10% of these neurons are cholinergic neurons, and in rat 30-50% are cholinergic. Ch2 corresponds to the vertical nucleus of the diagonal band. Over 50% of these neurons in both rat and primate are cholinergic. This region also includes neurons in areas previously called "vertical limb" and "pars angularis of the diagonal band." Ch1 and Ch2 project principally to the hippocampus and hypothalamus. Ch3 corresponds to the horizontal nucleus of the diagonal band and projects to the olfactory bulb. Most of these neurons are cholinergic. This area also includes the "preoptic magnocellularis nucleus" which bridges the gap between the horizontal limb and the nucleus basalis. Ch4 corresponds to the nucleus basalis (nucleus basalis of Meynert in primate). The majority of these neurons, 90%, are cholinergic. This area also includes the "substantia innominata," which forms a ventral band to the anterior commissure, the "entopeduncular nucleus" and cells in the globus pallidus. Neurons in this area project to the entire cortex and the amygdala. Ch4 can also be divided into four subdivisions based on the target of the projections even though the connection patterns may overlap. Cells in the anteromedial region project to the medial aspect of the cerebral hemispheres. The anterolateral neurons are the major source of cholinergic projections to the frontoparietal opercular area and amygdala. The intermediate cholinergic neurons send input to the dorsal prefrontal, insular, posterior parietal, inferotemporal and peristriatal areas. The posterior division projects to the superior temporal cortex and adjacent areas. This topographic orientation of the projections of the nucleus basalis Ch4 was first described by Divac (1975) and has since been studied by numerous investigators.

The brainstem cholinergic system, described by Mesulam et al. (1983b) as the pontomesencephalic reticular formation, is denoted as Ch5 and Ch6. These areas include cells in the pedunculopontine nucleus, nucleus cuneiformis, the parabrachial nucleus and the caudal end of the substantia nigra Ch5, as well as neurons in the periventricular gray Ch6. There is a minor projection to the telencephalic structures, including cortex, from this system.

EFFECTS OF LESIONS OF THE BASAL FOREBRAIN

Several questions remain despite this extensive research to map out the basal forebrain cholinergic system. Perhaps the most puzzling is how to explain the existence of cortical ChAT activity following extensive lesions of the basal forebrain (Lehmann et al., 1980). (A decrease of 80% of AChE activity was also found by Wenk et al. (1980) after lesioning the basal forebrain.) The existence of cholinergic markers in the cortex following lesions has been explained in many ways: by incomplete lesions, by the existence of other subcortical neurons projecting to the cortex (Mesulam and Mufson, 1980; Wenk et al., 1980), and by cortical innervation originating in the peripheral parasympathetic ganglia which enters the cortex via its pial surface (Fibiger, 1982). A more controversial explanation is the postulated existence of cholinergic neurons in the cortex. Studies by Green et al. (1970) and Hebb et al. (1963) indicate that 30% of the ChAT activity remains following cortical undercutting. Intrinsic cortical cholinergic neurons would explain this and would also explain the release of ACh found by Phillis (1968) following thalamic stimulation. Johnston et al. (1981) made kainate lesions in the dorsolateral parietal cortex and found a 29% reduction of ChAT activity. He reported that 70% of the cortical cholinergic innervation came from "pallidal perikarya" and that the remaining 30% came from a minor, but significant, intrinsically organized cortical system. These neurons were found in all layers of the prefrontal and parietal cortex and appeared to be small fusiform cells with vertical orientation (Eckenstein and Thoenen, 1983). Eckenstein and Thoenen (1983) specifically described fusiform cells of approximately 10 μM size in layers II-VI, with a slight enrichment in layer II.

Kimura et al. (1981) provided evidence against the existence of cortical cholinergic neurons in the cat using PAP and improved fixation techniques to differentiate ChAT positive cells.

Some cholinergic neurons stain only lightly, which might explain why they could have been missed in early studies (Kimura et al., 1981; Armstrong et al., 1983; Eckenstein and Sofroniew, 1983; Saper, 1984). Fusiform, cholinergic, cortical cells were also found by Houser et al. (1983, 1985) using a sensitive double-bridge labeling technique. Mesulam et al. (1984) suggested that there might be major species differences in the distribution of cortical cholinergic cells. Using similar techniques he found cortical cholinergic cells in the rat, but could find only moderately to lightly AChE-reactive cells in layer VI of the macaque.

There is somewhat greater agreement as to where the basal forebrain cholinergic fibers terminate. Houser et al. (1983) found that all layers have cholinergic fibers, which create a meshwork. The horizontally arranged fibers are in layers I and VI, while the vertically arranged fibers are in layers II-V. Saper (1984) and Kristt et al. (1985) found the highest concentration of fibers in layer V and the deepest part of layer VI. Layers I and III were found to have moderate densities of terminations.

There is also considerable agreement that while the neurons in the basal forebrain have widespread projections, the projections of individual cells are limited to restricted areas of cortex not more than 1 to 1.5 mm in diameter (Price and Stern, 1983).

ROLES OF ACh AND GLUT IN INDUCTION OF CONDITIONING AND LTP

A number of experimental models have been used to study the roles of ACh and Glut in learning more directly. Of these models, the most widely used are conditioning and LTP. LTP has been defined as a rapidly produced form of neuronal potentiation that lasts for more than 10 min after its induction (Brown et al. 1988). This type of potentiation is characterized by an enhancement of the efficacy of synaptic transmission which depends on postsynaptic factors, such as the presence of increased concentrations of Ca^{++}, for its induction.

ACh and the Chemical Induction of LTP

Acetylcholine itself can be used to induce a long lasting potentiation of neural excitability. Because it has several characteristics resembling those described above, it may be viewed as a chemically induced form of LTP (LTP_c).

When applied extracellularly to cortical neurons, ACh alone produces an increase in discharge and a transient increase in input resistance (Krnjević et al., 1971; Woody et al., 1976). The effects of ACh applied in this manner last for less than five minutes (Woody et al., 1976; Woody et al., 1978), and are prevented by extracellular application of atropine (Swartz and Woody, 1979).

If, however, while applying ACh extracellularly, one injects sufficient depolarizing current intracellularly to discharge the cell repeatedly, a long-lasting increase in input resistance and potentiation of neural excitability are observed. This enduring potentiation defines the basis of this type of LTP_c. Interestingly, with LTP_c of this type, there is no associated persistent increase in spontaneous firing.

Because of the need for depolarization-induced discharge to induce persistent potentiation, one may assume that increased intracellular concentrations of Ca^{++} are necessary for the induction of LTP_c as well as for LTP. Depolarization can promote Ca^{++} entry into the cell by a number of different mechanisms, as discussed further below. Ca^{++} , in turn, appears necessary for many molecular actions needed to induce and maintain persistent changes in channel proteins within nerve membranes. These requirements for Ca^{++} are not, however, confined to LTP or to LTP_c. Katz and Miledi (1968) showed years ago that calcium was needed for synaptic potentiation at the neuromuscular junction. Moreover, a direct demonstration of the need for calcium entry for the production of one form of associative conditioning was provided by Connor and Alkon (1984) in the type B photoreceptor of *Hermissenda.*

Although atropine blocks induction of LTP_c by ACh, it does not prevent its maintenance or intracellular expression (Swartz and Woody, 1979). After the induction of LTP_c, the persistence of increases in input resistance and excitability to intracellularly injected depolarizing current lasts for periods of over one hour (Woody et al., 1976, 1978). LTP_c thus meets the same criterion for persistence as does electrically induced LTP (LTP_e) described by Brown et al. (1988).

Dykes and colleagues (Metherate et al., 1987; Metherate et al., 1988a,b) showed that ACh plus glutamate enhanced neuronal excitability as did ACh plus stimulation of the cell's receptive field. This form of LTP_c also lasted for over an hour. Richardson and DeLong (1988) suggested that stimulation of the nucleus basalis of Meynert might lead to a comparable potentiation by causing a release of ACh together with an increase in firing.

A comparable LTP_c of neural excitability, with an underlying increase in input resistance, can be produced by intracellular application of cyclic GMP (cGMP) (Woody et al., 1978). Again, while cGMP plus concomitantly increased firing leads to persistence of the potentiation, the spontaneous firing of the cells is not persistently increased after LTP_c is produced. This lack of increased activity is potentially of importance because, as will be seen, it is isomorphic with what is found in the same cortical cells after behavioral conditioning. Thus, the mechanisms underlying LTP_c may be related to mechanisms underlying learning. The relationship between LTP_e and learning has yet to be established (Brown et al., 1988).

As might be expected, neither the induction, maintenance, nor intracellular expression of LTP_c induced by cGMP is prevented by extracellular application of atropine (Swartz and Woody, 1979).

Mechanisms of Action of ACh

The mechanisms of action of ACh may help us to distinguish differences between LTP_e and LTP_c and better establish the relationship of LTP_c to learning. For example, LTP_c (but not LTP_e) is associated with an increase in input resistance, and such changes can lead to an enhancement of synaptic transmission (Woody, 1982b; Holmes and Woody, 1989). A change in input resistance implies a change in membrane conductance. Cyclic nucleotide-induced changes in ionic conductances, such as might be produced by ACh or cGMP, are thought to be mediated through protein kinases that phosphorylate (or, sometimes, dephosphorylate) the proteins that form channels across nerve membranes. To examine this possibility we injected cyclic GMP dependent protein kinase (cGPK) intracellularly into neurons of the motor cortex of cats. Injection of the active kinase led to production of an increase in resistance and excitability similar to that seen with applications of ACh and cGMP (Woody et al., 1986a). Injections of heat-inactivated cGPK did not produce these effects, nor did injections of calcium, calcium-calmodulin dependent protein kinase (CalCAM PK), or cyclic AMP (Woody et al., 1984a; Woody and Gruen, 1986, 1988). CalCAM PK produced a small, transient increase in input resistance (of a few seconds duration) when applied together with depolarization-induced discharge, the latter to permit calcium entry. Injection of cAMP and calcium produced decreases in resistance and excitability.

Attempts were next made to measure directly the changes in conductance produced by ACh. Methodologies were developed to permit use of single electrode voltage-clamp (SEVC) techniques to measure currents *in vivo* in cortical neurons of conscious cats (Woody et al., 1985). By using this SEVC technique, it was possible to demonstrate that extracellular applications of acetylcholine or intracellular applications of cGPK produced decreases in a transient, depolarization induced outward current (Woody and Gruen, 1987). This current was defined as an A-current (gK_A) on the basis of its voltage dependency and its reduction by 3- and 4-aminopyridine (Woody et al., 1989). A decrease in gK_A could easily account for the increased neural excitability to depolarizing inputs (Pay and Woody 1988, 1989). Whether late components of the A-current are partially active at rest or whether the changes in input resistance are mediated by other currents, e.g., M-current, Na-current, etc., remains to be determined.

BEHAVIORAL CONDITIONING AND ITS RELATIONSHIP TO LTP_c AND ACh

Investigations of Pavlovian conditioning of a behavioral eyeblink response have suggested that mechanisms underlying conditioning might be similar to those underlying LTP_c . After conditioning, we found that cells of the motor cortex developed increased excitability and increased input resistance but no increase in spontaneous rates of discharge (Woody et al., 1970; Woody and Black-Cleworth, 1973). The changes occurred selectively in the cells that projected (polysynaptically) to the blink musculature involved in production of the CR, and lasted for over a month (Brons and Woody, 1980). As different types of conditioned facial responses were learned, different classes of motor projective cells underwent changes in excitability (Woody and Engel, 1972). The increases in neural excitability were correlated with increased probabilities of discharge in response to the CS. These discharges, which occurred with a timing appropriate for conduction between the cortex and facial musculature, initiated the conditioned behavioral response (Woody, 1982a). Morphologic analysis of the neurons of the motor cortex studied, using intracellular recording and marking techniques, indicated that the majority were layer V pyramidal cells (Sakai et al., 1978; Sakai and Woody, 1980; Woody et al., 1984b). Similar neurons responded to ACh, cGMP and cGPK with virtually identical, long lasting increases in neural excitability (Woody and Gruen, 1986, 1988). (As was noted earlier, numerous portions of the basal forebrain cholinergic system were found to terminate in layer V (Saper 1984; Kristt et al., 1985).)

Glut and the Electrical Induction of LTP_e

The role of glutamate and NMDA receptors in the electrical induction of LTP_e has been recently reviewed by Brown et al. (1988). Ca^{++} entry can result from a voltage-dependent, depolarizing activation of the glutamate-occupied NMDA receptor-ionophore (Dingledine, 1983). Ca^{++} entry may also conceivably arise by depolarization sufficient to activate other calcium channels, or concentrations of Ca^{++} may be increased by its release from internal stores, as by activation of the inositol triphosphate pathway. When applications of glutamate to NMDA receptors are accompanied by postsynaptic depolarizations sufficient to produce calcium entry, long-term potentiation of afferent induced EPSPs (LTP_e)

can be produced. This effect is reminiscent of the effect of depolarization-induced spike discharge described above.

Hypothetically, a long-lasting increase in a synaptic conductance could directly underlie the potentiation of the EPSP. Baranyi and colleagues measured changes in synaptic conductances of cortical cells following application of protein kinase C (PKC) activators using SEVC techniques (Baranyi et al., 1987; Baranyi et al., 1988). Like changes in PSPs produced by LTP, these changes lasted for over an hour.

LTP_e could also arise from potentiated or uncovered postsynaptic receptors. That mechanism has been reviewed elsewhere in detail (Baudry and Lynch, 1984). Expression of LTP_e depends on a presynaptic factor as well (Malinow et al., 1989). Thus, more than one mechanism underlies LTP_e.

Because inhibitors of CalCAM PKII and PKC inhibit induction (but not maintenance or expression) of LTP_e when applied directly intracellularly (Malinow et al., 1989), the postsynaptic substrates on which these agents act are implicated as supporting the induction of LTP_e. Note, however, that intracellular application of CalCAM PK in neocortical neurons does not produce an effect comparable to LTP_c (Woody et al., 1984a). Also, although intracellular application of activators of PKC produces an increased neuronal excitability as well as a potentiation of EPSPs (Baranyi et al., 1987, 1988), these changes are associated with increases in spontaneous discharge and significant increases in input resistance are not consistently observed.

Glut and the Acceleration of Behavioral Conditioning

Preliminary results suggest that cortical release of glutamate may underlie an acceleration of the rate of behavioral conditioning ($COND_b$) resulting from coapplication of electrical stimulation of the hypothalamus (HS) with delivery of USs used to produce Pavlovian conditioning (Cooper and Woody, 1983; Kim et al., 1983; Woody et al., 1983).

Voronin and colleagues observed that associative delivery of HS plus US (with a CS) could increase the rate of Pavlovian conditioning (Voronin et al., 1975). Our experiments (Kim et al., 1983) used a click CS followed by glabella tap US plus four brief electrical pulses to the lateral hypothalamus to produce rapid blink conditioning. With this procedure, animals learned the Pavlovian blink CR in 10 to 20 pairings as opposed to the 750 to 1000 pairings required when the same CS and US were given without added hypothalamic stimulation. We noted that hypothalamic stimulation successful in producing such effects also produced short-latency activation of neurons of the motor cortex whose activity and excitability increased to support development of the CR (Woody et al., 1983). That short-latency activation was found to be suppressed selectively by glutamate diethyl ester (GDEE) as opposed to atropine (Cooper and Woody, 1983).

Glutamate and Artificial Conditioning ($COND_a$)

Glutamate can be used as a kind of US to produce conditioning of single cortical neurons (Bures and Buresova, 1967). We applied glutamate iontophoretically in combination with click CS and tap US to produce rapid artificial conditioning of single cortical cells (Woody et al., 1984c). In further experiments we recorded intracellularly from single cortical units and obtained baseline measurements of electrical properties in bridge mode and then during single electrode voltage clamp (SEVC) (Woody et al., 1987). Next, glutamate was applied iontophoretically through an immediately adjacent extracellular micropipette while applying the CS and US. Then additional measurements were obtained with SEVC and bridge mode readings. When glutamate application followed the US, the neurons developed increased activity in response to the CS after ten pairings. When glutamate was applied before the CS, they did not. After this type of conditioning, increases in excitability and input resistance were observed, similar to those found behaviorally and after application of ACh. Also, gK_A was found to be decreased.

DIFFERENCES BETWEEN EFFECTS OF ACh AND GLUT AND BETWEEN LTP_c, LTP_e, $COND_b$ AND $COND_a$

As summarized above, changes in neuroelectric properties with LTP_c produced by ACh, cGMP and cGPK mirror the changes produced by $COND_b$ and $COND_a$. Specifically, there occur a long lasting increase in neural excitability and a decrease in gK_A, yet no accompanying increase in spontaneous discharge is seen. LTP_e and applications of PKC produce a potentiation of synaptic potentials *with or without* accompanying increases in postsynaptic neural excitability, and, when measured, rates of spontaneous discharge are usually increased. Additionally, no consistent increases in input resistance have been found with LTP_e or with application of PKC. There is with LTP_e a characteristic specificity of the synaptic input whose conductance is potentiated. Unless postsynaptic changes in membrane conductance were confined to selected spine processes, it seems unlikely that postsynaptic changes in any conductances except synaptic ones could be so highly specific. This degree of specificity is by no means isomorphic with that of learning and conditioning, which have distinct generalization gradients (Woody, 1982b).

Studies by Iriki et al. (1989) suggest that some forms of neocortical LTP_e affect layer III cells selectively. Other forms of cortical plasticity such as heterosynaptic facilitation and long lasting potentiation involve layer V as well as layer III cells (Baranyi and Feher, 1981a,b). Thus, there appear to be several different forms of neocortical neuronal potentiation.

Perhaps the most significant difference between LTP_e and conditioning lies in the paradigms by which they are typically produced. Generally, LTP_e is induced by higher rates of stimulation than those used to induce conditioning, even when LTP_e is induced by associative pairing of afferent inputs to produce the right combination of glutamate release and postsynaptic depolarization. COND is produced by low frequency associative stimulation.

Our evidence suggests that ACh plus depolarization-induced calcium entry (the latter possibly promoted by the action of glutamate on quisqualate/kainate receptors and affecting the rate of the adaptive process) can lead to LTP_c and COND involving a decreased gK_A, an increased input resistance due to a decrease of a steadily active membrane conductance, and perhaps an increase in synaptic conductance when Glut acts as well at NMDA receptors. cGPK and PKC appear to mediate these changes. Applications of glutamate without ACh may lead to LTP_e and selective changes in synaptic conductances. PKC appears to mediate induction of some of these changes (Baranyi et al 1987, 1988) and may also support consolidation of some neuronal changes underlying both COND and LTP (Alkon et al., 1983).

REFERENCES

Alkon, D.L., Acosta-Urquidi, J., Olds, J., Kuzma, G. and Neary, J. (1983): Protein kinase injection reduces voltage-dependent potassium currents. *Science* 219:303-306

Armstrong, D.M., Saper, C.B., Levey, A.I., Wainer, B.H. and Terry, R.D. (1983):

Distribution of cholinergic neurons in rat brain: demonstrated by the immunocytochemical localization of choline acetyltransferase. *J. Comp. Neurol.* 216:53-68

Baranyi, A. and Feher, O. (1981a): Intracellular studies on cortical synaptic plasticity. Conditioning effect of antidromic activation on test-EPSPs. *Exp. Brain Res.* 41:124-134

Baranyi, A. and Feher, O. (1981b): Long-term facilitation of excitatory synaptic transmission in single cortical neurons of the cat producd by repetitive pairing of synaptic potentials and action potentials following intracellular stimulation. *Neurosci. Lett.* 23:303-308

Baranyi, A., Szente, M.B. and Woody, C.D. (1987): Intracellular injection of phorbol ester increases the excitability of neurons of the motor cortex of awake cats. *Brain Res.* 424:396-401

Baranyi, A., Szente, M.B. and Woody, C.D. (1988): Activation of protein kinase C induces long-term changes of postsynaptic currents in neocortical neurons. *Brain Res.* 440:341-347

Bartus, R.T., Flicker, C., Dean, R.L., Pontecorvo, M., Figueiredo, J.C. and Fisher, S.K. (1985): Selective memory loss following nucleus basalis lesions: long term behavioral recovery despite persistent cholinergic deficiencies. *Pharmacol. Biochem. Behav.* 23:125-135

Baudry, M. and Lynch, G. (1984): The biochemistry of memory: a new and specific hypothesis. *Science* 224:1057-163

Brons, J. F. and Woody, C.D. (1980): Long-term changes in excitability of cortical neurons after Pavlovian conditioning and extinction. *J. Neurophysiol.* 44:605-615

Brown, T.H., Chapman, P.F., Kairiss, E.W. and Keenan, C.L. (1988): Long-term synaptic potentiation. *Science* 242:724-728

Bures, J. and Buresova, O. (1967): Plastic changes of unit activity based on reinforcing properties of extracellular stimulation of single neurons. *J. Neurophysiol.* 30:98-113

Campbell, L.B., Hanin, I. and Jenden, D.J. (1970): Gas chromatographic evaluation of the effects of some muscarinic and antimuscarinic drugs on acetylcholine levels in rat brain. *Biochem. Pharmacol.* 19:2053-2059

Collerton, D. (1986): Cholinergic function and intellectual decline in Alzheimer's disease. *Neurosci.* 19:1-28

Connor, J.A. and Alkon, D.L. (1984): Light- and voltage-dependent increases of calcium ion concentration in molluscan photoreceptors. *J. Neurophysiol.* 51:745-52

Cooper, J.R., Bloom, F.E. and Roth, R.H. (1986): *The Biochemical Basis of Neuropharmacology*. New York: Oxford University Press

Cooper, P.H. and Woody, C.D. (1983): Effects of L-glutamate and L-glutamic acid diethyl ester (GDEE) on the response of cortical units to hypothalamic stimulation. *Soc. Neurosci. Abstr.* 9:330

Csaky, T.Z., ed., (1979): *Cutting's Handbook of Pharmacology/The Actions and uses of Drugs*. USA: Appleton Century Crofts

Davies, P. (1985): A critical review of the role of the cholinergic system in human memory and cognition. *Ann. N.Y. Acad. Sci.* 444:212-217

Deutsch, J.A. (1971): The cholinergic synapse and the site of memory. *Science* 174:788-794

Dingledinc, R. (1983): N-Methyl aspartate activates voltage-dependent calcium conductance in rat hippocampal pyramidal cells. *J. Physiol.* 343:385-405

Divac, I. (1975): Magnocellular nuclei of basal forebrain project to neocortex, brain stem, and olfactory bulb. Review of some functional correlates. *Brain Res.* 93:385-398

Divac, I. (1981): Cortical projections of the magnocellular nuclei of the basal forebrain: a reinvestigation. *Neurosci.* 6:983-984

Drachman, D.A. and Leavitt, J. (1974): Human memory and the cholinergic system. A relationship to aging? *Arch. Neurol.* 30:113-121

Dunnet, S. (1985): Comparative effects of cholinergic drugs and lesions of nucleus basalis or fimbria fornix on delayed matching in rats. *Psychopharmacol.* 87:357-363

Eckenstein, F. and Sofroniew, M.V. (1983): Identification of central cholinergic neurons containing both choline acetyltransferase and acetylcholinesterase and of central neurons containing only acetylcholinesterase. *J. Neurosci.* 3:2286-2291

Eckenstein, F. and Thoenen, H. (1983): Cholinergic neurons in the rat cerebral cortex demonstrated by immunohistochemical localization of choline acetyltransferase. *Neurosci. Lett.* 36:211-215

Fibiger, H.C. (1982): The organization and some projections of cholinergic neurons of the mammalian forebrain. *Brain Res. Revs.* 4:327-388

Green, J.R., Halpern, L.M. and van Niel, S. (1970): Choline acetylase and acetylcholine-esterase changes in chronic isolated cerebral cortex of cat. *Life Science* 9:481-488

Hebb, C.O., Krnjević, K. and Silver, A. (1963): Effect of undercutting on the acetylcholinesterase and choline acetyltransferase activity in the cat's cerebral cortex. *Nature* (Lond.) 198:692

Hepler, D.J., Olton, D.S., Wenk, G.L. and Coyle, J.T. (1985): Lesions in nucleus basalis magnocellularis and medial septal area of rats produce qualitatively similar memory impairments. *J. Neurosci.* 4:866-873

Holmes, W.R. and Woody, C.D. (1989): Effects of uniform and non-uniform synaptic 'activation-distributions' on the cable properties of modeled cortical pyramidal neurons. *Brain Res.* 505:12-22

Hoover, D.B., Muth, E.A. and Jacobwitz, D.M. (1978): A mapping of the distribution of acetylcholine, choline acetyltransferase and acetylcholinesterase in discrete areas of rat brain. *Brain Res.* 153:295-306

Houser, C.R., Crawford, G.D., Barber, R.P., Salvaterra, P.M. and Vaughn, J.E. (1983): Organization and morphological characteristics of cholinergic neurons: an immunocytochemical study with a monoclonal antibody to choline acetyltransferase. *Brain Res.* 266:97-119

Houser, C.R., Crawford, G.D., Salvaterra, P.M. and Vaughn, J.E. (1985): Immunocytochemical localization of choline acetyltransferase in rat cerebral cortex: a study of cholinergic neurons and synapses. *J. Comp. Neurol.* 234:17-34

Iriki, A., Pavlides, C., Keller, A. and Asanuma, H. (1989): Long-term potentiation of motor cortex. *Science* 245:1385-1387

Johnston, M.V., McKinney, M. and Coyle, J.T. (1979): Evidence for a cholinergic projection to neocortex from neurons in basal forebrain. *Proc. Natl. Acad. Sci.* 76:5392-5396

Johnston, M.V., McKinney, M. and Coyle, J.T. (1981): Neocortical cholinergic innervation: a description of extrinsic and intrinsic components in the rat. *Exp. Brain Res.* 43:159-172

Katz, B. and Miledi, R. (1968): The role of calcium in neuromuscular facilitation. *J. Physiol.* 195:481-92

Kievit, J. and Kuypers, H. G. (1975): Basal forebrain and hypothalamic connections to frontal and parietal cortex in the Rhesus monkey. *Science* 187:660-662

Kim, E. H.-J., Woody, C. D. and Berthier, N. E. (1983): Rapid acquisition of conditioned eye blink responses in cats following pairing of an auditory CS with glabella tap US and hypothalamic stimulation. *J. Neurophysiol.* 49:767-779

Kimura, H., McGeer, P., Peng, F. and McGeer, E. (1980): Choline acetyltransferase-containing neurons in rodent brain demonstrated by immunohistochemistry. *Science* 208:1057-1059

Kimura, H., McGeer, P. L., Peng, J. H. and McGeer, E. G. (1981): The central cholinergic system studied by choline acetyltransferase immunohistochemistry in the cat. *J. Comp. Neurol.* 200:151-201

Kodama, S. (1929): Pathologisch-anatomische Untersuchungen mit Bezug auf die Sogemanten Basalganglien und ihre Adnexe. *Neurol. Psychiat. Abh.* 8:1-20

Kristt, D.A., McGowan Jr., R.A. Martin-Mackinnon, N. and Solomon, J. (1985): Basal forebrain innervation of rodent neocortex: studies using acetylcholinesterase histochemistry, Golgi and lesion strategies. *Brain Res.* 337:19-39

Krnjević, K. and Phillis, J.W. (1963): Acetylcholine-sensitive cells in the cerebral cortex. *J. Physiol.* 166:296-327

Krnjević, K., Pumain, R. and Renaud, L. (1971): The mechanism of excitation by acetylcholine in the cerebral cortex. *J. Physiol.* 215:247-68

Lehmann, J. and Fibiger, H.C. (1978): Acetylcholinesterase in the substantia nigra and caudate-putamen of the rat: properties and localization in dopaminergic neurons. *J. Neurochem.* 30:615-624

Lehmann, J., Nagy, J. I., Atmadja, S. and Fibiger, H.C. (1980): The nucleus basalis magnocellularis: the origin of a cholinergic projection to the neocortex of the rat. *Neurosci.* 5:1161-1174

Levey, A.I., Wainer, B.H., Mufson, E.J. and Mesulam, M.-M. (1983): Co-localization of acetylcholinesterase and choline acetyltransferase in the rat cerebrum. *Neurosci.* 9:9-22

Lewis, P.R. and Schon, F.E.G. (1975): The localization of acetylcholinesterase in the locus coeruleus of the normal rat and after 6-hydroxydopamine treatment. *J. Anat.*120:373-385

Lewis, P.R. and Shute, C.C.D. (1967): The cholinergic limbic system: projections to hippocampal formation, medial cortex, nuclei of the ascending cholinergic reticular system, and the subfornical organ and supra-optic crest. *Brain* 90:521-540

Malinow, R., Schulman, H. and Tsien, R. (1989): Inhibition of postsynaptic PKC or CaMKII blocks induction but not expression of LTP. *Science* 245: 862-866

Martindale, W. (1982): *The Extrapharmacopoeia.* Reynolds, J.E.F., ed. London: Pharmaceutical Press

McGeer, P. L., McGeer, E. G., Fibiger, H. C. and Wickson, V. (1971): Neostriatal choline acetylase and cholinesterase following selective brain lesions. *Brain Res.* 35:308-314

McGeer, P. L., McGeer, E. G., Singh, V. K. and Chase, W. H. (1974): Choline acetyltransferase localization in the central nervous sytem by immunohistochemistry. *Brain Res.* 81:373-379

Mesulam, M.-M. and Mufson, E. J. (1980): The rapid anterograde transport of horseradish peroxidase. *Neurosci.* 5:1277-1286

Mesulam, M.-M., Mufson, E. J., Levey, A. I. and Wainer, B. H. (1983a): Cholinergic innervation of cortex by the basal forebrain: cytochemistry and cortical connections of the septal area, diagonal band nuclei, nucleus basalis (substantia innominata), and hypothalamus in the rhesus monkey. *J. Comp. Neurol.* 214:170-197

Mesulam, M.-M., Mufson, E.J., Wainer, B.H. and Levey, A.I. (1983b): Central cholinergic pathways in the rat: an overview based on alternative nomenclature (Ch1-Ch6). *Neurosci.* 10:1185-1201

Mesulam, M.-M., Mufson, E.J., Levey, A.I. and Wainer, B.H. (1984): Atlas of cholinergic neurons in the forebrain and upper brainstem of the macaque based on monoclonal choline acetyltransferase immunohistochemistry and acetylcholinesterase histochemistry. *Neurosci.* 12:669-686

Metherate, N., Tremblay, N. and Dykes, R.W. (1987): Acetylcholine permits long-term enhancement of neuronal responsiveness in cat primary somatosensory cortex. *Neurosci.* 22:75-81

Metherate, N., Tremblay, N. and Dykes, R.W. (1988a): The effects of acetylcholine on response properties of cat somatosensory cortical neurons. *J. Neurophysiol.* 59:1231-1252

Metherate, N., Tremblay, N. and Dykes, R.W. (1988b): Transient and prolonged effects of acetylcholine on responsiveness of cat somatosensory cortical neurons. *J. Neurophysiol.* 59:1253-1276

Pay, R.G. and Woody, C.D. (1988): Conditioning-like operations arising from stimulation of voltage-dependent adaptive properties of a neuronal membrane current. *Soc. Neurosci. Abstr.* 14:276

Pay, R.G. and Woody, C.D. (1989): After hyperpolarization (AHP) changes and voltage-addressable information processing derived from simulated effects of gK_A^+. *Soc. Neurosci. Abstr.* 15:1309

Perry, E.K., Perry, R.H., Smith, C.J., Porohit, D., Bonham, J., Dick, D.J., Candy, J.M., Edwardson, J.A. and Fairbairn, A. (1986): Cholinergic receptors in cognitive disorders. *Le Journal Canadien des Sciences Neurologiques* 13: 521-527

Phillis, J. W. (1968): Acetylcholine release from the cerebral cortex: its role in cortical arousal. *Brain Res.* 7:378-389

Price, J. L. and Stern, R. (1983): Individual cells in the nucleus basalis-diagonal band complex have restricted axonal projections to the cerebral cortex in the rat. *Brain Res.* 269:352-356

Richardson, R.T. and DeLong, M.R. (1988): A reappraisal of the functions of the nucleus basalis of Meynert. *Trends Neurosci.* 11:264-267

Rossier, J. (1981): Serum monospecificity: a prerequisite for reliable immunohistochemical localization of neuronal markers including choline acetyltransferase. *Neurosci.* 6:989-991

Sakai, M., Sakai, H. and Woody, C.D. (1978): Sampling distribution of morphologically identified neurons of the coronal-pericruciate cortex of awake cats following intracellular injection of HRP. *Brain Res.* 152:329-333

Sakai, H. and Woody, C.D. (1980): Identification of auditory responsive cells in coronal-pericruciate cortex of awake cats. *J. Neurophysiol.* 44:223-231

Saper, C.B. (1984): Organization of cerebral cortical afferent systems in the rat. II. Magnocellular basal nucleus. *J. Comp. Neurol.* 222:313-342

Shute, C.C.D and Lewis P.R. (1967): The ascending cholinergic reticular system: neocortical, olfactory and subcortical projections. *Brain* 90:497-520

Swartz, B.E. and Woody, C.D. (1979): Correlated effects of acetylcholine and cyclic guanosine monophosphate on membrane properties of mammalia neocortical neurons. *J. Neurobiol.* 10:465-488

Voronin, L.L., Gerstein, G., Kudriashov, I. E. and Ioffe, S. V. (1975): Elaboration of a conditioned reflex in a single experiment with simultaneous recording of neural activity. *Brain Res.* 92:385-403

Weiner, N. (1980): Atropine, scopolamine, and related antimuscarinic drugs. In: *The Pharmacological Basis of Theraputics*. Goodman, L., Gilman, A., eds. New York: MacMillan 120-137

Wenk, H., Volker, B. and Meyer, U. (1980): Cholinergic projections from magnocellular nuclei of the basal forebrain to cortical areas in rats. *Brain Res.*

Rev. 2:295-316

Woody, C.D. (1982a): Acquisition of conditioned facial reflexes in the cat: cortical control of different facial movements. *Fed. Proc.* 41:2160-2168

Woody, C. D. (1982b): *Memory, Learning, and Higher Function: A Cellular View.* New York: Springer-Verlag

Woody, C.D., Alkon, D.L. and Hay, B. (1984a): Depolarization-induced effects of Ca^{2+}-calmodulin-dependent protein kinase injection, in vivo, in single neurons of cat motor cortex. *Brain Res.* 321:192-197

Woody, C.D., Baranyi, A., Szente, M.B., Gruen, E., Holmes,W., Nenov, V. and Strecker, G.J. (1989): An aminopyridine sensitive, early outward current recorded in vivo in neurons of the precruciate cortex of cats using single electrode voltage clamp techniques. *Brain Res.* 480: 72-81

Woody, C.D., Bartfai, T., Gruen, E. and Nairn, A. (1986a): Intracellular injection of cGMP-dependent protein kinase results in increased input resistance in neurons of the mammalian motor cortex. *Brain Res.* 386:379-385

Woody, C.D., Birt, D. and Gruen, E. (1987): In vivo effects of Pavlovian conditioning on currents measured in neurons of the motor cortex of awake cats with single electrode voltage clamp techniques. *Soc. Neurosci. Abstr.* 13:609

Woody, C.D. and Black-Cleworth, P. (1973): Differences in excitability of cortical neurons as a function of motor projection in conditioned cats. *J. Neurophysiol.* 36:1104-1116

Woody, C.D., Carpenter, D.O., Gruen, E. Knispel, J.D., Crow, T.W. and Black-Cleworth, P. (1976): Persistent increases in membrane resistance of neurons in cat motor cortex. *AFRRI Scientific Report* Feb. 1-31

Woody, C.D. and Engel, J. Jr. (1972): Changes in unit activity and thresholds to electrical microstimulation at coronal-pericruciate cortex of cat with classical conditioning of different facial movements. *J. Neurophysiol.* 35:230-241

Woody, C.D. and Gruen, E. (1986): Responses of morphologically identified cortical neurons to intracellularly injected cyclic AMP. *Exp. Neurol.* 91:596-612

Woody, C.D. and Gruen, E. (1987): Acetylcholine reduces net outward currents measured in vivo with single electrode voltage clamp techniques in neurons of the motor cortex of cats. *Brain Res.* 424:193-198

Woody, C.D. and Gruen, E. (1988): Evidence that acetylcholine acts in vivo in layer V pyramidal cells of cats via cyclic GMP and a cyclic GMP-dependent protein kinase to produce a decrease in an outward current. In: *Neurotransmitters and Cortical Function.* Avoli, M., Reader, T.A., Dykes, R.W. and Gloor, P. (Eds.), New York: Plenum Press, pp. 313-319

Woody, C.D., Gruen, E. and McCarley, K. (1984b): Intradendritic recordings from neurons of the motor cortex of cats. *J. Neurophysiol.* 51:925-938

Woody, C.D., Gruen, E., Sakai, H., Sakai, M. and Swartz, B. (1986b): Responses of morphologically identified cortical neurons to intracellularly injected cyclic GMP. *Exp. Neurol.* 91:580-595

Woody, C.D., Kim, E.J.-H. and Berthier, N.E. (1983): Effects of hypothalamic stimulation on unit responses recorded from neurons of sensorimotor cortex of awake cats during conditioning. *J. Neurophysiol.* 49:780-791

Woody, C.D., Nenov, V., Gruen, E. and Donley, P. (1985): A voltage-dependent, 4-aminopyridine sensitive, outward current studied *in vivo* in cortical neurons of awake cats by voltage squeeze techniques. *Soc. Neurosci. Abstr.* 11:955

Woody, C.D., Oomura, Y., Gruen, E., Miyake, J. and Nenov, V. (1984c): Attempts to rapidly condition increased activity to click in single cortical neurons of awake cats using glabella tap and iontophoretically applied glutamate. *Soc. Neurosci. Abstr.* 10:25

Woody, C.D., Swartz, B.E. and Gruen, E. (1978): Effects of acetylcholine and cyclic GMP on input resistance of cortical neurons in awake cats. *Brain Res.* 158:373-395

Woody, C.D., Vassilevsky, N.N. and Engel, J. Jr. (1970): Conditioned eye blink: unit activity at coronal-precruciate cortex of the cat. *J. Neurophysiol.* 33:851-864

Acetylcholine Modulation of Cellular Excitability Via Muscarinic Receptors: Functional Plasticity in Auditory Cortex

John H. Ashe and Norman M. Weinberger

INTRODUCTION

In recent years substantial advancement has occurred toward understanding integrative functions of the nervous system. Acetylcholine (ACh), dopamine (DA), norepinephrine (NE), and serotonin (5-HT), are substances that have gained general recognition as neurotransmitters in the sense of having a direct influence on the magnitude of membrane potential. These substances are now also characterized as *neuromodulators*, a designation which encompasses observations of complex electrophysiologic and metabolic effects in target neurons that occur in addition to, or are independent of, simple excitatory and inhibitory changes in the membrane potential (for reviews, see Dismukes, 1979; Kupfermann, 1979; Daly et al., 1980; Kaczmarek and Levitan, 1987).

The more prominent features of neuromodulator action include: (1) effects that are slow to develop and much longer-lasting than those of conventional neurotransmitters—the combination of ACh with nicotinic receptors of the neuromuscular junction is prototypic and (2) effects that may have little or no consequence on the magnitude of the membrane potential in and of themselves, but that nonetheless modify the outcome of subsequent synaptic input (Kupfermann, 1979; Libet, 1979a; Moises et al., 1979). The important finding relevant to conceptual formulations is that neuromodulatory action is predominantly involved in the production of a lasting modification of the state of reactivity of the neuron (Daly et al., 1980). It is likely that neuromodulation is of fundamental importance for an understanding of integrative functions of the nervous system and the maintenance of synaptic activity (e.g., extended period for temporal summation and changes in the electrotonic constants of the membrane). Advancement of knowledge concerning behavioral and neuronal modification may be accelerated substantially by an understanding of basic processes subserving neuromodulation and synaptic plasticity (Kupfermann, 1979; Daly et al., 1980; Kaczmarek and Levitan, 1987).

The physiological significance of cholinergic neurotransmission has received broad attention because of the involvement of ACh in a wide range of nervous system functions. Cholinergic activity is involved in transmission and integration at autonomic ganglia, and with the control of peripheral organs including heart, lung, trachea and gut (Karczmar et al., 1986). In the brain, ACh has been implicated in the control of states of arousal (Mitchell, 1963; Jasper, 1969), and central regulation of arterial pressure (Brezenoff, 1984). In addition, ACh has been implicated in various cognitive functions. Human and animal studies indicate a particularly important role for ACh in learning and memory (McDonough and Penetar, 1983; Bartus et al., 1987) and in the cognitive dysfunction that accompanies disorders such as Alzheimer's disease (for review, see Collerton, 1986).

The present chapter is concerned with the neuromodulatory actions of ACh in auditory cortex plasticity and learning. The chapter is quite selective; it focuses on the proposal that acetylcholine promotes the acquisition and storage of information in sensory cortex, and further presents an intended heuristic model for how this may occur. We believe that this topic is of special interest in view of the demonstrated importance of ACh and neuronal modulation in states of behavioral arousal, learning and memory, and mental disorders, as well as general nervous system function. We will discuss the electrophysiological data leading to this position with concentration on recent results obtained from auditory cortical neurons. These data indicate that physiological plasticity in auditory cortex can be revealed as highly specific changes in the frequency receptive fields of single neurons. Receptive field changes can be produced by acoustic stimuli used in a classical conditioning paradigm, and by application of muscarinic receptor agonists, or blockers of acetylcholinesterase. Receptive field plasticity is often expressed as a modification of responses to the best frequency, or to a selected frequency, e.g., to the tone used as a conditioned stimulus (CS), or both.

We believe that the actions of ACh in auditory cortex encompass and typify mechanisms that may lead to general principles that are important for the understanding of (1) the observations that individual transmitters produce their effects by engaging more than one type of specific receptor, (2) the functional significance of multiple receptors and receptor mechanisms in the nervous system, and (3) the extent and function of the aforementioned in the acquisition and storage of information. In the following sections we will briefly review (a) the distribution of cholinoceptive neurons in cortex, (b) evidence for a distinctive function for mechanisms mediated by muscarinic receptors, and the need to pursue research designed to elucidate the role of subtypes of the muscarinic receptor in regulating neuronal plasticity, (c) the function of muscarinic mechanisms in auditory receptive field plasticity, and (d) a working model of adaptive information processing in auditory cortex.

ANATOMICAL CONSIDERATIONS

Distribution of Cholinergic and Cholinoceptive Neurons

Suitable techniques for the morphological visualization and identification of markers of CNS cholinergic systems have been pursued for many years, essentially beginning with histochemical studies of the distribution of acetylcholinesterase (AChE) (Koelle and Friedenwald, 1949; Shute and Lewis, 1963; Shute and Lewis, 1967). However, histochemical identification of AChE has been found to be an inadequate technique for selective and specific identification of cholinergic neurons. AChE is widespread and enzyme activity has been found in non-cholinergic, non-cholinoceptive, and nonneuronal cells (Welsch and Pearse, 1969; Butcher and Bilezikjian, 1975). More recent investigations of the distribution of cholinergic cell bodies and terminals have used immunohistochemical techniques with monoclonal antibodies for visualization of choline acetyltransferase (ChAT), the enzyme that catalyzes the synthesis of ACh (Kimura et al., 1981; Houser et al., 1983; Mesulam et al., 1983b; Levey et al., 1984; Houser et al., 1985). ChAT has been found to be a highly reliable marker of cholinergic cell bodies and terminals. Data obtained with ChAT immunohistochemistry, with results obtained with fiber tracing methods, have led to apparent consensus regarding the existence of a strong cholinergic projection to the cerebral cortex from the basal forebrain. Cell bodies are located chiefly in the nucleus basalis (Lehmann et al., 1980; Johnston et al., 1981; Mesulam et al., 1983a; Mesulam et al., 1983b; Rye et al., 1984).

With regard to the existence of intrinsic (intracortical) cholinergic neurons in cerebral cortex, results from recent studies applying sensitive immunohistochemical techniques have shown the presence of ChAT in small neurons (presumably interneurons) distributed throughout all layers of cortex (Eckenstein and Sofroniew, 1983; Houser, et al., 1983; Eckenstein and Baughman, 1984; Houser, et al., 1985). Neurophysiological data suggest that intracortical cholinergic neurons may function as inhibitory interneurons (Phillis and York, 1968; McCormick and Prince, 1986b). Thus, cholinergic fibers (afferent and intrinsic) in the neocortex appear diffusely throughout all cortical layers; however, as indicated from higher ChAT concentrations, the levels of ACh are apparently higher in layers I, II, and IV (Beesley and Emson, 1975; Campbell et al., 1987).

Within the auditory system, the evidence suggests the existence of either cholinergic or cholinoceptive neurons at all levels (Godfrey and Matschinsky, 1981; Kimura, et al., 1981; Altschuler et al., 1985; Mesulam, 1988). These data suggest a wide functional role for ACh throughout the auditory system; and at the cortical level ACh is also capable of interaction within a large number of cells that have been demonstrated to be cholinoceptive. However, recent histochemical evidence suggests that glutamate is the transmitter for direct activation of neocortical neurons by medial geniculate projections to auditory cortex (Popowitz et al., 1988), whereas ACh functions to modulate the rate and pattern of cellular discharge (McKenna et al., 1988; Ashe et al., 1989; McKenna et al., 1989).

In addition to histochemical evidence, we have recently obtained physiological and pharmacological data that indicate auditory cortical neurons receive glutamatergic synaptic input. Intracellular recordings from guinea pig auditory cortical neurons maintained *in vitro* indicate that these cells receive a mixed pattern of synaptic excitation and inhibition (Fig. 1). The response consists of a sequence of an early EPSP followed by an IPSP, late EPSP, and late IPSP. The two EPSPs are mediated by an excitatory amino acid transmitter that is in all probability glutamate. Furthermore, the nature of the postsynaptic receptors engaged by the transmitter differ with regard to their sensitivity to excitatory amino acid antagonists. The amplitude of the early EPSP is selectively suppressed by quisqualate/kainate receptor antagonist DNQX (6,7-dinitroquinoxaline-2,3-dione) (Honore et al., 1988). In contrast, the late EPSP is selectively blocked by APV (2-amino-5-phosphonovaleric acid), an antagonist of NMDA type receptors that has little effect on quisqualate/kainate receptors (Watkins and Olverman, 1987) or the early EPSP in auditory cortical neurons (Fig. 2). Thus, neurons of the guinea pig auditory cortex are excited by an amino acid neurotransmitter that can activate both quisqualate/kainate and NMDA type receptors.

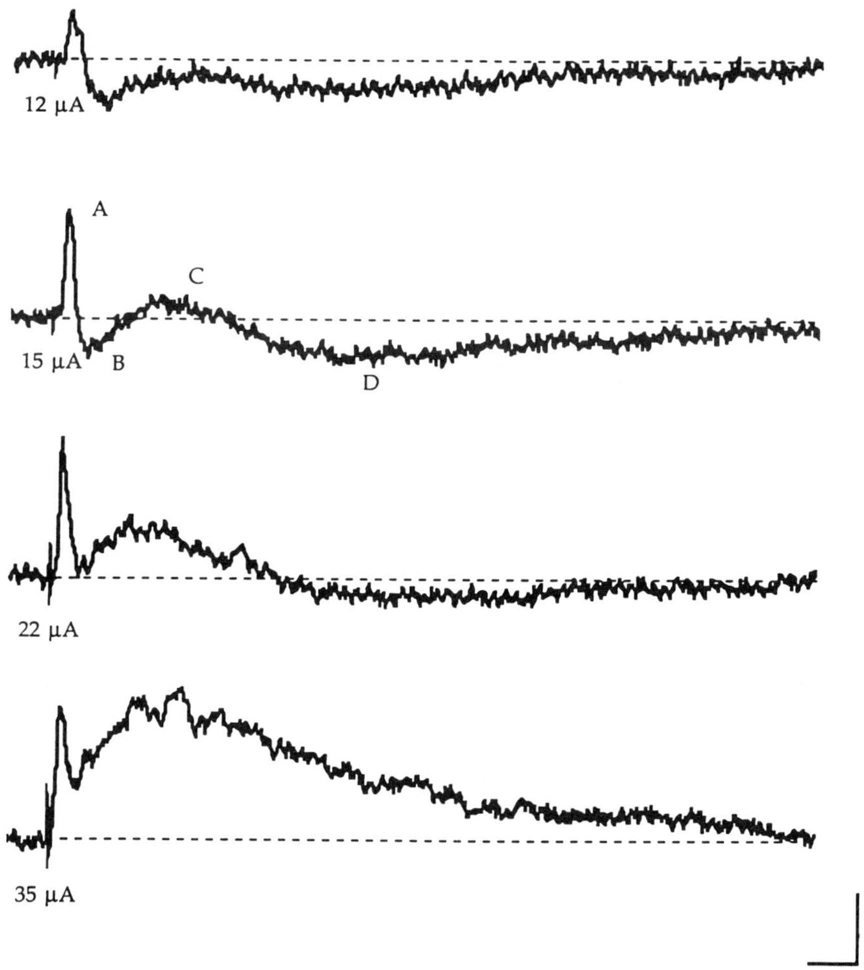

Figure 1. Intracellular recordings of synaptic responses elicited from guinea pig neocortex neurons maintained *in vitro*. The synaptic profile elicited by a single stimulus pulse of varying intensities to the underlying white matter consists of four components; a fast onset EPSP (A) that is followed by an IPSP (B), late EPSP (C), and late IPSP (D). Calibration: 5 mV, 25 msec.

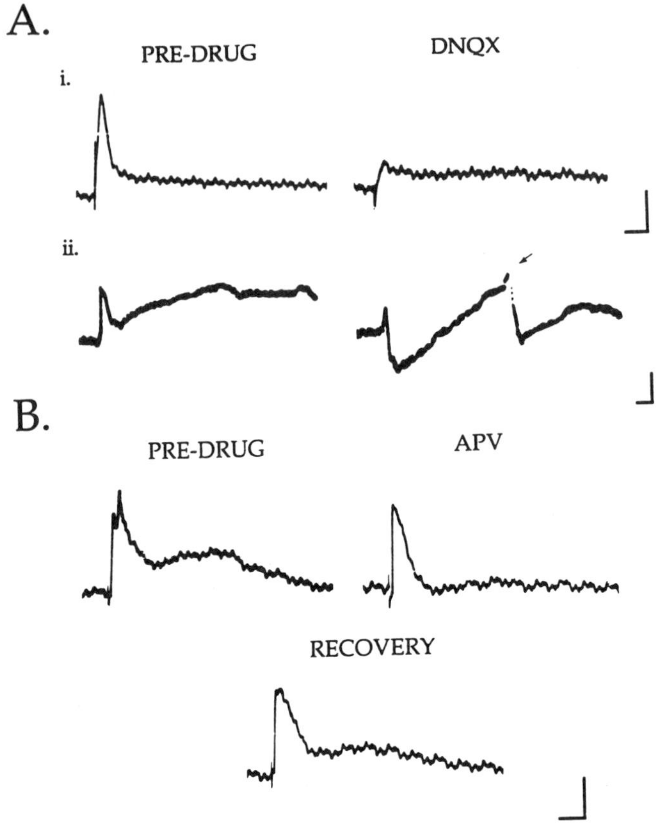

Figure 2. Differential effects of excitatory amino acid antagonists on the early and late EPSPs recorded from guinea pig neocortex neurons maintained *in vitro*. A. i and ii. Intracellular recordings from two different cells that responded to stimulation of adjacent gray matter with early and late EPSPs. Following microtopical application of the quisqualate/kainate antagonist DNQX (0.2 μl, 12 μM) the amplitude of the early EPSP is greatly reduced, however, the amplitude of the late EPSP is essentially unaffected. In ii the reduction in amplitude of the early EPSP unmasks the early IPSP. (The arrowhead indicates an action potential elicited by the late EPSP). Calibrations: (i) 10 mV, 20 ms; (ii) 5 mV, 10 ms.

In B the effect of the NMDA antagonist, APV (0.2 μl, 100 μM) on the amplitude of the early and late EPSP was tested. Microtopical application of APV resulted in strong suppression of the amplitude of the late EPSP with virtually no effect on the early EPSP. APV suppression of the late EPSP was partially reversed by 40 minutes of wash in drug free medium. Calibration 10 mV, 20 ms.

Identification and Distribution of Muscarinic Receptors

Although there is a population of nicotinic binding sites in neocortex (Boksa and Quirion, 1987; Deutch et al., 1987; Araujo et al., 1988; Parkinson et al., 1988; Prusky et al., 1988), there is little evidence for a neuromodulatory function. The overwhelming body of data regarding neuromodulatory actions of ACh has been concerned with the analysis of the consequences of activation of the muscarinic ACh receptor (mAChR). This is especially true for modulatory functions of ACh and its involvement in learning and memory processes (see Woody, this volume). Muscarinic binding sites are particularly concentrated in cerebral cortex (Kobayashi et al., 1978), and their concentration in cortex is considerably greater than that of nicotinic binding sites (Parkinson et al., 1988).

Furthermore, activation of mAChRs leads to several intracellular and membrane effects mediated via phospholipid and cyclic nucleotide metabolism (Gil and Wolfe, 1985; El-Fakahany et al., 1988). Modifications of phospholipid and cyclic nucleotide metabolism is of special interest, as these intracellular messengers have been also implicated in long-lasting changes in neuronal excitability and learning and memory (Akers and Routtenberg, 1987; Baranyi et al., 1988a; Baranyi et al., 1988b; Lovinger and Routtenberg, 1988; Nicoll, 1988).

Characterization of Subtypes of Muscarinic Receptors: Molecular biological and pharmacological criteria have now provided evidence for at least four types of mAChRs in the nervous system that are likely to have physiological significance (Marchi and Raiteri, 1985; Mash and Potter, 1986; Hammer et al., 1986; Bonner et al., 1987; Waelbroeck et al., 1987; Brann et al., 1988; Bonner, 1989). However, out of these four mAChRs, physiological responses mediated by those mAChR, generally termed M_1 and M_2, have been the most extensively studied to date (Brown et al., 1980; Ashe and Yarosh, 1984; McCormick and Prince, 1985; Newberry et al., 1985; Egan and North, 1986; Müller and Misgeld, 1986; Bradshaw et al., 1987; Yarosh and Ashe, 1987; Dutar and Nicoll, 1988a; Mochida and Kobayashi, 1988; Swanson and Phillis, 1988; Yarosh et al., 1988; Yarosh et al., 1988).

Early indication that the muscarinic ACh receptor may exist in several forms was suggested on the basis of comparing the ability of diverse cholinergic *agonists* to stimulate receptors associated with either autonomic ganglia or effector cells of the lower esophageal sphincter muscle (Goyal and Rattan, 1978). Concentrations of the muscarinic agonist McN-A-343 effective for eliciting end-organ responses mediated by way of sympathetic ganglia were lower than concentrations effective for stimulating cells of the lower esophageal sphincter muscle. On the other hand, the muscarinic agonists such as bethanechol, methacholine (MCh), muscarine, and carbachol, were more effective for stimulation of cells of the lower esophageal sphincter muscle. On the basis of these observations, it was proposed that mAChRs associated with autonomic ganglia be classified as M_1 and those mAChRs of the lower esophageal sphincter be classified as M_2 (Goyal and Rattan, 1978). This distinction was subsequently adopted by investigators utilizing ligand binding techniques to study and classify the binding characteristics of specific muscarinic agonists or antagonists (Hammer and Giachetti, 1982).

Heterogeneity of mAChRs has been further investigated with radioligand binding of agonists (Birdsall et al., 1976; Birdsall et al., 1978). It was found that the binding of agonists in rat cortex was complex but could be explained by suggesting at least three subtypes of mAChRs to which agonists bind with low affinity (L), high affinity (H) and super-high affinity (SH) (Birdsall et al., 1976; Birdsall et al., 1978). Comparable results were obtained by other investigators along with evidence for regional differences in the affinities of agonists for mAChRs in brain (Ellis and Hoss, 1980). However, an alternative explanation for the heterogeneity of agonist binding was recognized, namely, that these differences could represent conformational changes that occurred with the coupling of receptors to effector mechanisms. An additional complication was the negative results obtained from experiments using muscarinic *antagonists* such as atropine, scopolamine and propylbenzilylcholine, rather than agonists; it was suggested that there was only a single class of mAChR (Yamamura and Snyder, 1974; Birdsall et al., 1976; Hulme et al., 1978). An alternative explanation for the negative results obtained with these agents, not recognized until later, was that these antagonists were simply non-selective for subtypes of the mAChR.

The possibility that some muscarinic *antagonists* were able to discriminate between subtypes of the mAChR was suggested by the finding that 4-DAMP (4 - diphenyl-acetoxy-N-methyl piperidine methiodide) showed a tenfold difference in affinity for mAChRs located in heart or ileum (Barlow et al., 1976). Subsequently, the binding profile of another muscarinic antagonist, pirenzepine, provided even stronger evidence that the mAChR may exist in several forms (Hammer et al., 1980). The binding of pirenzepine was determined indirectly from competition experiments against the non-selective muscarinic antagonists, ^{3}H-propylbenzilylcholine or ^{3}H-N-methylscopolamine. Pirenzepine displayed high affinity for sites in the cerebral cortex and hippocampus, intermediate affinity for sites in medulla-pons, salivary glands and lacrimal glands and low affinity for muscarinic binding sites in heart and smooth muscle. Heart, smooth muscle and the parotid and lacrimal glands were areas in which pirenzepine recognized a relatively uniform population of mAChRs, whereas pirenzepine binding was heterogeneous within other areas (Hammer et al., 1980). Thus, pirenzepine identified multiple binding sites both within and across different tissues. The finding of regional variation in the affinity of pirenzepine for mAChRs in brain and peripheral tissues has been repeatedly confirmed (Watson et al., 1982; Luthin and Wolfe, 1984; Giraldo et al., 1985; Watson et al., 1986). The binding profile of pirenzepine has formed the basis of initial classification of mAChRs into M_1 and M_2 subtypes which corresponded to binding sites exhibiting high and low affinity for pirenzepine, respectively (Hammer and Giachetti, 1982).

Gallamine, a neuromuscular blocking agent, has also been shown to have antimuscarinic effects at many other sites and to be a useful pharmacological tool for the study of the M_2 receptor (Riker and Wescoe, 1951; Bird and Aghajanian, 1976; Clark and Mitchelson, 1976; Ashe and Yarosh, 1984). In general, the binding profile of gallamine at the mAChR is opposite to that of pirenzepine. Gallamine has a high affinity for muscarinic sites in brainstem and cardiac muscle, and low affinity for muscarinic sites in forebrain and exocrine glands (Ellis and Hoss, 1982; Stockton et al., 1983; Price et al., 1986). Competition studies with ^{3}H-pirenzepine indicate that gallamine exhibits low and high affinity, respectively, for the M_1 and M_2 sites that are defined by the pirenzepine binding profile (Burke, 1986). However, the exact nature of gallamine binding to the mAChR is not at all clear. Binding of gallamine to mAChRs has been reported to be competitive, allosteric, or both (Ellis and Hoss, 1982; Dunlap and Brown, 1983; Stockton et al., 1983; Ellis and Lenox, 1985a; Hammer et al., 1986). Whether one observes competitive or allosteric interactions with the receptor may depend upon the antagonists used in competition studies (Ellis and Lenox, 1985b) and/or concentration factors (Dunlap and Brown, 1983; Burke, 1986). Also related to the issue of allosteric interactions are the observations that gallamine, at concentrations sufficient to block muscarinic postsynaptic potentials, results in membrane depolarization and an increase in input resistance (Yarosh et al., 1990).

Development of the M_2 muscarinic antagonist AF-DX-116 { 11-([2- [(diethylamino)methyl]-1-piperidinyl] acetyl)-5, 11-dihydro-6H-pyrido [2,3-b] [1,4] benzodiazepine-6-one } (Engel et al., 1987), a synthetic analogue of pirenzepine, has been helpful in eliminating the problems in interpretation that may be associated with gallamine, i.e., whether binding is non-competitive, competitive or allosteric. The binding profile of AF-DX 116 is nearly identical to that of gallamine, but unlike gallamine, AF-DX 116 appears to interact *only* in a *competitive* manner with the mAChR (Hammer et al., 1986); also, unlike gallamine, it has no effect upon membrane potential or input resistance (Yarosh et al., 1990).

Ligand binding studies with AF-DX 116 have provided additional evidence for the heterogeneity of mAChRs. AF-DX 116 binds with high affinity to M_2 receptors (Hammer et al., 1986). However, AF-DX 116 has a greater binding affinity for those M_2 receptors located in cardiac tissue and cerebellum than it does with those M_2 receptors in exocrine glands (Barlow and Shepherd, 1986; Hammer et al., 1986; Doods et al., 1987; Giraldo et al., 1987). Thus, it appears that the M_2 class of muscarinic receptors may be further subdivided, and that AF-DX 116 has its greatest specificity for the "cardiac-type" M_2 receptor (Barlow and Shepherd, 1986; Hammer et al., 1986; Doods, 1987; Giraldo et al., 1987; Micheletti et al., 1987). The "cardiac-type" M_2 receptor has been strongly implicated in neuron-neuron synaptic transmission (Mochida and Kobayashi, 1988; Yarosh et al., 1988).

In neocortex, autoradiographic visualization of mAChRs indicates a laminar variation in the density of the M_1 and M_2 subtypes. M_1 and M_2 receptors are found in all cortical layers; however, the M_1 receptor subtype is more concentrated in superficial layers (layers I-II), whereas the density of the M_2 subtype is greater in deeper layers (Spencer et al., 1986; Mash et al., 1988).

The physiological significance of multiple receptors for a single transmitter may very likely be that the nervous system utilizes different receptors under different operating conditions. This idea was originally explored with studies of the cholinergic responses of Renshaw cells

(Eccles et al., 1954; Curtis and Ryall, 1966a; Curtis and Ryall, 1966b) and neurons of sympathetic ganglia (Eccles and Libet, 1961; Trendelenburg, 1966; Haefely, 1974). These cells respond to released ACh with generation of fast and slow synaptic excitation mediated by nicotinic and muscarinic receptors respectively. Nicotinic receptors have been associated with fast phasic type functions, whereas muscarinic responses are associated with slow tonic functions. Thus, there appears to be a significant relationship between the nature of receptors engaged and functional outcome. One particularly exciting example of what may be an emerging general principle of receptor subtype gating of function comes from recent studies of long-term potentiation (LTP). Induction of LTP at the Schaffer collateral-commissural CA1 synapses in hippocampus by repetitive activation requires processes gated by the N-methyl-D-aspartate (NMDA) type of glutamate receptor (for reviews, see Collingridge and Bliss, 1987; Gustafsson and Wigstrom, 1988). However, the maintenance of LTP does not involve potentiation of membrane responses elicited by the direct action of glutamate at NMDA receptors (Muller et al., 1988). Rather responses to glutamate at the quisqualate type excitatory amino acid receptor are potentiated for periods of hours. Thus, it appears that the processes of *induction* and *maintenance* of LTP, although involving the same neurotransmitter, are compartmentalized and governed by the nature of the receptor. (For data and theory concerning the separation of the processes of induction and maintenance of physiological plasticity in auditory cortex during behavioral learning, see Diamond and Weinberger, 1989).

In certain regions of the hippocampus and other regions of the brain, ACh may be allowing the NMDA pathways to turn on more easily by increasing membrane resistance and slightly depolarizing the cell. Thus, ACh may not be absolutely necessary for plasticity, but may facilitate plasticity and as such would be importantly related to the *induction* rather than to the *maintenance* of plasticity. In CA3 cells, a muscarinic action of ACh suppresses the development of LTP (Williams and Johnston, 1988). However, mechanisms of induction of LTP at the mossy fiber-CA3 pyramidal cell synapse differ from those in other regions of the hippocampal formation in that NMDA receptors are not involved (Monaghan and Cotman, 1985; Harris and Cotman, 1986).

A very similar receptor-regulated separation of function is apparent in cholinergic transmission involving nicotinic and muscarinic receptors. Receptor regulated partition of function may extend beyond the nicotinic/muscarinic dichotomy to include subtypes of the muscarinic receptor. There is an abundance of evidence for muscarinic involvement in learning, and recent evidence suggests a differential involvement of mAChR subtypes. It has been suggested that functions such as memory and cognitive processes that involve the neocortex and hippocampus are mediated by M_1 receptors, and that these M_1 receptors are located postsynaptically (Cortes et al., 1986). On the other hand, the nucleus basalis region contains predominantly M_2 receptors, and it has been suggested that cortical projections from this region have presynaptic muscarinic receptors regulated by the M_2 subtype (Cortes et al., 1986). The M_1 muscarinic receptor antagonist pirenzepine induces dose-dependent deficits in passive avoidance and spatial learning in rats (Hagan et al., 1987; Hunter and Roberts, 1988; Worms et al., 1989). Unfortunately, these studies did not provide a direct comparison of subtype-selective antagonists. Thus the relative contributions of processes mediated by M_1 and M_2 receptors remain to be determined. However, studies that have measured a range of CNS effects mediated by muscarinic receptors suggest an important and possibly selective role for processes mediated by M_1 mAChRs. That is, intraventricular administration of pirenzepine was found to be fifty times more potent for blockade of one-trial passive avoidance learning than for blockade of agonist-induced (oxotremorine) hypothermia and tremor (Caulfield et al., 1983). It appears that a broader understanding of cholinergic function requires a fine grain analysis of the components of muscarinic transmission, the dynamics of these interactions, and functional significance to behavioral regulation. That is, the question is not merely to determine whether neuromodulation takes place, but to understand the functional role of neuromodulation.

Summary: Overall, the studies with antagonists support a regional difference in the ratio of M_1 to M_2 muscarinic binding sites in brain. Furthermore, it has been suggested that functions such as memory may depend more heavily upon activation of postsynaptic M_1 receptors than M_2 in neocortex and hippocampus. However, at this time it is difficult to reach any firm conclusions regarding the relative, or selective, involvement of these receptor subtypes in memory. In future experiments it will be necessary to consider the actions of pharmacological agents selective for either the M_1 or M_2 mAChR within the same experiment.

FUNCTIONAL ACTIONS OF ACh IN BRAIN

Electrophysiological approaches have been used extensively to study the actions of ACh on membrane potentials and firing rates of brain neurons. In general, the effect of exogenously applied ACh is predominantly, but not exclusively, membrane depolarization and/or acceleration of discharge rates. ACh has been reported to modify cellular activity in several cortical and subcortical areas of brain. The modulatory effects of ACh are sensitive to blockade by muscarinic antagonists, but are relatively insensitive to nicotinic antagonists, indicating that the predominant modulatory action of ACh in the brain is on mAChRs.

Exogenous Cholinergic Agonists In Vitro

The effects of exogenous cholinergic agonists on membrane potential and membrane conductance have been examined utilizing *in vitro* preparations which provide a situation appropriate for resolution of the mechanisms that underlie synaptic phenomena. Furthermore, *in vitro* studies are particularly useful for the analysis of neurotransmitter action and receptor function as they are amenable to the control of several experimental variables, particularly the concentration of agonists and antagonists delivered to the tissue.

The muscarinic actions of ACh have been studied using preparations from various brain regions including medial and lateral geniculate (McCormick and Prince, 1987), thalamic nucleus reticularis (McCormick and Prince, 1986a), nucleus parabrachialis (Egan and North, 1986), hippocampus (Ben-Ari et al., 1981; Benardo and Prince, 1981; Dodd et al., 1981; Benardo and Prince, 1982b; Segal, 1982; Cole and Nicoll, 1984b), cingulate gyrus (McCormick and Prince, 1985; McCormick and Prince, 1986b), and auditory cortex (Metherate et al., 1989b). In all of these investigations the actions of cholinergic agonists have been sensitive to blockade by non-selective muscarinic antagonists, such as atropine and scopolamine, and in some cases the differential action of selective muscarinic antagonists also has been demonstrated.

Application of ACh to neurons of guinea pig cingulate cortex results in both an initial membrane hyperpolarization and slower developing membrane depolarization (McCormick and Prince, 1985; McCormick and Prince, 1986b). These changes in membrane potential appear to be muscarinic because they can be blocked by the non-selective muscarinic antagonists atropine and scopolamine, but are unaffected by nicotinic antagonists. However, following exposure to the selective antagonist pirenzepine, only membrane hyperpolarization is observed, suggesting the block of mAChRs that produced depolarization. Thus, in cingulate cortex, muscarinic depolarization appears to be associated with an M_1 receptor subtype, and may be distinct from that subtype mediating membrane hyperpolarization. ACh-induced hyperpolarization is blocked by manipulations that either prevent synaptic transmission or reduce postsynaptic GABAergic activity, i.e., exposure to bicuculline, picrotoxin, tetrodotoxin and low Ca^{++}, and high Mn^{++}. These data were taken as an indication of the involvement of M_2 receptors located on inhibitory interneurons in the production of ACh-induced hyperpolarization, which has also been suggested to be the case for agonist-induced hyperpolarization in the dorsal lateral geniculate nucleus of the cat (McCormick and Prince, 1987; McCormick and Pape, 1988). To determine the exact nature of the mAChR involved in ACh-induced hyperpolarization, however, will require experiments that specifically consider the sensitivity of membrane hyperpolarization to M_2 antagonists such as gallamine, and especially AF-DX 116.

The results of other investigations suggest that ACh-induced hyperpolarization in the CNS may be associated with the M_2 receptor subtype. In nuclei reticularis and parabrachialis, ACh produces membrane hyperpolarization with an accompanying increase in membrane conductance which appears to be the result of an increase in K^+ conductance (Egan and North, 1986; McCormick and Prince, 1986a). Muscarinic agonists mimic ACh-induced hyperpolarization, which is blocked by non-selective muscarinic antagonists. Manipulations that block synaptic transmission fail to alter muscarinic hyperpolarization, suggesting that the cholinergic agonists exert a direct action on the neurons from which recordings are obtained. In contrast to the sensitivity of agonist-induced hyperpolarization to low concentrations of non-specific muscarinic antagonists, concentrations of pirenzepine greater than 300 nM were necessary to block muscarine-induced hyperpolarization in neurons of nucleus parabrachialis (Egan and North, 1986), and pirenzepine at concentrations as high as 100 μM did not block the ACh-induced hyperpolarization in nucleus reticularis neurons (McCormick and Prince, 1986a). These findings were interpreted as indication that activation of mAChRs of the M_2 subtype can result in hyperpolarization of CNS neurons. However, results of direct tests with M_2 antagonists have yet to be reported.

Neurons of rat and guinea-pig hippocampal formation respond to ACh and other muscarinic agonists to produce a membrane depolarization characterized by slow onset and long duration (Benardo and Prince, 1981; Dodd et al., 1981; Segal, 1982; Cole and Nicoll, 1984a; Cole and Nicoll, 1984b). Depolarization is accompanied by an increased input resistance and is antagonized by atropine (Benardo and Prince, 1981; Dodd et al., 1981; Segal, 1982; Cole and Nicoll, 1984b). Also, hyperpolarization accompanied by a decrease in resistance has been observed to precede the depolarization (Benardo and Prince, 1981; Benardo and Prince, 1982a; Benardo and Prince, 1982c; Segal, 1982), but whether the hyperpolarization is the result of the direct action of ACh on the pyramidal neurons, or whether it is due to activation of inhibitory interneurons by ACh is not clear (Benardo and Prince, 1982c; Segal, 1982). In addition, muscarinic depolarization is apparently insensitive to blockade by gallamine (Cole and Nicoll, 1984b). Slow muscarinic depolarization produced by carbachol has been reported to be sensitive to blockade by pirenzepine suggesting involvement of a mAChR of the M_1 subtype (Müller and Misgeld, 1986).

Endogenous Acetylcholine In Vitro

Although the effects of exogenous cholinergic agonists have been extensively studied in the CNS, direct investigation of the role of ACh in synaptic transmission has been more difficult. Unequivocal evidence for cholinergic mediated synaptic potentials in the brain has been reported only recently (Cole and Nicoll, 1983; Cole and Nicoll, 1984a). Electrical stimulation of afferent cholinergic fibers in the hippocampal slice, presumably derived from the medial septum, produces a slow depolarization in CA1 pyramidal neurons which meets criteria for synaptic responses (Cole and Nicoll, 1983; 1984a; 1984b). The slow depolarization is blocked by tetrodotoxin and cadmium, suggesting that it was dependent on the propagation of action potentials and calcium, and is enhanced by anticholinesterases and reduced by the muscarinic antagonist atropine, indicating an involvement of muscarinic receptors. The slow cholinergic EPSP recorded from hippocampal neurons is strikingly similar to the slow muscarinic EPSP that has been recorded in mammalian sympathetic ganglia and extensively characterized in terms of electrogenesis, pharmacology, and plasticity (Libet, 1979b; Brown and Adams, 1980; Ashe and

Libet, 1981; Ashe and Yarosh, 1984). Comparable slow EPSPs can be elicited from area CA3 pyramidal neurons (Müller and Misgeld, 1986) and dentate granule cells (Gribkoff and Ashe, 1984; Müller and Misgeld, 1986).

Although there has not been a detailed comparative examination of the action of selective muscarinic antagonists on cholinergic synaptic responses in hippocampus, the evidence to date suggests that the slow EPSP is associated with an M_1 receptor subtype. The slow EPSP of guinea pig dentate granule cells and CA3 pyramidal neurons is blocked by the M_1 antagonist pirenzepine (0.1-1μM) (Müller and Misgeld, 1986).

In addition to ACh-induced changes in resting membrane potential and synaptic potentials, muscarinic regulation of K^+ conductances serves as an important regulatory mechanism on the excitability of the neuron, e.g., the voltage dependent K^+ current termed the M-current, and the slow after hyperpolarization (AHP) elicited by a series of action potentials. However, whether muscarinic regulation of neuronal excitability occurs by way of one or more cellular effector mechanisms has not yet been resolved. The M-current is a voltage dependent muscarine sensitive K^+ current that is slowly turned on by membrane depolarization (Brown, 1988), and the AHP is a slow calcium-activated K^+ conductance that is elicited by a series of action potentials and depressed by several cholinergic agonists (Benardo and Prince, 1982c; Cole and Nicoll, 1984a; Madison et al., 1987). The M-current and AHP are both increased by afferent activity, i.e., they reduce cellular discharge. Consequently, their reduction by ACh at muscarinic receptors increases the output of cells that are activated in the presence of ACh, or the long-term consequences of activation of muscarinic receptors. Thus, ACh, acting through muscarinic receptors, can have a profound effect on cellular excitability and responses to afferent input.

Carbachol-induced suppression of the slow AHP recorded from dentate and CA3 is insensitive to pirenzepine at concentrations that are sufficient to block the muscarinic s-EPSP (Müller and Misgeld, 1986). Thus, these results indicate a differential effect of pirenzepine on muscarinic regulation of cellular excitability, and it has been proposed that the action of cholinergic agonists on the slow AHP is associated with an M_2 receptor subtype. On the other hand, it has been reported that agonist blockade of the slow AHP, recorded from CA1 pyramidal cells, is insensitive to the M_2 antagonist gallamine (Cole and Nicoll, 1984b). Whether the discrepancy in results obtained from areas CA1 and CA3 represents regional differences, or the presence of another mAChR subtype (M_3 or M_4), has yet to be clarified.

Summary: Long duration changes in membrane potential, such as those that occur via muscarinic mechanisms, may provide a substrate particularly suited for development of long-lasting changes in cellular excitability, and may account for the well-known involvement of ACh in modulation of excitability of inputs releasing other neurotransmitters and learning and memory. The involvement of muscarinic receptors in these phenomena is most likely initiated by modulation of K^+ conductances and serves as an important regulatory mechanism on the excitability of the neuron. However, the data suggest that in various regions of the CNS muscarinic responses are being mediated by subtypes of the receptor. The M_1 sites appear to be associated with a membrane depolarization that is the result of a direct activation of postsynaptic M_1 receptors, whereas there is evidence that muscarinic regulated membrane hyperpolarization may involve interceding interneurons activated by M_2 receptors.

Pharmacological Characterization: Exogenous ACh In Vivo

The predominant effect of iontophoretic or micropressure application ACh is to increase spontaneous and/or evoked discharge rate, although decreases in rate are also observed in the same studies. These data will not be discussed in the present chapter. There are several excellent reviews of this material, and the reader is refered to these sources (Dykes et al., 1988; Krnjevic, 1987, 1988).

In the auditory cortex, ACh is reported to have an excitatory effect upon both background discharges and responses to species-specific vocalizations in the awake, restrained monkey (Foote et al., 1975). More recently, we have investigated the effects of muscarinic agonists in auditory cortex. Cholinergic agents were applied to single neurons in auditory cortex of a waking cat while recording responses to controlled tones (McKenna et al., 1988). Our results indicate that neurons throughout auditory field A1 are susceptible to discharge modification by exposure to exogenous ACh or acetyl-β-methacholine (MCh), an agonist at the muscarinic receptor. These agents have the ability to produce complex, dose-dependent modification of the spontaneous discharge rate of single cortical neurons, as well as their response to activation by afferents conveying acoustic information from the environment. The complexity associated with cortical processing of acoustic information, as well as the complexity of ACh in auditory cortex, is illustrated by the observations that neither ACh nor MCh produce uniform effects on the discharge rate. Our results clearly demonstrated that the action of either ACh or MCh may result in the modification of spontaneous and evoked activity. Moreover, modification of spontaneous and evoked activity can be independent of each other within a neuron. Consequently, the relation between changes in spontaneous and evoked discharge rate is complex, and such that knowledge of the magnitude and direction of change in discharge rate of one is of little help in predicting the magnitude or direction of change of the other. Further indication of the complexity of cholinergic influence in auditory cortex are the observations that either ACh or MCh modify evoked activity in a manner more subtle than simple increase or decrease in discharge rate during an acoustic stimulus. The most pronounced effect was a modification of the short latency, brief duration "onset" response to an acoustic stimulus. The onset response was typically facilitated, and ACh or MCh were equally effective for modifying the "onset" response to an acoustic stimulus. On the other hand, neuronal discharge that immediately follows the "onset" and precedes stimulus offset, the "through" (sustained) component was more likely to be modified by MCh than ACh.

To date there have been only a few studies of the involvement of muscarinic subtypes in regulation of the discharge of cortical neurons (Bradshaw et al., 1987; Rascol and Lamour, 1988; Swanson and Phillis, 1988; Metherate et al., 1989a, in press). The effects of muscarinic antagonists have been studied on cholinoceptive cells of the parietal cortex of the rat (Bradshaw et al., 1987; Swanson and Phillis, 1988). These studies suggest that functionally different muscarinic receptors may be found at the level of the cortex, and that the complex effect of ACh is mediated, at least in part, via M_1 and M_2 muscarinic receptors. Gallamine (Swanson and Phillis, 1988) and pirenzepine (Bradshaw et al., 1987; Swanson and Phillis, 1988) both suppress cell discharge induced by iontophoretic application of muscarinic agonists. However, gallamine was found to be a more effective and consistent inhibitor of spontaneous firing than pirenzepine. Interestingly, stimulation of nucleus basalis magnocellularis (NBM) elicited both short and long latency excitations. Short latency excitations were actually enhanced by either agent, whereas long latency excitation was more effectively antagonized by gallamine than pirenzepine. These results suggest that the various muscarinic agonists studied might act through different receptor mechanisms.

ACh Modification of Sensory Cortical Receptive Fields

In sensory neocortex, the effects of ACh on receptive fields have been studied in visual, somatosensory, and auditory regions (Sillito and Kemp, 1983; Sato et al., 1987; Ashe et al., 1989; Lamour et al., 1988; McKenna et al., 1989; Metherate and Weinberger, 1989). In visual cortex of barbiturate anesthetized cats, iontophoretic application of ACh could either increase or decrease the rate of discharge evoked by receptive field stimulation with optimal stimuli. The predominant effect of ACh was to facilitate visual responses to optimal stimuli without modification of major receptive field parameters such as orientation or direction selectivity (Sillito and Kemp, 1983). However, they also reported some opposite effects of ACh. In contrast there are reports that ACh in visual cortex increases responses to both optimum and non-optimum stimuli, often accompanied by reduced selectivity (Sato et al., 1987).

In the somatosensory cortex of anesthetized cat and rat, ACh modulation of responses to cutaneous stimulation is mainly excitatory, may have persistent effects, and can reveal receptive fields not observed under control conditions (Donoghue and Carroll, 1987; Metherate et al., 1987; Lamour et al., 1988; Metherate et al., 1988a; Metherate et al., 1988b). In rat, ACh generally facilitates responses to tactile stimulation in supra- and infra-granular layers but tends to suppress responses in middle lamina (Donoghue and Carroll, 1987). It has been suggested that ACh can reduce weak sensory inputs while preserving strong inputs, possibly producing contrast effects supplementary to known lateral inhibitory effects (Donoghue and Carroll, 1987). This action could promote selective information processing.

The effects of ACh on receptive field organization have also been studied in auditory cortex in awake, rather than in anesthetized, animals (Ashe et al., 1989; McKenna et al., 1989; Metherate and Weinberger, 1989). Results suggest that the prior findings, in the anesthetized animal, are part of a larger, more complex picture for several reasons. While ACh does produce facilitation of responses to optimal receptive field stimulation, discharges may also be depressed (McKenna et al., 1988; Metherate et al., 1988a); see also (Sillito and Kemp, 1983; Sato et al., 1987). In auditory cortex, ACh can have opposite effects on different components of the response to tone within the same neuron, at the same time; e.g., depress onset responses while facilitating offset responses (McKenna et al., 1988). These results highlight the fact that the full effect of ACh is likely to be expressed over groups, or networks of neurons that may include interneurons as well as projection neurons, and complexities due to functional distinctions between muscarinic subtypes.

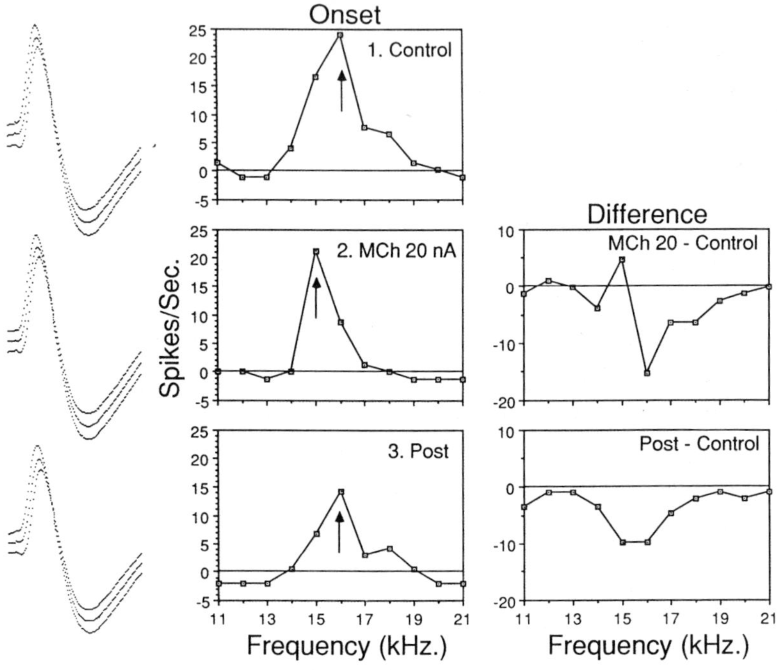

Figure 3. Shift in frequency tuning induced by muscarinic agonist. Shown are data for a single cell in primary auditory cortex of waking cat. During application of the muscarinic agonist MCh, the BF (arrow) shifts from 16.0 kHz (Control) to 15.0 kHz (MCh 20nA), with BF recovery 5 min later (Post). Difference function shows increased response to 15.0 kHz with reduced response to the original BF (16.0 kHz), higher frequencies, and small reduction at 14.0 kHz. Single unit waveforms (mean ±SD) for each period show stability throughout testing. Reprinted with permission of Alan R. Liss, Inc. from Ashe et al. (1989): Cholinergic modulation of frequency receptive fields in auditory cortex: II. Frequency-specific effect of anticholinesterases provide evidence for a modulatory action of endogenous ACh. *Synapse* 4:44-54.

Furthermore, ACh, acting via muscarinic receptors, can produce various types of systematic modifications of receptive fields. Thus, muscarinic agonists can increase or decrease frequency selectivity (i.e., "narrow" or "broaden" the bandwidth of frequency tuning). Muscarinic agonists can also alter the frequency tuning of cortical cells by *shifting the best frequency (BF)* to a previously less effective frequency (Fig. 3). This is produced by simultaneously decreasing the response to the original BF and increasing the response to the new BF. Such systematic alterations of receptive fields suggest that the facilitatory and suppressive effects of ACh reflect organized changes in the excitability of neurons within a cortical network.

ACh is known to be released in cerebral cortex under physiological conditions in unanesthetized animals (Mitchell, 1963; Jasper, 1969). Thus, it is of interest that the effects of exogenous ACh, including shifts in receptive fields, also can be produced by the application of *anticholinesterases* (Ashe et al., 1989) (Fig. 4). These findings suggest that endogenous ACh can alter the tuning of single neurons in auditory cortex, and may function in a manner analogous to that observed with exogenous ACh. All of these effects of ACh can also be produced by the muscarinic agonist MCh, and can be blocked by atropine, indicating a strong involvement of muscarinic receptors (McKenna et al., 1989). At this time, the contribution of muscarinic subtypes in sculpturing the complex effect of ACh on response patterns and shifts in tuning curves are unknown; we have begun to explore this issue (Metherate et al., 1989a).

In addition, the pairing of ACh and a single tone results in a frequency-specific change in the frequency receptive fields of single neurons in auditory cortex; the maximum change in tuning is at the frequency previously paired with ACh (Metherate and Weinberger, 1989). These findings show that the presence of increased levels of ACh at or near a cortical neuron during a period of excitation with an acoustic stimulus results in plasticity that can be specific to that stimulus. This is consistent with the possibility that cortical ACh is involved in the frequency-specific receptive field plasticity that is induced by conditioning (Diamond and Weinberger, 1986; Weinberger and Diamond, 1987). The ability of muscarinic agonists to substitute for ACh in this pairing specific effect has not yet been explored. However, the frequency-specific change in the frequency receptive field is blocked by atropine, which once again implicates muscarinic receptors.

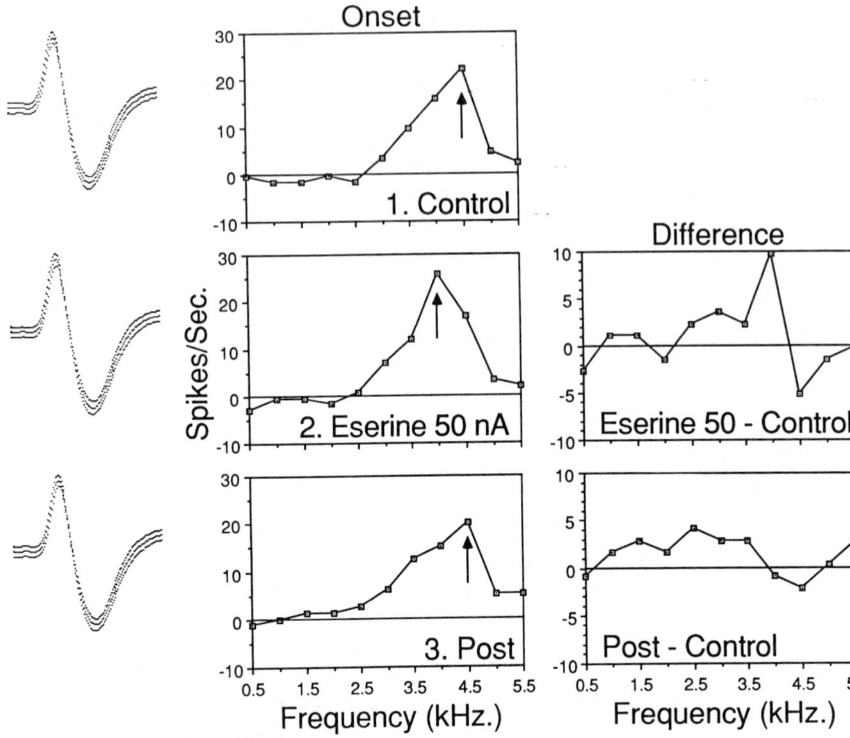

Figure 4. Shift in frequency tuning induced by an anticholinesterase. Data depicted are for a single cell in primary auditory cortex of waking cat. The cholinesterase blocker eserine produces a shift in tuning with a new best frequency, similar to that produced by muscarinic agonists (e.g., Fig. 3). The original best frequency was 4.5 kHz (Control); responses to this frequency decreased during application of the cholinesterase blocker while responses to 4.0 kHz increased to the extent that it became the new best frequency (Eserine 50 nA). Recovery was observed 3 min later (Post). Difference function shows eserine increased response to 4.0 kHz (BF during drug) and decreased response to the original BF. Corresponding single unit waveforms (mean ± SD) show no change during application of eserine. Reprinted with permission of Alan R. Liss, Inc. from Ashe et al. (1989): Cholinergic modulation of frequency receptive fields in auditory cortex: II. Frequency-specific effect of anticholinesterases provide evidence for a modulatory action of endogenous ACh. *Synapse* 4:44-54.

Summary: Muscarinic agonists and anticholinesterases can facilitate responses to sensory stimuli, and can also produce response suppression. Simultaneous opposite effects can result in a *shift* of tuning to a new best frequency. The effects of muscarinic agonists cannot, therefore, be viewed as simply facilitatory or as simply increasing "signal-to-noise." Rather, it seems likely that a comprehensive understanding must await parametric studies in which the interactions of (a) concentration of agonist, (b) stimulus intensity and (c) stimulus frequency are completely determined. The findings of increased and decreased response within the same neuron for (a) spontaneous vs. evoked activity, (b) different components of evoked, or (c) different frequencies may be related to previous reports (see above) that ACh, acting at muscarinic receptors, can hyperpolarize or depolarize the membrane potential; these effects are atropine-sensitive, suggesting mediation by muscarinic receptors.

Acetylcholine in Cortical Plasticity and Learning

Several lines of evidence suggest an important role for ACh in cortical plasticity involved in learning. At the psychological level, cholinomimetics and antagonists modify learning and memory in a variety of tasks and species (for reviews, see Deutsch and Rogers, 1979; Gold and Zornetzer, 1983; McDonough and Penetar, 1983). Furthermore, experimentally-produced deficits of learning and memory following lesions of the nucleus basalis can be reversed by systemic administration of the anticholinesterase physostigmine (Murray and Fibiger, 1985). Concern regarding the function of ACh in the cerebral cortex has intensified with the finding that Alzheimer's disease appears to critically involve a significant reduction in cortical ACh (Collerton, 1986). Several laboratories have reported major effects of ACh in cortical plasticity as related to major learning paradigms, e.g., classical conditioning. For example, classical conditioning procedures are reported to increase the excitability in neurons projecting to facial musculature involved in eyeblink or nose-twitch conditioned responses in the cat (Woody, 1988). Application of ACh to the relevant cortical area also results in an atropine-sensitive increase in neuronal excitability which appears to be a consequence of increased membrane resistance (Woody et al., 1978; Swartz and Woody, 1979).

In somatosensory cortex of the rabbit, acquisition of a classically-conditioned flexion response is accompanied by an increased sensitivity of neurons to ACh and subsequent extinction of the conditioned response is correlated with a decreased effect of ACh applied to involved neurons

(Koshtoyants et al., 1981). During conditioning, the effects of an aversive unconditioned stimulus on neocortex may be mediated by endogenously released ACh. Thus, sequential pairing of an acoustic CS followed by direct application of ACh produces cellular discharge plasticity in which the effect of ACh "...is comparable to that of a natural electrodermal unconditioned stimulus" (Kopytova et al., 1981). Similar effects have been found for instrumental conditioning (Andrianov, 1982).

Physiological plasticity in the frontal cortex of the anesthetized rat during conditioning also appears to depend on the presence of cortical ACh. Thus, learning-induced event-related slow potentials, which are components of the electroencephalogram, requires intact input from the nucleus basalis (Pirch et al., 1986). Associatively-induced plasticity at the level of single neurons also involves cortical ACh: (i) local application of atropine suppresses neuronal conditioned responses, (ii) kainic acid lesions of the nucleus basalis cause a decrease in the probability of obtaining such plasticity, and (iii) nucleus basalis neurons exhibit conditioned changes in discharge rate (Rigdon and Pirch, 1988).

In summary, behavioral, physiological and pharmacological evidence implicates cortical acetylcholine in physiological plasticity and learning.

A MODEL OF MUSCARINIC FUNCTION IN RECEPTIVE FIELD PLASTICITY

In the previous sections, we have summarized evidence that ACh, acting on mAChRs within the auditory cortex, modulates the processing of acoustic information. Further, the modulatory action of ACh appears to be highly specific. Rather than simply producing a general change in the responses of cells to auditory stimuli, muscarinic agonists change the detailed patterning of responses and can produce systematic shifts in the receptive fields for frequency information; that is, appropriate activation of mAChRs can "retune" cortical neurons. That these specific and pronounced modulatory effects of ACh occur endogenously is supported by the observations that agents that block acetylcholinesterase produce changes similar to those obtained with exogenous application of muscarinic agonists.

Plasticity of receptive fields induced by cholinergic agents bears a striking resemblance to the systematic modifications of receptive fields which develop in auditory cortex during learning, as when an auditory stimulus is used as a signal in classical conditioning (Diamond and Weinberger, 1986; Weinberger and Diamond, 1987; Diamond and Weinberger, 1989).

The combined findings with agents that modify cholinergic transmission and learning suggest that ACh may play an important role in learning. In order to integrate these findings and to provide a framework to both encourage and guide future research into the modulatory actions of neurotransmitters in sensory cortical plasticity, we have formulated a preliminary model of receptive field plasticity. At this juncture, we provide a brief review of the relevant findings from our studies of learning in the auditory system followed by a succinct description of the model. A more detailed account of this model has been discussed elsewhere (Weinberger et al., 1990a; Weinberger et al., 1990b).

Learning-Induced Physiological Plasticity in the Auditory System

In order to determine if the actual neurophysiological coding of stimuli is altered by its acquired signal value, we first had to develop a behavioral preparation in which (a) the stimulus is controlled at the receptor level, (b) sensory feedback from learned responses cannot influence the relevant neuronal activity, (c) validation of acquired signal value is provided behaviorally, and (d) sensory neuronal responses can be recorded continually without artifact during the acquisition phase of learning. All of these criteria were satisfied by recording the pupillary dilation conditioned response in cats under neuromuscular blockade. This CR exhibits all of the major features of other conditioned responses. Of particular interest and advantage, acquisition is extremely rapid, consistent conditioned responses being present in 5-10 trials and asymptote in 20-30 trials. This is sufficiently rapid to permit simultaneous recording of single neuron discharges during acquisition, even after a preceding sensitization control phase. These behavioral findings have been replicated repeatedly over the past 15 years (Oleson et al., 1972; Oleson et al., 1973; Weinberger et al., 1973; Oleson et al., 1975; Weinberger et al., 1975; Ashe et al., 1978a; Ashe et al., 1978b; Cooper et al., 1978; Ryugo and Weinberger, 1978; Weinberger et al., 1984; Diamond and Weinberger, 1986; Diamond and Weinberger, 1989).

Following these behavioral experiments which established that pupillary conditioning obeys the same descriptive laws as do other conditioned responses, we performed studies in which neurophysiological responses to acoustic conditioned stimuli were recorded at various levels of the auditory system during conditioning.

Lack of Plasticity in the Cochlea: The receptor potential (cochlear microphonic) is unaffected by learning at the same time that behavioral learning (pupillary dilation) develops (Ashe et al., 1975). Thus, descending peripheral gating of auditory information does not appear to be involved, and these results supported the conclusion that plasticity in auditory cortex and thalamus is endogenous.

Acquisition, Discrimination and Retention of Plasticity: Primary auditory cortex rapidly develops discharge plasticity, as recorded in the discharges of neuronal clusters, to the conditioned stimulus during simple acquisition, two-tone discrimination, and discrimination reversal. Retention of frequency discrimination in the auditory cortex was obtained for seven days, the longest period tested (Oleson et al., 1975). More recent studies in which continual recordings were obtained from one neuron per training session replicated and extended the findings, showing extremely rapid development of discharge plasticity (e.g., 10-20 trials) (Diamond and Weinberger, 1984; Weinberger, et al., 1984).

Differential Plasticity in the Thalamic Auditory System: The obligatory thalamic gateway to the auditory cortex contains morphologically-distinct nuclei in which two functions are compartmentalized; the lemniscal, ventral medial geniculate nucleus (MGv) is tonotopically-organized and provides precise information to restricted areas of auditory cortex. In contrast, the magnocellular medial geniculate nucleus (MGm) is not tonotopic and provides diffuse input to upper and lower lamina of all auditory cortical fields. By recording from neuronal "clusters" simultaneously in both nuclei, we discovered a parallel difference in plasticity: the MGv exhibits no change in discharges to a CS during learning; in contrast, the MGm rapidly develops physiological plasticity during conditioning (Ryugo and Weinberger, 1978). These findings were again extended to single neurons, revealing associatively-induced plasticity in as few as 3-5 trials (Weinberger, 1982).

Long Term Potentiation in MGm: To further characterize possible loci of plasticity, we studied long-term potentiation (LTP, previously found only in hippocampus) in the medial geniculate. We found LTP (field potential) in the MGm (Gerren and Weinberger, 1983). Moreover, we extended these studies to the level of single cells and discovered that the field potential LTP was based on reduced latency of discharge, greater number of spikes per test stimulus, and less temporal variability (Weinberger, 1982). These effects lasted as long as recording was continued, up to an hour.

CS-Specific Receptive Field Plasticity: The transformations of information processing due to learning cannot be studied by using only the CS or a small number of different stimuli. Thus, we combined approaches from two fields of study, sensory physiology and the neurophysiology of learning. We determined the effects of learning on the frequency receptive fields (RF) of single neurons (one cell per training session) before and after various phases of classical conditioning in cats under neuromuscular blockade. We discovered that learning-induced plasticity to the CS in secondary and ventral ectosylvian auditory fields of the cat actually reflects a highly specific change in the frequency receptive fields of single neurons—the greatest effect is at the frequency of the conditioned stimulus. Furthermore, the receptive fields are stable in the absence of conditioning, and the changes in receptive fields are maintained unless the behavioral learning is altered by extinction, in which case the neural changes also revert to pre-conditioning status. These effects were found both for narrowly and broadly-tuned cells (Diamond and Weinberger, 1986; Diamond and Weinberger, 1989).

Receptive Field Plasticity in Primary Auditory Cortex: In order to determine the degree of generality of associatively-induced frequency-specific plasticity of receptive fields, studies were extended to waking, undrugged adult guinea pigs. Recordings were obtained from primary, tonotopic auditory fields. We found that classical conditioning induced facilitation at the frequency of the CS, usually with a simultaneous decrease in response to one or more adjacent frequencies. Moreover, these specific changes in frequency RF could be so large that conditioning produced a new best frequency, that of the conditioned stimulus (Figs. 5 and 6).

Thus, CS-specific RF plasticity is general over orders of mammals, type of preparation (undrugged vs. muscle-blocked) and type of auditory cortex (primary vs. secondary).

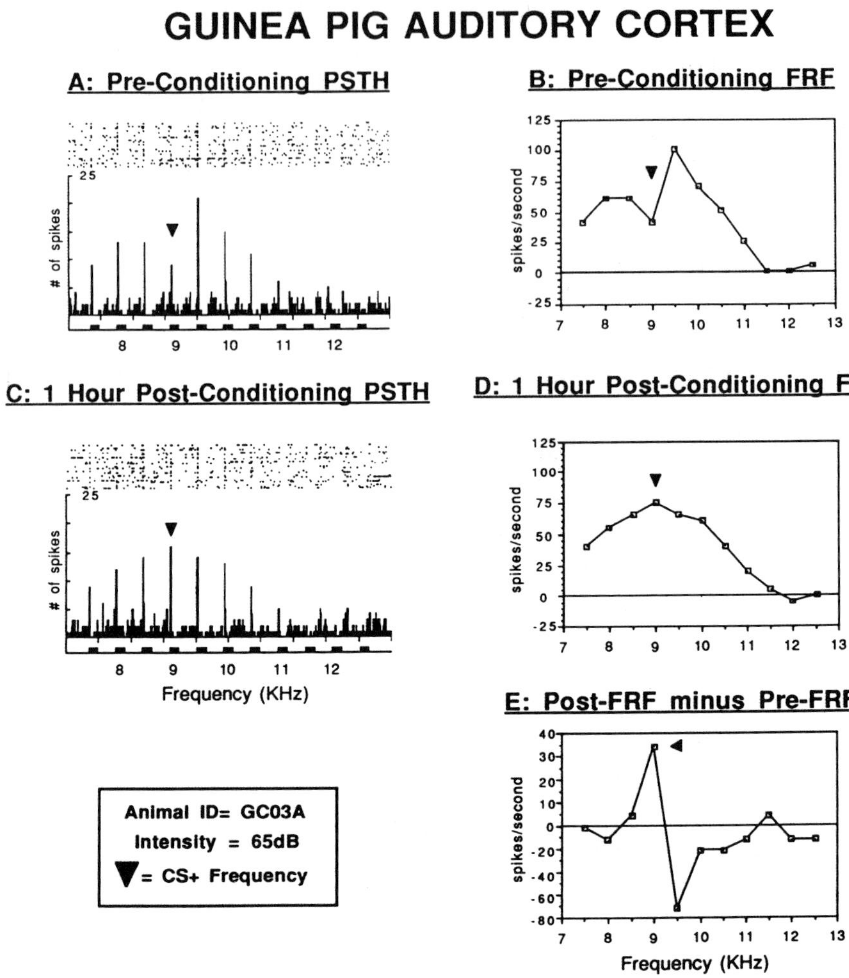

Figure 5. CS-Specific Receptive Field Plasticity in Guinea Pig. Post stimulus time histograms (PSTH) A, before and C, 1 hour after classical conditioning using 9.0 kHz (arrowhead) as the CS; corresponding quantified frequency response at 65db, B and D, respectively. The BF before conditioning was 9.5 kHz, the BF after conditioning was the CS frequency. E, effect of training (difference function); note the increased response to the CS frequency and decreased responses to the previous BF and, to a lesser extent, adjacent higher frequencies. Reprinted with permission of World Scientific Publishing Co. from Weinberger N.M. et al. (1990a): Retuning auditory cortex by learning: a preliminary model of receptive field plasticity. *Concepts in Neuroscience*, vol. 1, no. 1.

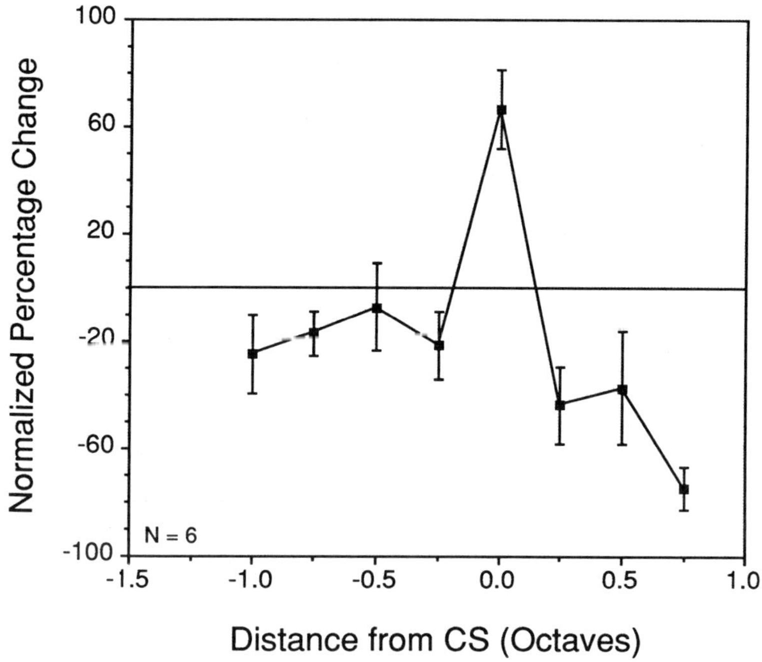

Figure 6. Group data for CS-specific receptive field plasticity in the guinea pig anterior tonotopic field. Group mean (±SE) normalized change in frequency response due to conditioning, expressed as distance from CS frequency (octaves). Note facilitation at CS frequency and decreased response at several other frequencies. Side-band suppression may be limited to frequencies lower or higher than the frequency of the CS within an animal (e.g., see Fig. 5) accounting for higher variance at side-bands. The basis for greatest reduction of side-band responses to frequencies higher than the CS frequency is currently unknown. Reprinted with permission of World Scientific Publishing Co. from Weinberger N.M. et al. (1990a): Retuning auditory cortex by learning: a preliminary model of receptive field plasticity. *Concepts in Neuroscience*, vol. 1, no. 1.

A Model of Adaptive Information Processing in Auditory Cortex

Although theoretical developments would benefit from additional neurobiological data, there are now a very large number of separate neuroanatomical, neurophysiological, neuropharmacological and behavioral findings relevant to cortical plasticity and information processing. It is an appropriate time to initiate attempts to relate these data to each other. Our model, preliminary as it is, provides a basis for formulating theory-driven experiments. It should have heuristic value regardless of the fate of our particular current hypotheses.

Components of the Model: The core of the model is that physiological plasticity in auditory cortex results from the coordinated action of *three systems*, each unique but complementary. These systems are characterized with respect to two dimensions: (1) degree of specificity of auditory information conveyed, and (2) extent of physiological plasticity during learning. Each system has a root nucleus that is the basis of its projection to auditory cortex (Fig. 7).

VENTRAL MEDIAL GENICULATE NUCLEUS: AUDITORY-LEMNISCAL, PRECISE PROJECTION TO AUDITORY CORTEX, NON-PLASTIC: This system projects precise information about the physical parameters of sound to auditory cortex in a point-to-point, tonotopic manner. Several laboratories have consistently failed to obtain discharge plasticity in the MGv (Weinberger and Diamond, 1987).

MAGNOCELLULAR MEDIAL GENICULATE NUCLEUS: AUDITORY-NONLEMNISCAL, DIFFUSE PROJECTIONS TO AUDITORY CORTEX, PLASTIC: This system is concerned with information about the acquired significance of acoustic stimuli, but not about the precise physical parameters of sound. Its neurons are broadly tuned to frequency, and are bimodal, i.e., respond to somatosensory or noxious input as well as auditory input (Poggio and Mountcastle, 1960; Erickson et al., 1964; Wepsic, 1966; Lund and Webster, 1967). This is likely to be the basis for CS-UCS convergence and associative plasticity in the MGm. It is not definitely known whether plasticity in the MGm is purely local or "projected" to this nucleus, but MGm input to auditory cortex must reflect the discharge plasticity that rapidly develops in response to the CS during conditioning. The MGm projects diffusely to all auditory cortical fields (Winer et al., 1977). Replicable findings from several laboratories demonstrate that the MGm does develop discharge plasticity during classical conditioning (Weinberger and Diamond, 1987).

NUCLEUS BASALIS OF MEYNERT: NON-AUDITORY, CHOLINERGIC PROJECTIONS TO THE CEREBRAL CORTEX: Neurons in the NBM respond to sensory stimulation in behaving animals, but they are polymodal and definitely

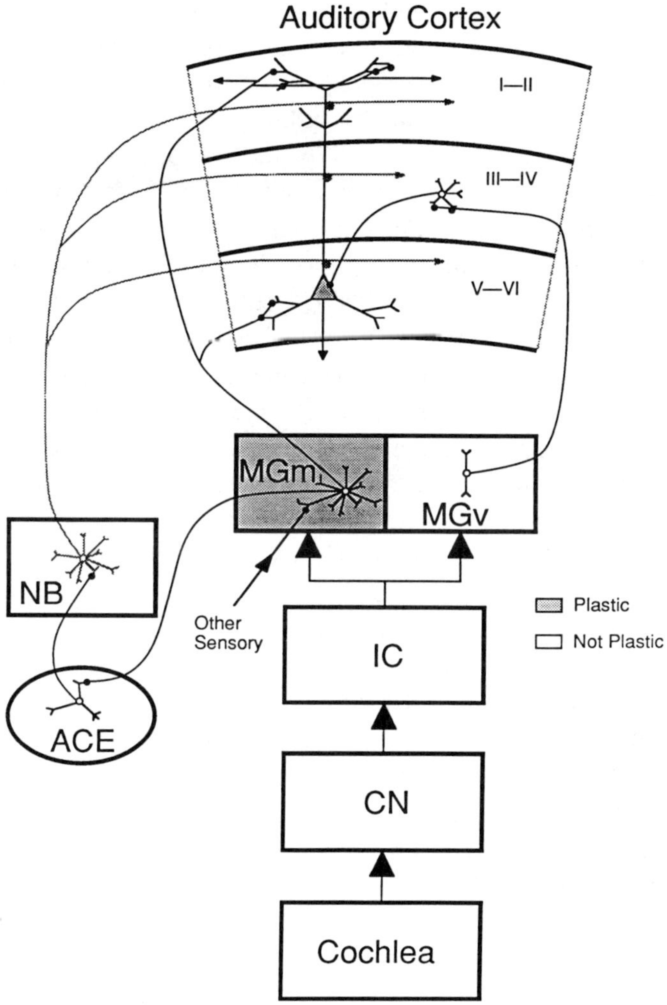

Figure 7. Schematic representation of the model for adaptive information processing in auditory cortex. Shown are the major components of the model, a greatly abbreviated diagram of the lower auditory system, and their interconnections—not to scale. Abbreviations: ACE, central nucleus of amygdala; CN, cochlear nucleus; IC, inferior colliculus; MGm, magnocellular medial geniculate nucleus; MGv, ventral medial geniculate nucleus; NB, nucleus basalis of Meynert. Roman numerals refer to cortical laminar zones. Grey tone indicates probable site of local plasticity. Reprinted with permission of World Scientific Publishing Co. from Weinberger, N.M. et al. (1990a): Retuning auditory cortex by learning: a preliminary model of receptive field plasticity. *Concepts in Neuroscience*, vol. 1, no. 1.

are not restricted to acoustic stimuli (Richardson et al., 1988). Its cortical projections are global, extend across most of the cortical mantle and are not confined to auditory cortex. NBM neurons appear to develop discharge plasticity during learning although the data are not extensive (Burton et al., 1976; Mora et al., 1976; Rolls et al., 1979).

The full consequences of the neuromodulatory action of muscarinic responses in auditory cortex must be considered in the context of cortical anatomy. It appears that the majority of cholinergic synapses are located on the dendritic shafts of pyramidal (P) cells (Houser et al., 1985) such that an ACh-induced increase in input resistance would be to increase the time and space constants of P cells (Shepherd, 1988). Thus, other synaptic inputs would be integrated over a longer time, providing additional opportunity for temporal summation. Also, a given synaptic input would produce a larger voltage change in the postsynaptic target following ACh-induced increased input resistance. Therefore, ACh could "amplify" the effects of MGm input on distal dendrites, increasing its influence on the probability of discharge of a P cell.

As discussed above, ACh can increase and decrease responses within the same neuron such that there are differential effects on spontaneous versus evoked activity and different components of evoked activity. Recent intracellular data from our laboratories indicate that ACh and MCh can modify the excitability of neurons of guinea pig auditory cortex maintained *in vitro* (Metherate et al., 1989b). Fig. 8 illustrates the finding that application of MCh can result in an increase in input resistance with an accompanying long latency, long duration membrane depolarization. These effects, as well as similar effects produced by ACh, are mediated by muscarinic receptors as they are readily blocked by atropine. Membrane depolarization occurs in the majority of cells exposed to ACh or MCh. However, in several cells we have observed that a substantial change in input resistance can occur without any change in membrane potential, indicating that these two events may not be tightly coupled. Also, in preliminary studies we have found that ACh can facilitate responses elicited by iontophoretic application of glutamate.

AUDITORY CORTEX: At this time, there is no conclusive evidence as to the cortical cell types that develop associative plasticity. Pyramidal cells are likely to be some if not all of this population because the laminar

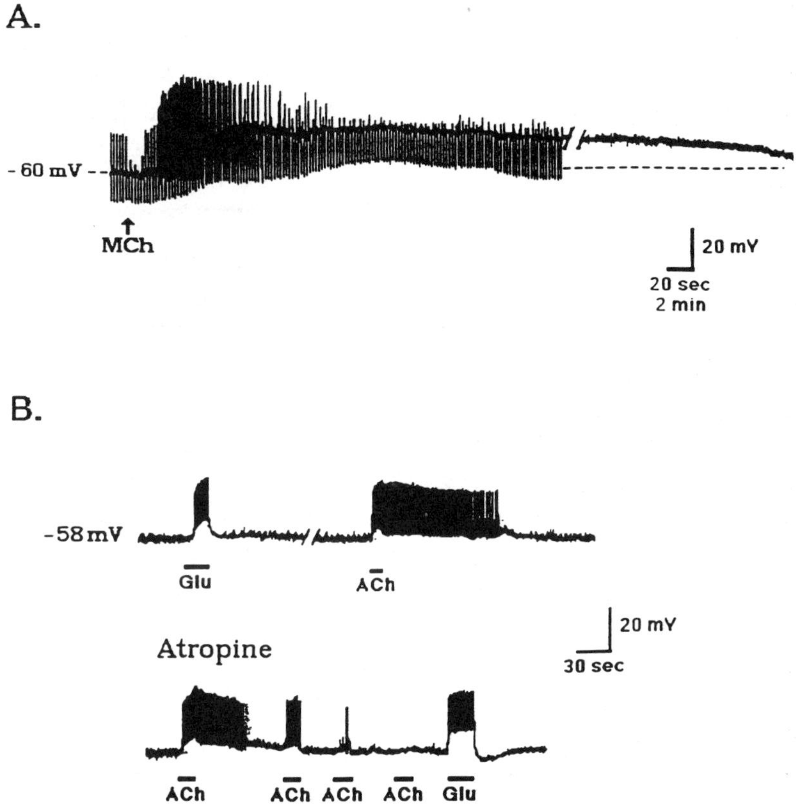

Figure 8. Intracellular recordings of the effect of muscarinic agonists on membrane potential of guinea pig auditory cortex neurons *in vitro*. A: Application of MCh, by microdrop (at arrowhead: 0.5 μl of 0.4M) depolarized the membrane potential and modified the responses to constant current (0.4 nA, 200 msec), hyperpolarizing transmembrane pulses indicating an increase in input resistance (transient negative-going deflections of the membrane potential). [Positive-going transient deflections that occur before MCh are off-spikes produced by the current pulses.] MCh-induced depolarization elicited firing of the cell which is intermixed with off-spikes elicited by the current pulses. B: The effect of atropine on membrane depolarization produced by iontophoretic application of glutamate (100 nA) and ACh (50 nA). Upper trace: Responses before atropine. Lower trace: Responses obtained following microdrop application of atropine (0.3 μl of 0.1mM) which was given at the beginning of the trace. Note gradual reduction in the amplitude of membrane depolarization elicited by ACh. In contrast, membrane depolarization elicited by glutamate is not reduced. Reprinted with permission of World Scientific Co. from Weinberger, N.M. et al. (1990a): Retuning auditory cortex by learning: a preliminary model of receptive field plasticity. *Concepts in Neuroscience*, vol. 1, no. 1.

distribution of plasticity is consistent with pyramidal cell involvement (Diamond and Weinberger, 1984) and microelectrode recordings are heavily biased toward largest neurons, i.e., P cells. These data are only suggestive and correlative anatomical-physiological studies of plasticity in cortex are needed.

AMYGDALA: A link between conditioning-dependent plasticity in the magnocellular medial geniculate body and the nucleus basalis may be provided via the central nucleus of the amygdala (ACE). Several lines of evidence are consistent with this possibility. First, the MGm projects to the ACE (Kapp et al., 1984; LeDoux et al., 1985). Second, amygdala-dependent behavioral conditioned responses to acoustic (but not visual) stimuli are abolished by lesions of the MGm (LeDoux et al., 1984; Jarrell et al., 1986a; Jarrell et al., 1986b). Third, lesions of auditory cortex do not alter such conditioned responses (LeDoux et al., 1984). Fourth, the ACE projects to the NBM (Krettek and Price, 1978; Price and Amaral, 1981; Russchen et al., 1985). Fifth, neurons in the NBM respond selectively to stimuli (conditioned stimuli or unconditioned stimuli) that activate ACE cells (DeLong, 1971; Burton et al., 1976; Mora et al., 1976; Richardson, et al., 1988). Therefore, learning-induced changes in response to acoustic stimuli in the MGm may produce changes in NBM discharge via the amygdala.

Modification of Synaptic Strengths: Given the foregoing, we propose that the frequency-specific information provided by the MGv to pyramidal cells is modulated by the auditory-significant information provided by the MGm. From this point of view, the pyramidal cells of auditory cortex are the first neurons in which information about both the frequency and the acquired signal value or significance of the same stimulus come together.

During classical conditioning, the MGv output to the cortex does not change because neurons in this lemniscal nucleus do not develop discharge plasticity. However, as discussed below, the synaptic strengths of MGv effects on pyramidal neurons are modified during learning; inputs that carry CS frequency information are strengthened, while non-active inputs (those for other frequencies not presented as the CS) are weakened.

The MGm excitatory effects on pyramidal cells should increase across trials since neurons in this nucleus do develop physiological plasticity during conditioning.

The NBM is hypothesized to play a critical role in amplifying the MGm effects to induce long-term changes in synaptic strengths. That is, by releasing ACh in the auditory cortex, the NBM serves as the "record now" mechanism for long term memory. This increased release of ACh is presumably due to the conditioned increase in MGm discharge via the MGm → amygdala → NBM circuit. Evidence that is consistent with this schema is that NBM neurons appear to increase their discharge to stimuli having motivational significance (Richardson et al., 1988).

Such NBM action could also be accomplished by other influences. For example, since learning is not limited to a pulse of experience for a single modality, other sensory input to the amygdala could promote information storage of auditory input. Similarly, a significant auditory stimulus could incite the NBM to release ACh so that any or all other sensory inputs currently being processed in the cerebral cortex are stored. Further, the "contents" of non-sensory regions of the cortex could be stored as a consequence of the global release of ACh, wherever it acts on muscarinic receptors. Changes in synaptic strengths are hypothesized to depend on two modified Hebbian rules (Baranyi and Szente, 1988; Frégnac et al., 1988; Gustafsson and Wigstrom, 1988; Reiter and Stryker, 1988).

(I) If the postsynaptic cell is active when pre-synaptic input is present then synaptic strength is *increased.*

(II) If the postsynaptic cell is active when pre-synaptic input is absent then synaptic strength is *weakened.* The term "active" refers to a state of increased excitability, not restricted to cellular discharge.

We add one corollary: the amount of change in synaptic strength is directly proportional to the degree of postsynaptic excitability.

Sequence of Events: The acquisition of information about the physical parameters and the behavioral significance of an acoustic stimulus, including CS-specific changes in frequency receptive fields, could come about as follows.

(a) The *MGv* specifies the physical (e.g., frequency) parameters, providing such information to pyramidal cells (and others not considered here) whose current receptive field includes the frequency of the conditioned stimulus. Output of the MGv to the auditory cortex is not changed during learning but its effect on pyramidal cells is changed.

(b) The *MGm* specifies the importance of the stimulus. The first neural change during conditioning is hypothesized to be the induction of plasticity due to convergence of CS and UCS inputs in this nucleus. Effectively, its output message to the auditory cortex is the equivalent of the presence of the UCS) moved up in time so that it coincides with the presence of the CS rather than with the presence of the UCS. In short, the MGm mechanism converts a non-auditory UCS which occurs following the CS into an auditory-coded representation of the anticipated UCS. The auditory modality-specific nature of the MGm means that there is a general increase in pyramidal cell excitability within and between all auditory cortical fields; our concern at this point is with primary tonotopic auditory cortex.

There is convergence of the MGv input (from neurons responding to the frequency of the conditioned stimulus) with the MGm increase in excitability. Convergence occurs only for a subset of auditory cortical pyramidal cells, that is, for those neurons that receive input from the CS frequency. Presynaptic inputs initiated either indirectly via stellate cells or directly from the MGv will be strengthened, according to Rule (I). In contrast, by Rule (II) all other presynaptic inputs, for frequencies not present as the conditioned stimulus, will be weakened (Fig. 9).

However, by themselves, MGm inputs are likely to produce only a small increase in pyramidal cell excitability because of their distal location on dendrites, as explained above. Corollary (A) suggests that an amplification of the MGm effect would produce larger changes in the synapses that are concerned with frequency information. We suggest that the role of ACh is to amplify the MGm effects.

(c) The *nucleus basalis of Meynert facilitates* synaptic transmission in auditory cortex. The full consequences of the neuromodulatory action of responses mediated by mAChRs in the auditory cortex must be considered in the context of cortical anatomy. As pointed out previously, the majority of cholinergic synapses appear to be located on the dendritic shafts of pyramidal cells (Houser et al., 1985) such that an ACh-induced increase in input resistance would be to increase the time and space constants of pyramidal cells (Shepherd, 1988). Thus, other synaptic inputs would be integrated over a longer time, providing additional opportunity for temporal summation. Furthermore, a given synaptic input would produce a larger voltage change in the post-synaptic target following ACh-induced increased input resistance. Thus, ACh could "amplify" the effects of MGm input on distal dendrites, increasing its excitatory effects on pyramidal cells.

The model suggests that the NBM provides a cascade of modulation. That is, the NBM increases release of ACh in response to the plasticity that is rapidly expressed in the magnocellular medial geniculate nucleus during conditioning. This occurs via the amygdala, which is "driven" by the MGm. This release of ACh in the auditory cortex would produce increased input resistance, including effects on the dendrites of pyramidal cells. As pointed out above, increased input resistance would produce an increase in the time constant and effectively increase the length constant of the target neurons. Consequently, weak excitatory MGm inputs would be amplified. Thus, the MGm input to pyramidal cell dendrites would increase post-synaptic excitability and thus provide the basis for changing the strength of inputs concerned with frequency information.

The role of the NBM and cortical ACh is also hypothesized to provide for long-term effects of learning. Muscarinic actions of ACh have been implicated in intracellular and membrane changes that could serve as bases for long-term alterations in excitability (Libet, Kobayashi and Tanaka, 1975; Brown and Adams, 1987; Dutar and Nicoll, 1988b; Libet et al., 1975). A large number of reviews have provided evidence for such changes in long-term synaptic plasticity and learning (e.g., Hawkins and Kandel, 1984; Lynch, 1986; Alkon, 1988; Disterhoft et al., 1988; Nelson and Routtenberg, 1988; Woody, 1988).

Effects whose duration lasts minutes would likely alter the responses of target neurons (i.e., pyramidal cells) to acoustic input on subsequent trials. The putative role of ACh is of particular importance in this regard because of the hypothesized sequence of events within a learning experience, e.g., conditioning trial. According to the model, the mobilization of the nucleus basalis and subsequent release of ACh would take place following increased discharges in the magnocellular medial geniculate nucleus. Therefore, on the first trial in which this occurs, the release of ACh would likely occur shortly after the output of the MGm reaches the auditory cortex; consequently, the increased ACh release may not be particularly effective in facilitating MGm effects on target cells on that trial. But long-term effects of ACh acting at muscarinic synapses could provide an altered state of the target neurons so that MGm actions on subsequent trials would be facilitated.

Predictions: The model at this stage is clearly preliminary and oversimplified. A discussion of its omissions and other problems has been presented elsewhere (Weinberger et al., 1990a; Weinberger et al., 1990b) and the interested reader may consult those publications. For present purposes it is sufficient to simply state that we believe that the model captures an essential feature – that the basis for sensory (and perhaps other) cortical plasticity requires the convergence of *three* types of systems: (1) sensory (stimulus) specific, (2) sensory-adjunct (plastic) and (3) neuromodulatory (i.e., ACh based on the basal forebrain cholinergic system).

Certain predictions follow from the model. We present two major predictions here, for heuristic purposes.

First, impairment of any one of the three systems, e.g., by lesions of the MGv, MGm, or NBM, will interfere with receptive field plasticity during learning. The type of degradation would be expected to depend

---

Figure 9. Schematic representation of hypothesized changes in synaptic strengths due to classical conditioning. Depicted is a pyramidal cell in primary auditory cortex that receives lemniscal frequency input from the ventral medial geniculate nucleus (MGv); inputs from three frequencies ("1,2,3") that converge on this cell are shown, synapsing on the shaft of the apical dendrite. Also converging on this cell are connections from the magnocellular medial geniculate nucleus (MGm) to the distal apical dendrites in cortical layer I (and also the basilar dendrites), and afferents from the basal nucleus of Meynert (NBM) to the apical dendritic shaft. The synapses from the MGv are represented by filled circles of various sizes, with synaptic strengths proportional to their diameters. The "best frequency" (BF) is that frequency having the greatest synaptic strength for a cell. **Top:** Preconditioning situation, in which the order of synaptic strengths of frequency input is 3>2>1. **Bottom:** Postconditioning situation, following classical conditioning in which frequency #2 had been employed as the conditioned stimulus ("CS"). The effects of classical conditioning are shown as if synaptic strengths for the frequency used as the CS were incremented by two arbitrary units (dot diameters) while synaptic strengths to the other frequencies (i.e., #1 and #3) were decreased by one unit. Post-conditioning, the order of synaptic strengths has changed to 2>3>1. Note that the best frequency of this cell was altered from frequency #3 to frequency #2. These changes would produce organized receptive field effects due to associative learning, i.e., increased response to the CS frequency and decreased responses to adjacent frequencies. Reprinted with permission of World Scientific Publishing Co. from Weinberger, N.M. et al. (1990a): Retuning auditory cortex by learning: a preliminary model of receptive field plasticity. *Concepts in Neuroscience*, vol. 1, no. 1. *See page 227*

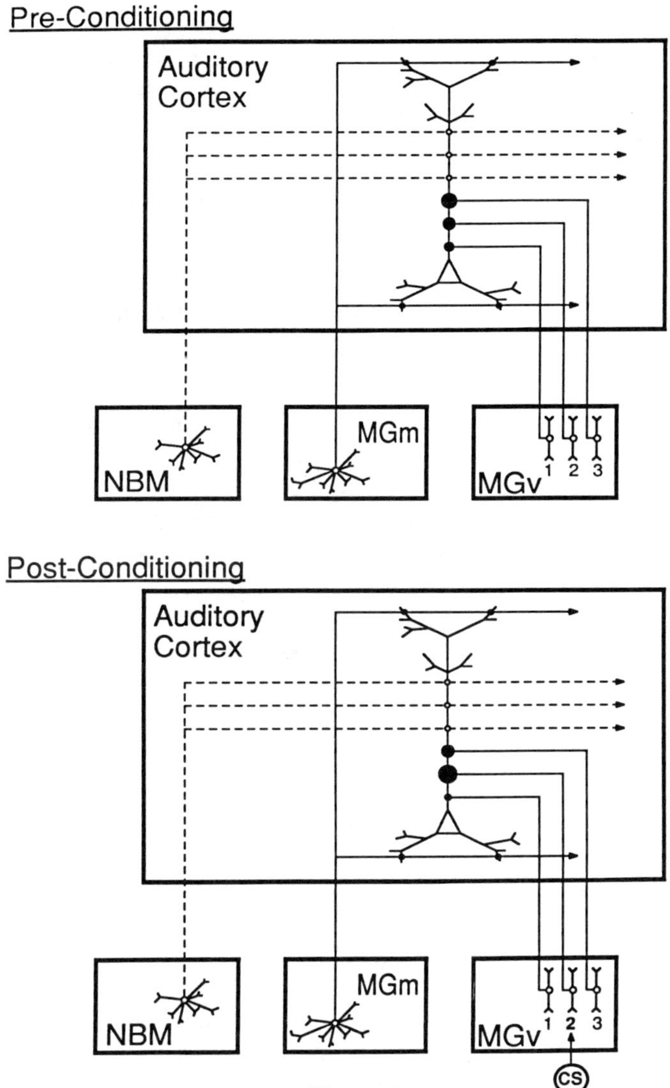

Figure 9.

upon which system is impacted. For example, lesions of the BFCS are likely to prevent long-term plasticity of receptive fields. Destruction of the MGv should prevent precise frequency information from reaching the auditory cortex so that frequency-selectivity may be precluded altogether. MGm lesions should prevent plasticity both because of direct effects of MGm influences at the cortex and because of indirect effects due to inability of acoustic meaning to trigger the BFCS via the amygdala.

Direct tests are possible by means of the various techniques available to produce lesions. Additionally, impairment of the BFCS influence on the auditory cortex may be accomplished by the direct application of anticholinergic agents to the auditory cortex, including specific blockers of mAChR, e.g., M_1 and M_2 receptors.

Second, frequency representation across primary auditory cortex should be changed by learning. Specifically, the frequency map should show an increase in the number of neurons (and thus the amount of cortical area) for which the best frequency is the frequency used as the conditioned stimulus. Because of the need to obtain data from the entire frequency representation, a test of this prediction will be very difficult. Perhaps newer techniques for imaging entire cortical areas can be applied to this problem.

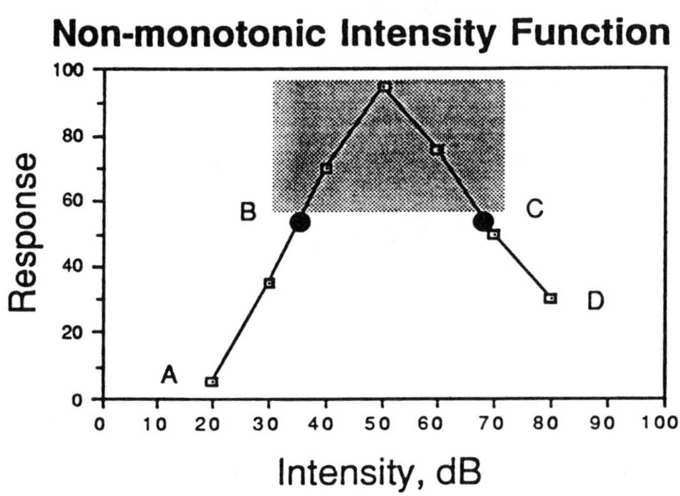

Figure 10. A schematic non-monotonic intensity function for a single neuron. The effects of increasing intensity depend upon the "location" of the neuron on its intensity function. For example, an acoustic stimulus of 35 db would elicit responses of about 55 on an arbitrary scale of 0–100, and the cell would be "located" at point B. Any increase of intensity would result in an increase in response (gray area) provided that the increase of intensity was not too great; any intensity greater than 70 db would drive the neuron below point C, resulting in a decrease in response. Note that no change in the response of the cell would occur if the intensity increase moves the neuron to point C. If a cholinergic agent alters the intensity function of a cortical neuron, then the effect on discharge rate would depend upon whether or not the neuron had a non-monotonic intensity function, the cells initial place on this function, and the amount of change in effective intensity related to the slope(s) of the function.

CONCLUDING COMMENTS: BEHAVIORAL IMPLICATIONS OF MUSCARINIC ACTIONS IN SENSORY CORTEX

In this final section, we suggest a possible muscarinic role in the processing of information and in behavioral performance. While our comments are somewhat speculative, it is hoped that they are sufficiently interesting to promote accelerated inquiry into the role of the BFCS in behavior.

The effects of muscarinic agents in sensory cortex have not yet been fully characterized. In our view, a full understanding of cholinergic actions on cortical sensory processing requires a comprehensive analysis of possible interactions among stimulus parameters (e.g., intensity, frequency) concentrations of ACh, and behavioral state. Studies of ACh in visual and somatosensory cortex, using anesthetized preparations, have emphasized the facilitation of information processing (Sillito and Kemp, 1983; Sato et al., 1987; Metherate, 1988a,b). This has obvious implications for perceptual and behavioral functions. However, it seems likely that the role of ACh is not restricted to facilitation, particularly in the unanesthetized animal.

As summarized above, and reported in detail elsewhere (Ashe et al., 1989; McKenna et al., 1989), we have found specific alterations of frequency receptive fields in auditory cortex of waking animals. These include increased frequency selectivity, decreased selectivity and systematic shifts in receptive field tuning, involving simultaneous suppression of response to the original best frequency and facilitation of response to the new best frequency. Taken together, the actions of muscarinic agonists in auditory cortex cannot be simply characterized as facilitation of responses to environmental stimuli.

Response facilitation is often viewed as beneficial, whereas decreased selectivity may be thought to be deleterious for adaptive behavior. However, quantitative behavioral studies suggest that the role of sensory cortical neurons in behavioral performance cannot be independent of the ongoing interactions between an organism and the environment.

One of the best-documented relevant behavioral effects is that of the Yerkes-Dodson Law, or the "inverted U curve of arousal." Briefly, the relationship between arousal level and performance in a wide range of tasks is that of a non-monotonic function; increasing arousal produces more effective behavior (e.g., attention, perception, etc.) up to a maximum; thereafter, increasing arousal generally leads to impairment of behavioral performance (for reviews, see Kahneman, 1973; Eysenck, 1982). Thus, depending upon the initial level of arousal and the amount of arousal increment, the result can be increased, decreased, or even leave no change in response. A function of this type may be very closely related to the level of ACh in neocortex, because release of ACh appears to be an increasing function of behavioral arousal (Jasper, 1969). Therefore, it is possible that as arousal increases, and ACh levels increase, the effects on neuronal processing of information will depend on the initial, baseline position of the organism on the inverted U curve. A given amount of ACh might either facilitate, suppress, or have no detectable effect on a cells response to a stimulus if that cell has a non-monotonic intensity function and if ACh affects that function (Fig. 10). The effects of ACh on intensity functions have not been determined in studies of receptive field modification. However, based upon the effects of ACh on receptive fields, we have proposed a "muscarinic intensity model" in which ACh mimics an increase in stimulus intensity (Ashe et al., 1989). Additionally, preliminary findings support this model (Metherate et al., 1989a).

Furthermore, there may well be an interaction between the task demands and the effects of arousal and/or ACh. For example, an increase in stimulus selectivity would be adaptive for tasks benefitting from narrowed attention and decreased distractibility (e.g., detection of a known target) but would be maladaptive for tasks that require divided attention (e.g., monitoring multiple targets). Shifts in receptive fields may be adaptive for situations in which shifts of attention are required. In other words, the relationship between cholinergic modulation of sensory cortical neuronal responses to stimuli and adaptive information processing may not be deduced only on the basis of the type of change in neuronal response, but rather, may also require knowledge of the current environmental demands on an organism.

If this proves to be the case, then it should be possible to relate cholinergic modulation of sensory cortical processing and behavioral adaptation in a comprehensive manner. Cholinergic facilitation may be the dominant mode that is detectable in animals under general anesthesia but may be only part of the larger role of endogenous ACh in the processing of information in sensory cortex. Resolution of this issue will await the results of appropriate experiments involving simultaneous measures of neuronal and behavioral responses to controlled stimulation and environmental demands.

Many studies have demonstrated that the responses of neurons in sensory neocortex are systematically altered (increased or decreased response to stimuli) during learning, particularly by associative processes (Weinberger and Diamond, 1987). Such changes in auditory cortex actually reflect associative modification of frequency receptive fields that are specific to the tone that acquires signal value during classical conditioning (Diamond and Weinberger, 1986; Weinberger and Diamond, 1987). Furthermore, during behavioral "extinction" the receptive field modifications are eliminated. Learning-induced frequency-specific receptive field plasticity develops as rapidly as has been measured, e.g., a few minutes (for review, see Weinberger and Diamond, 1987). Because of the similarity of the changes in frequency receptive fields induced by muscarinic agonists or anticholinesterases to those observed during learning, it is possible that one role of endogenous ACh, acting at muscarinic receptors, is to reshape cortical sensory receptive fields which are basically plastic, in accordance with environmental stimuli that are currently of behavioral significance.

ACKNOWLEDGMENTS

This research has been supported by ONR N-00014-87-K-0433, ONR N-00014-84-K-0391, DAMD 17-85-C-5072, NSF PRM-8200575, the Monsanto Company, and The Center for the Neurobiology of Learning and Memory.

REFERENCES

Akers, R.F. and Routtenberg, A. (1987): Calcium-promoted translocation of protein kinase C to synaptic membranes: relation to the phosphorylation of an endogenous substrate (protein F1) involved in synaptic plasticity. *J. Neurosci.* 7:3976-3983

Alkon, D.L. (1988): Conservation of cellular mechanisms for models of learning and memory. In: *Mechanisms of Conditioning and Behavioral Plasticity.* Woody, C.D., Alkon, D.L. and McGaugh, J.L., eds. New York: Plenum Publishing

Altschuler, R.A., Kachar, B., Rubio, J.A., Parakkal, M.H. and Fex, J. (1985): Immunocytochemical localization of choline acetyltransferase-like immunoreactivity in the guinea pig cochlea. *Brain Res.* 338:1-11

Andrianov, V.V. (1982): Neurotransmitters and plasticity of cortical neurons during behavioral acts. *Neurosci. Behav. Physiol.* 12:145-147

Araujo, D.M., Lapchak, P.A., Collier, B. and Quirion, R. (1988): Characterization of N-[^{3}H]methylcarbamylcholine binding sites and effect of N-methylcarbamylcholine on acetylcholine release in rat brain. *J. Neurochem.* 51:292-2999

Ashe, J.H., Cassady, J.M. and Weinberger, N.M. (1975): The relationship of the cochlear microphonic potential to the acquisition of a classically conditioned pupillary dilation response. *Behav. Biol.* 16:45-62

Ashe, J.H., Cooper, C.L. and Weinberger, N.M. (1978a): Mesencephalic multiple-unit activity during acquisition of conditioned pupillary dilation. *Brain Res. Bull.* 31:43-154

Ashe, J.H., Cooper, C.L. and Weinberger, N.M. (1978b): Role of the parasympathetic pupillomotor system in classically conditioned pupillary dilation in the cat. *Behav. Biol.* 23:1-13

Ashe, J.H. and Libet, B. (1981): Modulation of slow postsynaptic potentials by dopamine in rabbit sympathetic ganglion. *Brain Res.* 217:93-106

Ashe, J.H., McKenna, T.M. and Weinberger, N.M. (1989): Cholinergic modulation of frequency receptive fields in auditory cortex: II. Frequency-specific effects of anticholinesterases provide evidence for a modulatory action of endogenous ACh. *Synapse* 4:44-54

Ashe, J.H. and Yarosh, C.A. (1984): Differential and selective antagonism of the slow-inhibitory postsynaptic potential and slow-excitatory postsynaptic potential by gallamine and pirenzepine in the superior cervical ganglion of the rabbit. *Neuropharmacol.* 23:1321-1329

Baranyi, A. and Szente, M.B. (1988): Postsynaptic activity-dependent facilitation of excitatory synaptic transmission in the neocortex. In: *Cellular Mechanisms of Conditioning and Behavioral Plasticity.* Woody, C.D., Alkon, D.L. and McGaugh, J.L., eds. New York: Plenum Publishing

Baranyi, A., Szente, M.B. and Woody, C.D. (1988a): Activation of protein kinase C induces long-term changes of postsynaptic currents in neocortical neurons. *Brain Res.* 440:341-347

Baranyi, A., Szente, M.B. and Woody, C.D. (1988b): Intracellular injection of phorbol ester increases the excitability of neurons of the motor cortex of awake cats. *Brain Res.* 424:396-401

Barlow, R.B., Berry, K.J., Glenton, P.A.M., Nikolaou, N.M. and Soh, K.S. (1976): A comparison of affinity constants for muscarine-sensitive acetylcholine receptors in guinea-pig atrial pacemaker cells at twenty-nine degrees C and in ileum at twenty-nine degrees C and thirty-seven degrees C. *Brit. J. Pharmacol.* 58:613-620

Barlow, R. B. and Shepherd, M. K. (1986): A further search for selective antagonists at M_2-muscarinic receptors. *Brit. J. Pharmacol.* 71:362-364

Bartus, R.T., Dean, R.L. and Flicker, C. (1987): Cholinergic psychopharmacology: an integration of human and animal research on memory. In: *Psychopharmacology: The Third Generation of Progress*. Meltzer, H.Y., ed. New York: Raven Press

Beesley, P.W. and Emson, P.C. (1975): Distribution of transmitter related enzymes in the rat sensorimotor cortex. *Biochem. Soc. Trans.* 3:936-939

Ben-Ari, Y., Krnjević, K., Reinhardt, W. and Ropert, N. (1981): Intracellular observations on the disinhibitory action of acetylcholine in the hippocampus. *Neurosci.* 6:2475-2484

Benardo, L.S. and Prince, D.A. (1981): Acetylcholine induced modulation of hippocampal pyramidal neurons. *Brain Res.* 211:227-234

Benardo, L.S. and Prince, D.A. (1982a): Cholinergic excitation of mammalian hippocampal pyramidal cells. *Brain Res.* 249:315-331

Benardo, L.S. and Prince, D.A. (1982b): Cholinergic pharmacology of mammalian hippocampal pyramidal cells. *Neurosci.* 7:1703-1712

Benardo, L.S. and Prince, D.A. (1982c): Ionic mechanisms of cholinergic excitation in mammalian hippocampal pyramidal cells. *Brain Res.* 249:333-344

Bird, S.J. and Aghajanian, G.K. (1976): The cholinergic pharmacology of hippocampal pyramidal cells: a microiontophoretic study. *Neuropharmacol.* 15: 273-282

Birdsall, N.J.M., Burgen, A.S.V., Hiley, C.R. and Hulme, E.C. (1976): Binding of agonists and antagonists to muscarinic receptors. *J. Supramolecular Structure.* 4:367-371

Birdsall, N.J.M., Burgen, A.S.V. and Hulme, E.C.(1978): The binding of agonists to brain muscarinic receptors. *Mol. Pharmacol.* 14:723-736

Boksa, P. and Quirion, R. (1987): [^{3}H]N-methyl-carbamylcholine, a new radioligand specific for nicotinic acetylcholine receptors in brain. *Eur. J. Pharmacol.* 139:323-333

Bonner, T.I. (1989): The molecular basis of muscarinic receptor diversity. *Trends Neurosci.* 12:148-151

Bonner, T.I., Buckley, N.J. , Young, A.C. and Brann, M.R. (1987): Identification of a family of muscarinic acetylcholine receptor genes. *Science* 237:527-532

Bradshaw, C.M., Sheridan, R.D. and Szabadi, E. (1987): Involvement of M_1-muscarinic receptors in the excitation of neocortical neurones by acetylcholine. *Neuropharmacol.* 26:1195-1200

Brann, M.R., Buckley, N.J. and Bonner, T.I. (1988): The striatum and cerebral cortex express different muscarinic receptor mRNAs. *FEBS Lett.* 230:90-94

Brezenoff, H.E. (1984): Cardiovascular regulation by brain acetylcholine. *Fed. Proc.* 43:17-20

Brown, D. (1988): M-currents: an update. *Trends Neurosci.* 11:294-299

Brown, D.A. and Adams, P.R. (1980): Muscarinic suppression of a novel voltage-sensitive K^+ current in a vertebrate neurone. *Nature* 283:673-676

Brown, D.A. and Adams, P.R. (1987): Effect of phorbol dibutyrate on M-currents and M-current inhibition in bull frog sympathetic neurons. *Cell. Molec. Neurobiol.* 7:255-269

Brown, D.A., Forward, A. and Marsh, S. (1980): Antagonist discrimination between ganglionic and ileal muscarinic receptors. *Brit. J. Pharmacol.* 71:362-364

Burke, R.E. (1986): Gallamine binding to muscarinic M_1 and M_2 receptors, studied by inhibition of [^{3}H]pirenzepine and [^{3}H]quinuclidinyl benzilate binding to rat brain membranes. *Mol. Pharmacol.* 30:58-68

Burton, M.J., Rolls, E.T. and Mora, F. (1976): Effects of hunger on the responses of neurons in the lateral hypothalamus to the sight and taste of food. *Exp. Neurol.* 51:668-677

Butcher, L.L. and Bilezikjian, L. (1975): Acetylcholinesterase-containing neurons in the neostriatum and substantia nigra revealed after punctate intracerebral injection of di-isopropylflurophosphate. *Eur. J. Pharmacol.* 34:115-125

Campbell, M.J., Lewis, D.A., Foote, S.L. and Morrison, J.H. (1987): Distribution of choline acetyltransferase-, serotonin-, dopamine-beta-hydroxylase, tyrosine hydroxylase-immunoreactive fibers in monkey primary auditory cortex. *J. Comp. Neurol.* 261:209-220

Caulfield, M.P., Higgins, G.A. and Straughan, D.W. (1983): Central administration of the muscarinic receptor subtype-selective antagonist pirenzepine selectively impairs passive avoidance learning in the mouse. *J. Pharm. Pharmacol.* 35:131-132

Clark, A.L. and Mitchelson, F. (1976): The inhibitory effect of gallamine on muscarinic receptors. *Brit. J. Pharmacol.* 58:323-331

Cole, A.E. and Nicoll, R.A. (1983): Acetylcholine mediates a slow synaptic potential in hippocampal pyramidal cells. *Science* 221:1299-1301

Cole, A.E. and Nicoll, R.A. (1984a): Characterization of a slow cholinergic postsynaptic potential recorded in vitro from rat hippocampal pyramidal cells. *J. Physiol.* (Lond.) 352:173-188

Cole, A.E. and Nicoll, R.A. (1984b): The pharmacology of cholinergic excitatory responses in hippocampal pyramidal cells. *Brain Res.* 305:283-290

Collerton, D. (1986): Cholinergic functional and intellectual decline in Alzheimer's disease. *Neurosci.* 19:1-28

Collingridge, G.L. and Bliss, T.V.P. (1987): NMDA receptors: their role in long-term potentiation. *Trends Neurosci.* 10:288-293

Cooper, C.L., Ashe, J.H., and Weinberger, N.M. (1978): Effects of stimulus omission during habituation of the pupillary dilation reflex. *Physiol. Psychol.* 6:1-6

Cortes, R., Probst, A., Tobler, H.J. and Palacios, J.M. (1986): Muscarinic cholinergic receptor subtypes in the human brain. II. Quantitative autoradiographic studies. *Brain Res.* 362:239-253

Curtis, D.R. and Ryall, R.W. (1966a): The acetylcholine receptors of Renshaw cells. *Exp. Brain Res.* 2:66-80

Curtis, D.R. and Ryall, R.W. (1966b): The synaptic excitation of Renshaw cells. *Exp. Brain Res.* 2:81-96

Daly, J.W., Hoffer, B.J. and Dismukes, R.K. (1980): Mechanisms of regulation of neuronal sensitivity. *Neurosci. Res. Prog.* 17:331-456

DeLong, M.R. (1971): Activity of pallidal neurons during movement. *J. Neurophysiol.* 43:414-427

Deutch, A.Y., Holliday, J., Roth, R.H., Chun, L.L. and Hawrot, E. (1987): Immunohistochemical localization of a neuronal nicotinic acetylcholine receptor in mammalian brain. *Proc. Nat. Acad. Sci.* 84:8697-8701

Deutsch, J.A. and Rogers, J.B. (1979): Cholinergic excitability and memory: animal studies and their clinical implication. In: *Brain Acetylcholine and Neuropsychiatric Disease.* Davis, K.L. and Berger, P.A., eds. New York: Plenum Press

Diamond, D.M. and Weinberger, N.M. (1984): Physiological plasticity of single neurons in auditory cortex of the cat during acquisition of the pupillary conditioned response: II. Secondary field (AII). *Behav. Neurosci.* 98:189-210

Diamond, D.M. and Weinberger, N.M. (1986): Classical conditioning rapidly induces specific changes in frequency receptive fields of single neurons in secondary and ventral ectosylvian auditory cortical fields. *Brain Res.* 372:357-360

Diamond, D.M. and Weinberger, N.M. (1989): Role of context in the expression of learning-induced plasticity of single neurons in auditory cortex. *Behav. Neurosci.* 103:471-494

Dismukes, R.K. (1979): New concepts of molecular communication among neurons. *Behav. Brain Sci.* 2:409-448

Disterhoft, J.F., Coulter, D.A. and Alkon, D.L. (1988): Conditioning-specific biophysical alterations in rabbit hippocampus. In: *Cellular Mechanisms of Conditioning and Behavioral Plasticity.* Woody, C.D., Alkon, D.L. and McGaugh, J.L., eds. New York: Plenum Publishing

Dodd, J., Dingeldine, R. and Kelly, J.S. (1981): The excitatory action of acetylcholine on hippocampal neurones of the guinea pig and rat maintained *in vitro. Brain Res.* 207:109-127

Donoghue, J.P. and Carroll, K.L. (1987): Cholinergic modulation of sensory responses in rat primary somatic sensory cortex. *Brain Res.* 408:367-371

Doods, H.N., Mathy, M.J., Daivdesko, D., van Charldorp, K.J., de Jonge, A. and van Zwieten, P.A. (1987): Selectivity of muscarinic antagonists in radioligand in *in vivo* experiments for the putative M_1, M_2 and M_3 receptors. *J. Pharmacol. Exp. Ther.* 242:257-262

Dunlap, J. and Brown, J.H. (1983): Heterogeneity of binding sites on cardiac muscarinic receptors induced by the neuromuscular blocking agents gallamine and pancuronium. *Mol. Pharmacol.* 24:15-22

Dutar, P. and Nicoll, R.A. (1988a): Classification of muscarinic responses in hippocampus in terms of receptor subtypes and second-messenger systems:

electrophysiological studies in vitro. *J. Neurosci.* 8:4214-4224

Dutar, P. and Nicoll, R.A. (1988b): Stimulation of phosphatidylinositol (PI) turnover may mediate the muscarinic suppression of the M-current in hippocampal pyramidal cells. *Neurosci. Lett.* 85:89-94

Dykes, R.W., Metherate, R. and Tremblay, N. (1988): Cholinergic modulation of neuronal excitability in cat somatosensory cortex. In: *Neurotransmitters and Cortical Function: From Molecules to Mind.* Avoli, M., Reader, T.A., Dykes, R.W. and Gloor, P., eds. New York: Plenum Press

Eccles, J.C., Fatt, P. and Koketsu, K. (1954): Cholinergic and inhibitory synapses in a pathway from motor-axon collaterals to motoneurones. *J. Physiol.* (Lond.) 126:524-562

Eccles, R.M. and Libet, B. (1961): Origin and blockade of the synaptic responses of curarized sympathetic ganglia. *J. Physiol.* (Lond.) 157:484-503

Eckenstein, F. and Baughman, R.W. (1984): Two types of cholinergic innervation in cortex, one co-localized with vasoactive intestinal polypeptide. *Nature* 309:153-155

Eckenstein, F. and Sofroniew, M.V. (1983): Identification of central cholinergic neurons containing both choline acetyltransferase and acetylcholinesterase and of central neurons containing only acetylcholinesterase. *J. Neurosci.* 3:2286-2291

Egan, T.M. and North, R.A. (1986): Acetylcholine hyperpolarizes central neurones by acting on an M_2 muscarinic receptor. *Nature* 319:405-407

El-Fakahany, E.E., Alger, B.E., Lai, W.S., Pitler, T.A., Worley, P.F. and Baraban, J.M. (1988): Neuronal muscarinic responses: role of protein Kinase C. *FASEB Jour.* 2:2575-2583

Ellis, J. and Hoss, W. (1980): Analysis of regional variations in the affinities of muscarinic agonists in the rat brain. *Brain Res.* 193:189-198

Ellis, J. and Hoss, W. (1982): Competitive interaction of gallamine with multiple muscarinic receptors. *Biochem. Pharmacol.* 31:873-876

Ellis, J. and Lenox, R.H. (1985a): Characterization of the interacting of gallamine with muscarinic receptors from brain. *Biochem. Pharmacol.* 34:2214-2217

Ellis, J. and Lenox, R.H. (1985b): Quaternary forms of classical muscarinic antagonists distinguish subpopulations of muscarinic receptors: correlation with gallamine-defined subpopulations. *Biochem. Biophys. Res. Commun.* 126:1242-1250

Engel, W., Eberlein, W., Trummlitz, G. and Mihm, G. (1987): Pirenzepine and AF-DX 116, two structurally related antimuscarinics with opposite receptor selectivity. *Fed. Proc.* 46:2527-2528

Erickson, R.P., Jane, J., Waite, R. and Diamond, I.T. (1964): Single neuron investigation of sensory thalamus of the opossum. *J. Neurophysiol.* 27:1026-1047

Eysenck, M.W. (1982): *Attention and Arousal: Cognition and Performance.* New York: Springer-Verlag

Foote, S.L., Freedman, R. and Oliver, A.P. (1975): Effects of putative neurotransmitters on neuronal activity in monkey cortex. *Brain Res.* 86:229-242

Frégnac, Y., Shultz, D., Thorpe, S. and Bienenstock, E. (1988): A cellular analogue of visual cortical plasticity. *Nature* 333:367-370

Gerren, R. and Weinberger, N.M. (1983): Long term potentiation in the magnocellular medial geniculate nucleus of the anesthetized cat. *Brain Res.* 265:138-142

Gil, D.W. and Wolfe, B.B. (1985): Pirenzepine distinguishes between muscarinic receptor-mediated phosphoinositide breakdown and inhibition of adenylate cyclase. *J. Pharmacol. Exp. Ther.* 232:608-616

Giraldo, E., Hammer, R. and Ladinsky, H. (1987): Distribution of muscarinic receptor subtypes in rat brain as determined in binding studies with AF-DX 116 and pirenzepine. *Life Sci.* 40:833-840

Godfrey, D.A. and Matschinsky, F.M. (1981): Quantitative distribution of choline acetyltransferase and acetylcholinesterase activities in the rat cochlear nucleus. *J. Histochem. Cytochem.* 29:720-730

Gold, P.E. and Zornetzer, S.F. (1983): The mnemon and its juices: neuromodulation of memory processes. *Behav. Neurobiol.* 38:151-189

Goyal, R.K. and Rattan, S. (1978): Neurohumoral, hormonal and drug receptors for the lower esophageal sphincter. *Gastroenterol.* 74:598-619

Gribkoff, V.K. and Ashe, J.H., (1984): Stimulus-evoked slow depolarization of dentate granule cells *in vitro*: evidence for a slow muscarinic cholinergic EPSP. *Physiologist.* 27:233

Gustafsson, B. and Wigstrom, H. (1988): Physiological mechanisms underlying long-term potentiation. *Trends Neurosci.* 11:156-162

Haefely, W. (1974): Muscarinic postsynaptic events in the cat superior cervical ganglion in situ. *Naunyn-Schmiedeberg's Arch. Pharmacol.* 281:119-143

Hagan, J.J., Jansen, J.H. and Broekkamp, C.L. (1987): Blockade of spatial learning by the M_1 muscarinic antagonist pirenzepine. *Psychopharmacol.* 93:470-476

Hammer, R., Berrie, C.P., Birdsall, N.J.M., Burgen, A.S.V. and Hulme, E.C. (1980): Pirenzepine distinguishes between different subclasses of muscarinic receptors. *Nature.* 283:90-92

Hammer, R. and Giachetti, A. (1982): Muscarinic receptor subtypes: M_1 and M_2, biochemical and functional characterization. *Life Sci.* 31:2991-2998

Hammer, R., Giraldo, E., Schiavi, G.B., Monferini, E. and Ladinsky, H. (1986): Binding profile of a novel cardioselective muscarine receptor antagonist, AF-DX 116, to membranes of peripheral tissues and brain in the rat. *Life Sci.* 38:1653-1662

Harris, E.W. and Cotman, C.W. (1986): Long-term potentiation of guinea pig mossy fiber responses is not blocked by N-methyl-D-aspartate antagonists. *Neurosci. Lett.* 70:132-137

Hawkins, R.D .and Kandel, E.R. (1984): Steps toward a cell-biological alphabet for elementary forms of learning. In: *Neurobiology of Learning and Memory.*

Lynch, G., McGaugh, J.L. and Weinberger, N.M., eds. New York: Guilford Press

Honore, T., Davies, S.N., Drejer, J., Fletcher, E.J., Jacobsen, P., Lodge, D. and Nielsen, F.E. (1988): Quinoxalinediones: potent competitive non-NMDA glutamate receptor antagonists. *Science* 241:701-703

Houser, C.R., Crawford, G.D., Barber, R.P., Salvaterra, P.M. and E.V.J. (1983): Organization and morphological characteristics of cholinergic neurons: an immunocytochemical study with a monoclonal antibody to choline acetyltransferase. *Brain Res.* 266:96-119

Houser, C.R., Crawford, G.D., Salvaterra, P.M. and Vaughn, J.E. (1985): Immunocytochemical localization of choline acetyltransferase in rat cerebral cortex: a study of cholinergic neurons and synapses. *J. Comp. Neurol.* 234:17-34

Hulme, E.C., Birdsall, N.J.M., Burgen, A.S.V. and Mehta, P. (1978): The binding of antagonists to brain muscarinic receptors. *Mol. Pharmacol.*14:737-750

Hunter, A.J. and Roberts, F.F. (1988): The effect of pirenzepine on spatial learning in the Morris Water Maze. *Pharmacol. Biochem. Behav.* 30:519-523

Jarrell, T.W., Gentile, C.G., McCabe, P.M. and Schneiderman, N. (1986a): The role of the medial geniculate region in differential Pavlovian conditioning of bradycardia in rabbits. *Brain Res.* 374:126-136

Jarrell, T.W., Romanski, L.M., Gentile, C.G., McCabe, P.M. and Schneiderman, N. (1986b): Ibotenic acid lesions of the medial geniculate region prevent the acquisition of differential Pavlovian conditioning to acoustic stimuli in rabbits. *Brain Res.* 382:199-203

Jasper, H.H. (1969): Neurochemical mediators of specific and nonspecific cortical activation. In: *Attention in Neurophysiology.* Evans, C.R. and Mulholland, T.B., eds. New York: Appelton-Century-Crofts

Johnston, M.V., McKinney, M. and Coyle, J.T. (1981): Neocortical cholinergic innervations: a description of extrinsic and intrinsic components in the rat. *Exp. Brain Res.* 43:159-172

Kaczmarek, L.K. and Levitan, I.B. (1987): What is neuromodulation? In: *Neuromodulation: The biochemical control of neuronal excitability.* Kaczmarek, L.K. and Levitan, I.B., eds. New York: Oxford University Press

Kahneman, D. (1973): *Attention and Effort.* Prentice-Hall, New Jersey

Kapp, B.S., Gallagher, M., Applegate, C.D. and Frysinger, R.C. (1984): The amygdala central nucleus: contributions to conditioned cardiovascular responding during aversive Pavlovian conditioning in the rabbit. In: *Conditioning: Representation of Involved Neural Function.* Woody, C.D., ed. New York: Plenum Press

Karczmar, A.G., Koketsu, K. and Nishi, S. (1986): *Autonomic and Enteric Ganglia: Transmission and its Pharmacology.* New York: Plenum Press

Kimura, H., McGeer, P.I., Peng, J.H. and McGeer, E.G. (1981): The central cholinergic system studied by choline acetyltransferase immunohistochemistry in the cat. *J. Comp. Neurol.* 200:151-201

Kobayashi, R.M., Palkovits, M., Hruska, R.E., Roth-Schild, R. and Yamamura, H.I. (1978): Regional distribution of muscarinic cholinergic receptors in rat brain. *Brain Res.* 154:13-23

Koelle, G. B. and Friedenwald, J.S. (1949): A histochemical method for localizing cholinesterase activity. *Proc. Soc. Exp. Biol. Med.* 70:617-622

Kopytova, F.V., Mednikova, Y.S. and Rusinova, E.V. (1981): Analog of a conditioned reflex of sensomotor cortical units following microinjection of acetylcholine. *Neurosci. Behav. Physiol.* 11:213-220

Koshtoyants, O.K., Antipina, M.Y. and Kol'tsova, A.V. (1981): Changes in acetylcholine sensitivity of sensory-motor cortical neurons during extinction of a conditioned reflex. *Neurosci. Behav. Physiol.* 11

Krettek, J.E. and Price, J.L. (1978): Amygdaloid projections to subcortical structures within the basal forebrain and brainstem in the rat and cat. *J. Comp. Neurol.* 178:225-254

Krnjević, K. (1987): Role of acetylcholine in the cerebral cortex. In: *Neurobiology of Acetylcholine.* Dun, N.J. and Perlman, R.L., eds. New York: Plenum Press

Krnjević, K. (1988): Acetylcholine as transmitter in the cerebral cortex. In: *Neurotransmitters and Cortical Function: From Molecules to Mind.* Avoli, M., Reader, T.A., Dykes, R.W. and Gloor, P., eds. New York: Plenum Press

Kupfermann, I. (1979): Modulatory actions of neurotransmitters. *Ann. Rev. Neurosci.* 2:447-465

Lamour, Y., Dutar, P., Jobert, A. and Dykes, R.W. (1988): An iontophoretic study of single somatosensory neurons in rat granular cortex serving the limbs: a laminar analysis of glutamate and acetylcholine effects on receptive-field properties. *J. Neurophysiol.* 60:725-50

LeDoux, J.E., Ruggiero, D.A. and Reis, D.J. (1985): Projections to the subcortical forebrain from anatomically defined regions of the medial geniculate body in the rat. *J. Comp. Neurol.* 242:182-213

LeDoux, J.E., Sakaguchi, A. and Reis, D.J. (1984): Subcortical efferent projections of the medial geniculate nucleus mediate emotional responses to conditioned acoustic stimuli. *J. Neurosci.* 4:683-698

Lehmann, J., Nagy, J.I., Atmadja, S. and Fibiger, H.C. (1980): The nucleus basalis magnocellularis: the origin of a cholinergic projection to the neocortex of the rat. *Neurosci.* 5:1161-1174

Levey, A.I., Wainer, B.H., Rye, D.B., Mufson, E. J. and Mesulam, M.-M. (1984): Choline acetyltransferase-immunoreactive neurons intrinsic to rodent cortex and distinct from acetylcholinesterase-positive neurons. *Neurosci.* 13:341-353

Libet, B. (1979a): Neuronal communication and synaptic modulation: experimental evidence vs. conceptual categories. *Behav. Brain Sci.* 2:431-433

Libet, B. (1979b): Slow postsynaptic actions in ganglionic function. In: *Integrative Functions of the Autonomic Nervous System.* Brooks, C.M., Koizumi, K.

and Sato, A., eds. Tokyo: University of Tokyo Press

Libet, B., Kobayashi, H. and Tanaka, T. (1975): Synaptic coupling into the production and storage of a neuronal memory trace. *Nature* 258:155-157

Lovinger, D.M. and Routtenberg, A. (1988): Synapse-specific protein kinase C-activation enhances maintenance of long-term potentiation in rat hippocampus. *J. Physiol.* 400:321-333

Lund, R.D. and Webster, K.E. (1967): Thalamic afferents from the spinal cord and the trigeminal nucleus: an experimental anatomic study in the rat. *J. Comp. Neurol.* 130:313-328

Lynch, G. (1986): *Synapses, Circuits, and the Beginnings of Memory.* Cambridge, Mass.: MIT Press

Madison, D.V., Lancaster, B., and Nicoll, R.A. (1987): Voltage clamp analysis of cholinergic action in the hippocampus. *J. Neurosci.* 7:733-741

Marchi, M. and Raiteri, M. (1985): On the presence in the cerebral cortex of muscarinic receptor subtypes which differ in neuronal localization, function and pharmacological properties. *J. Pharmacol. Exp. Ther.* 235:230-233

Mash, D.C. and Potter, L.T. (1986): Autoradiographic localization of M_1 and M_2 muscarine receptors in the rat brain. *Neurosci.* 19:551-564

Mash, D.C., White, W.F. and Mesulam, M.-M. (1988): Distribution of muscarinic receptor subtypes within architectonic subregions of the primate cerebral cortex. *J. Comp. Neurol.* 278:265-274

McCormick, D.A. and Pape, H.-C. (1988): Acetylcholine inhibits identified interneurons in the cat lateral geniculate nucleus. *Nature* 334:246-248

McCormick, D.A. and Prince, D.A. (1985): Two types of muscarinic response to acetylcholine in mammalian cortical neurons. *Proc. Natl. Acad. Sci.* 82: 6344-6348

McCormick, D.A. and Prince, D.A. (1986a): Acetylcholine induces burst firing in thalamic reticular neurones by activating a potassium conductance. *Nature* 319:402-405

McCormick, D.A. and Prince, D.A. (1986b): Mechanisms of action of acetylcholine in the guinea-pig cerebral cortex *in vitro. J. Physiol.* (Lond.) 375: 169-194

McCormick, D.A. and Prince, D.A. (1987): Actions of acetylcholine in the guinea-pig and cat medial and lateral geniculate nuclei, *in vitro. J. Physiol.* (Lond.) 392:147-165

McDonough, J.H. and Penetar, D.M. (1983): The effects of cholinergic blocking agents and anticholinesterase compounds on memory, learning and performance. In: *Behavioral Models and the Analysis of Drug Action.* Spiegelstein, M.Y. and Levy, A., eds. Amsterdam: Elsevier

McKenna, T.M., Ashe, J.H., Hui, G. K. and Weinberger, N.M. (1988): Muscarinic agonists modulate spontaneous and evoked unit discharge in auditory cortex of cat. *Synapse* 2:54-68

McKenna, T.M., Ashe, J.H., and Weinberger, N.M. (1989): Cholinergic modulation of frequency receptive fields in auditory cortex: I. Frequency-specific effects of muscarinic agonists. *Synapse* 4:30-43

Mesulam, M.-M. (1988): Central cholinergic pathways; neuroanatomy and some behavioral implications. In: *Neurotransmitters and Cortical Function: From Molecules to Mind.* Avoli, M., Reader, T.A., Dykes, R.W. and Gloor, P., eds. New York: Plenum Press

Mesulam, M.-M., Mufson, E.J., Levey, A.I. and Wainer, B.H. (1983a): Cholinergic innervation of cortex by the basal forebrain: cytochemistry and cortical connections of the septal area, diagonal band nuclei, nucleus basalis (substantia innominata), and hypothalamus in the rhesus monkey. *J. Comp. Neurol.* 214:170-197

Mesulam, M.-M., Mufson, E.J., Wainer, B.H. and Levey, A.I. (1983b): Central cholinergic pathways in the rat: an overview based on an alternative nomenclature (Ch1-Ch6). *Neurosci.* 10:1185-1201

Metherate, R., Ashe, J.H., and Weinberger, N.M. (1989a): M_1 and M_2 muscarinic receptors mediate acetylcholine (ACh) modulation of auditory cortical neurons. *Soc. Neurosci. Abstr.* 15:409

Metherate, R., Ashe, J.H. and Weinberger, N.M. (in press): Acetylcholine modifies neuronal acoustic rate-level functions in guinea pig auditory cortex by an action at muscarinic receptors. *Synapse*

Metherate, R., Cox, C.L., Acosta, C.G. and Ashe, J.H., (1989b): Cholinergic agonists modify membrane potential and input resistance of auditory neocortical neurons *in vitro. FASEB Jour.* 3:A393

Metherate, R., Tremblay, N. and Dykes, R.W. (1987): Acetylcholine permits long-term enhancement of neuronal responsiveness in cat primary somatosensory cortex. *Neurosci.* 22:75-81

Metherate, R., Tremblay, N. and Dykes, R.W. (1988a): The effects of acetylcholine on response properties of cat somatosensory cortical neurons. *J. Neurophysiol.* 59:1231-1252

Metherate, R., Tremblay, N. and Dykes, R.W. (1988b): Transient and prolonged effects of acetylcholine on responsiveness of cat somatosensory cortical neurons. *J. Neurophysiol.* 59:1253-1276

Metherate, R. and Weinberger, N.M. (1989): Acetylcholine produces stimulus-specific receptive field alterations in cat auditory cortex. *Brain Res.* 480:372-377

Micheletti, R., Montagna, E. and Giachetti, A. (1987): AF-DX 116, a cardio-selective muscarinic antagonist. *J. Pharmacol. Exp. Ther.* 241:628-634

Mitchell, J. F. (1963): The spontaneous and evoked release of acetylcholine from the cerebral cortex. *J. Physiol.* (Lond.) 165:98-116

Mochida, S. and Kobayashi, H. (1988): Protein kinase C-activators mimic the M_2 muscarinic receptor-mediated effects on the action potential in isolated sympathetic neurons of rabbits. *Neurosci. Lett.* 86:201-206

Mochida, S. and Kobayashi, H. (1988): A novel muscarinic receptor antagonist

AF-DX 116 differentially blocks slow inhibitory and slow excitatory postsynaptic potentials in the rabbit sympathetic ganglia. *Life Sci.* 42:2195-2201

Moises, H.C., Woodward, D.J., Hoffer, B.J. and Freedman, R. (1979): Interactions of norepinephrine with Purkinje cell responses to putative amino acid neurotransmitters applied by microiontophoresis. *Exp. Neurol.* 64:493-515

Monaghan, D.T. and Cotman, C.W. (1985): Distribution of N-methyl-D-aspartate-sensitive L[^{3}H]Glutamate binding sites in rat brain. *J. Neurosci.* 5:2909-2919

Mora, F., Rolls, E.T. and Burton, M.J. (1976): Modulation during learning of the responses of neurons in the lateral hypothalamus to the sight of food. *Exp. Neurol.* 53:508-519

Muller, D., Joly, M. and Lynch, G. (1988): Contributions of quisqualate and NMDA receptors to the induction and expression of LTP. *Science* 242:1694-1697

Müller, W. and Misgeld, U. (1986): Slow cholinergic excitation of guinea pig hippocampal neurons is mediated by two muscarinic receptor subtypes. *Neurosci. Lett.* 67:107-112

Murray, C.L. and Fibiger, H.C. (1985): Learning and memory deficits after lesions of the nucleus basalis magnocellullaris: reversal by physostigmine. *Neurosci.* 14:1025-1032

Nelson, R.B. and Routtenberg, A. (1988): Contrasting roles of a brain-specific protein kinase C substrate: Has protein F1 evolved a new function in CNS of higher vertebrates? In: *Cellular Mechanisms of Conditioning and Behavioral Plasticity.* Woody, C.D., Alkon, D.L. and McGaugh, J.L., eds. New York: Plenum Publishing

Newberry, N.R., Priestley, T. and Woodruff, G.N. (1985): Pharmacological distinction between two muscarinic responses on the isolated superior cervical ganglion of the rat. *Eur. J. Pharmacol.* 116:191-192

Nicoll, R.A. (1988): The coupling of neurotransmitter receptors to ion channels in the brain. *Science* 241:545-551

Oleson, T.D., Ashe, J.H., and Weinberger, N.M. (1975): Modification of auditory and somatosensory system activity during pupillary conditioning in the paralyzed cat. *J. Neurophysiol.* 38:1114-1139

Oleson, T.D., Vododnick, D.S. and Weinberger, N.M. (1973): Pupillary inhibition of delay during Pavlovian conditioning in paralyzed cat. *Behav. Biol.* 8:337-346

Oleson, T.D., Westenberg, I.S. and Weinberger, N.M. (1972): Characteristics of the pupillary dilation response during Pavlovian conditioning in paralyzed cats. *Behav. Biol.* 7:829-840

Parkinson, D., Kratz, K.E. and Daw, N.W. (1988): Evidence for a nicotinic component to the actions of acetylcholine in cat visual cortex. *Exp. Brain Res.* 73:553-568

Phillis, J.W. and York, D.H. (1968): Pharmacological studies on a cholinergic inhibition in the cerebral cortex. *Brain Res.* 10:297-306

Pirch, J.H., Corbus, M.J., Rigdon, G.C. and Lyness, W.H. (1986): Generation of cortical event-related slow potentials in the rat involves nucleus basalis cholinergic innervation. *EEG Clin. Neurophysiol.* 63:464-475

Poggio, G.F. and Mountcastle, V.B. (1960): A study of the functional contributions of the lemniscal and spinothalamic systems to somatic sensibility. *Bull. Johns Hopkins Hosp.* 106:266-316

Popowitz, J.M., Larue, D.T. and Winer, J.A. (1988): Glutamate is a major transmitter in the rat medial geniculate body. *Soc. Neurosci. Abstr.* 14:490

Price, J. L. and Amaral, D.G. (1981): An autoradiographic study of the projections of the central nucleus of the monkey amygdala. *J. Neurosci.* 1:1242-1259

Price, M., Messer, W.S. and Hoss, W. (1986): Regional distribution of muscarinic receptors preferring gallamine in the rat brain. *Biochem. Pharmacol.* 35:4171-4176

Prusky, G.T., Shaw, C. and Cynader, M.S. (1988): The distribution and ontogenesis of [^{3}H]nicotine binding sites in cat visual cortex. *Brain Res.* 467:161-176

Rascol, O. and Lamour, Y. (1988): Differential effects of M_1 and M_2 muscarinic drugs on septohippocampal, hippocampal and cortical neurons in the rat. *Brain Res.* 446:303-313

Reiter, H.O. and Stryker, M.P. (1988): Neural plasticity without postsynaptic action potentials: less-active inputs become dominant when kitten visual cortical cells are inhibited. *Proc. Nat. Acad. Sci.* 85:3623-3627

Richardson, R.T., Mitchell, S.J., Baker, F.H. and DeLong, M.R. (1988): Responses of nucleus basalis of Meynert neurons in behaving monkeys. In: *Cellular Mechanisms of Conditioning and Behavioral Plasticity*. Woody, C.D., Alkon, D.L. and McGaugh, J.L., eds. New York: Plenum Press

Rigdon, G.C. and Pirch, J. (1988): Nucleus basalis involvement in conditioned neuronal responses in the rat frontal cortex. *J. Neurosci.* 6:2535-2542

Riker, W.F. and Wescoe, W.C. (1951): The pharmacology of Flaxedil with observations on certain analogues. *Ann. N. Y. Acad. Sci.* 54:373-392

Rolls, E.T., Sanghera, M.K. and Roper-Hall, A. (1979): The latency of activation of neurones in the lateral hypothalamus and substantia innominata during feeding in the monkey. *Brain Res.* 164:121-135

Russchen, F.T., Amaral, D.G. and Price, J.L. (1985): The afferent connections of the substantia innominata in the monkey, Macaca fascicularis. *J. Comp. Neurol.* 242:1-27

Rye, D.B., Wainer, B.H., Mesulam, M.-M. and Saper, C.D. (1984): Cortical projections arising from the basal forebrain: a study of cholinergic and noncholinergic components employing combined retrograde tracing and immunohistochemical localization of choline acetyl transferase. *Neurosci.* 13:627-643

Ryugo, D.K. and Weinberger, N.M. (1978): Differential plasticity of morphologically distinct neuron populations in the medial geniculate body of the cat during classical conditioning. *Behav. Biol.* 22:275-301

Sato, H., Hata, Y., Masui, H. and Tsumoto, T. (1987): A functional role of cholinergic innervation to neurons in the cat visual cortex. *J. Neurophysiol.* 58:765-780

Segal, M. (1982): Multiple actions of acetylcholine at a muscarinic receptor studied in the rat hippocampal slice. *Brain Res.* 246:77-87

Shepherd, G.M. (1988): *Neurobiology.* New York: Oxford University Press

Shute, C.C.D. and Lewis, P.R. (1963): Cholinesterase-containing systems of the brain of the rat. *Nature* 199:1160-1164

Shute, C.C.D. and Lewis, P.R. (1967): Ascending cholinergic reticular system: neocortical, olfactory and subcortical projections. *Brain* 90:497-521

Sillito, A.M. and Kemp, J.A. (1983): Cholinergic modulation of the functional organization of the cat visual cortex. *Brain Res.* 289:143-155

Spencer, D.G.J., Horvath, E. and Traber, J. (1986): Direct autoradiographic determination of M_1 and M_2 muscarinic acetylcholine receptor distribution in the rat brain: relation to cholinergic nuclei and projections. *Brain Res.* 380:59-68

Stockton, J.M., Birdsall, N.J.M., Burgen, A.S.V. and Hulme, E.C. (1983): Modification of the binding properties of muscarinic receptors by gallamine. *Mol. Pharmacol.* 23:551-557

Swanson, T.H. and Phillis, J.W. (1988): Effects of the muscarinic antagonists pirenzepine and gallamine on spontaneous and evoked responses of rat cerebral cortical neurones. *Brit. J. Pharmacol.* 94:192-198

Swartz, B.E. and Woody, C.D. (1979): Correlated effects of acetylcholine and cyclic guanosine monophosphate on membrane properties of mammalian neocortical neurons. *J. Neurobiol.* 10:465-488

Trendelenburg, U. (1966): Transmission of preganglionic impulses through the muscarinic receptors of the superior cervical ganglion of the cat. *J. Pharm. Exp. Ther.* 154:426-440

Waelbroeck, M., Gillard, M., Robberecht, P. and Christophe, J. (1987): Muscarinic receptor heterogeneity in rat central nervous system. I. Binding of four selective antagonists to three muscarinic receptor subclasses: a comparison with M_2 cardiac muscarinic receptors of the C type. *Mol. Pharmacol.* 32:91-99

Watkins, J.C. and Olverman, H.J. (1987): Agonists and antagonists for excitatory amino acid receptors. *Trends Neurosci.* 10:265-272

Watson, M., Roeske, W.R., Yamamura, H.I. (1986): [^{3}H pirenzepine and (-(-[^{3}H quinuclidinyl benzilate binding to rat cerebral cortical and cardiac muscarinic cholinergic sites. II. Characterization and regulation of antagonist binding to putative muscarinic subtypes. *J. Pharmacol. Exp. Ther.* 237:419-427

Weinberger, N.M. (1982): Sensory plasticity and learning: The magnocellular medial geniculate nucleus of the auditory system. In: *Conditioning: Representation of Involved Neural Function.* Woody, C.D., ed. New York: Plenum Press

Weinberger, N.M., Ashe, J.H., Metherate, R., McKenna, T.M., Diamond, D.M. and Bakin, J. (1990a): Retuning auditory cortex by learning: a preliminary model of receptive field plasticity. *Concepts in Neurosci.*

Weinberger, N.M., Ashe, J.H., Metherate, R., McKenna, T.M., Diamond, D.M., Bakin, J. and Cassady, J.M. (1990b): Neural adaptive information processing: a model of receptive field plasticity in auditory cortex during pavlovian conditioning. In: *Neurocomputation and Learning: Foundations of Adaptive Networks.* Moore, J., Gabriel, M., eds. Cambridge, Mass.: Bradford Books/MIT Press

Weinberger, N.M. and Diamond, D.M. (1987): Physiological plasticity in auditory cortex: rapid induction by learning. *Prog. Neurobiol.* 29:1-55

Weinberger, N.M., Hopkins, W. and Diamond, D.M. (1984): Physiological plasticity of single neurons in auditory cortex of the cat during acquisition of the pupillary conditioned response: I. Primary field (A1). *Behav. Neurosci.* 98:171-188

Weinberger, N.M., Oleson, T.D. and Ashe, J.H., (1975): Sensory system neural activity during habituation of the pupillary orienting reflex. *Behav. Biol.* 15:283-301

Weinberger, N.M., Oleson, T.D. and Haste, D. (1973): Inhibitory control of conditional pupillary dilation response in the paralyzed cat. *Behav. Biol.* 9:307-316

Welsch, U. and Pearse, A.G.E. (1969): Electron cytochemistry of BuChE and AChE in thyriod and parathyroid C cells, under normal and experimental conditions. *Histochemie.* 17:1-10

Wepsic, J.G. (1966): Multimodal sensory activation of cells in the magnocellular medial geniculate nucleus. *Exp. Neurol.* 15:299-318

Williams, S. and Johnston, D. (1988): Muscarinic depression of long-term potentiation in CA3 hippocampal neurons. *Science* 242:84-87

Winer, J.A., Diamond, I.T. and Raczwokswi, D. (1977): Subdivisions of the auditory cortex of the cat: the retrograde transport of horseradish peroxidase to the medial geniculate body and posterior thalamic nuclei. *J. Comp. Neurol.* 177:387-418

Woody, C.D. (1988): Is conditioning supported by modulation of an outward current in pyramidal cells of the motor cortex of cats? In: *Cellular Mechanisms of Conditioning and Behavioral Plasticity.* Woody, C.D., Alkon, D.L. and McGaugh, J.L. eds. New York: Plenum Press

Woody, C.D., Swartz, B.E. and Gruen, E. (1978): Effects of acetylcholine and cyclic GMP on input resistance of cortical neurons in awake cats. *Brain Res.* 158:373-395

Worms, P., Gueudet, C., Perio, A. and Soubrie, P. (1989): Systemic injection of pirenzepine induces a deficit in passive avoidance learning in rats. *Psychopharm.* 98:286-288

Yamamura, H.I. and Snyder, S.H. (1974): Muscarinic cholinergic binding in rat brain. *Proc. Natl. Acad. Sci.* 71:1725-1729

Yarosh, C.A., Acosta, C.G. and Ashe, J.H., (1988): Modification of nicotinic ganglionic transmission by muscarinic slow postsynaptic potentials in the *in vitro* rabbit superior cervical ganglion. *Synapse* 2:174-182

Yarosh, C.A. and Ashe, J.H., (1987): Antagonist discrimination of two muscarinic responses elicited by applied agonists and orthodromic stimuli in superior cervical ganglion of rabbit. *Neuropharmacol.* 26:1539-1560

Yarosh, C.A., Ashe, J.H. and Olito, A.C. (1990): Differential effects of the muscarinic M_2 antagonists AF-DX 116 and gallamine on single neurons of rabbit sympathetic ganglia. *Neuropharmacol.* in press

Yarosh, C.A., Olito, A.C. and Ashe, J.H., (1988): AF-DX 116: a selective antagonist of the slow inhibitory postsynaptic potential and methacholine-induced hyperpolarization in superior cervical ganglion of the rabbit. *J. Pharmacol. Exp. Ther.* 245:419-425

Basal Forebrain, Memory and Attention

David S. Olton, Gary L. Wenk, and Alicja M. Markowska

INTRODUCTION

A functional analysis of the basal forebrain (BF), which includes the medial septal area (MSA) and nucleus basalis magnocellularis (NBM), benefits from consideration of its anatomical and neurochemical characteristics. Anatomically, the MSA projects to the hippocampus (H) and the NBM projects to the frontal cortex (FC) (Wenk et al., 1980; Fibiger, 1982), areas that have been linked to memory and attention (Schacter, 1987; Squire, 1987; Olton et al., 1988). Neurochemically, a major transmitter of cells in these BF areas is acetylcholine (Johnston et al., 1979), a transmitter that has been closely linked with mnemonic functions (Bartus et al., 1985a). If the projections from the BF to the H and FC are necessary for the normal function of these target areas, then destruction of these projections should result in behavioral syndromes similar to those produced by direct disruption of the target areas.

As might be expected by this introduction, behavioral tests used to examine the consequences of BF lesions have often used procedures that are sensitive to H and FC damage. These tasks have been useful in describing the types of behavioral changes produced by BF lesions. The discussion of these results is organized around three questions, each of which is summarized briefly here. The rest of the paper provides the details of this analysis.

Do BF lesions produce cognitive impairments?

Destruction of the H and FC, two targets of BF projections, produce changes in a wide variety of tasks. The basic characteristics of the frontal syndrome (the impairments following lesions of the FC) and the hippocampal syndrome (the impairments following lesions of the H) are well documented. The H syndrome is usually ascribed to a failure of some kind of memory (Squire, 1987; Olton, 1989b), whereas the FC syndrome has had a variety of interpretations, all of which have emphasized its role in cognition of some kind (Kolb, 1984; Fuster, 1989; Olton, 1989a). If the projections from the BF to the H and to the FC are necessary for the normal functioning of the H and FC, then lesions of the cells that project from the BF to these target sites should impair the cognitive processes requiring normal function of these target sites, in turn producing a syndrome of behavior that reflects these cognitive impairments.

Do the projections from different subdivisions of the BF have different functions?

The BF is topologically organized so that cells in different areas of the BF have projections to different target sites. Of particular importance for the current analysis is the distinction between the projections from the NBM to the FC, and the projections from the MSA to the H. The H syndrome and the FC syndrome, resulting from lesions of these target areas, differ in some of their characteristics, data which has led in turn to different descriptions of the functions of these areas. If this neuroanatomical organization has functional implications, then lesions of the NBM and MSA should produce different syndromes of behavior, reflecting the different functions of their target sites.

Are the behavioral impairments following lesions of the BF due to involvement of the cholinergic cells, or might other neurotransmitters also be involved?

The MSA and the NBM contain both cholinergic and noncholinergic cells. The neurotoxins used to make the lesions have destroyed both populations of cells. Consequently, both cholinergic and noncholinergic damage may contribute to the behavioral impairments observed after these lesions. If the behavioral deficits produced after these neurotoxic lesions are due solely to involvement of the cholinergic system, then the magnitude of the behavioral impairment should always be highly correlated with the magnitude of cholinergic damage. If these deficits are influenced by damage to noncholinergic systems, then this correlation should be reduced by any manipulation that independently alters the destruction of the cholinergic and noncholinergic components of the BF.

Each of these questions will be addressed in turn below. The titles of the respective sections indicate the answers to them. Only a few examples of the relevant experiments are provided here because extensive reviews are already available (Olton and Wenk, 1987; Wenk and Olton, 1987; Fibiger, in press).

COGNITIVE IMPAIRMENTS FOLLOW BF LESIONS

Destruction of the hippocampus produces a substantial amnesic syndrome in all mammals, and destruction of the FC can influence mnemonic abilities (Kolb, 1984; Schacter, 1987; Fuster, 1989; Olton, 1989a,b). In rats, lesions of both areas produce a substantial impairment of choice accuracy in tasks that require recent memory. These tasks are all variations of a delayed conditional discrimination (DCD). At the beginning of each trial in a DCD, some information is presented to the animal. After a subsequent delay interval, which can vary in length, two or more alternative responses are provided to the animal. The response that is correct at the end of the delay depends on the information that was presented at the beginning of the delay. Consequently, the optimal strategy for the animal is to remember that information during the delay interval, and then choose the appropriate response.

Lesions of both the FC and H impair choice accuracy in a DCD, and the magnitude of this impairment is often related to the length of the delay. With a short delay, the lesion group may perform almost as accurately as controls. With a long delay, the lesion group may have a maximal impairment and perform at the level expected by chance. This pattern of results, with the magnitude of the impairment increasing with the length of the delay, is usually taken to indicate that the behavioral impairment in the DCD is due to a primary disruption of recent memory.

Neurotoxic lesions of the BF produce a consistent impairment in DCD tasks, which require recent memory. The magnitude of this impairment typically increases with longer delays.

One DCD used a discrete trial spatial delayed nonmatch-to-sample task in a T-maze (Hepler et al., 1985). At the beginning of each trial, only one arm was available to the rat. The rat entered the arm and obtained reinforcement there. After the delay interval, both arms were available to the rat. However, reinforcement was present only in the arm not entered prior to the delay, at the beginning of the trial. Consequently, the optimal strategy for the rat was to remember the arm entered at the beginning of each trial, prior to the delay, and when given a choice at the end of each trial after the delay, enter the opposite arm. At the end of postoperative testing, rats with BF lesions had normal choice accuracy with a 5-second delay, but had severely impaired choice accuracy with a one-minute delay.

Similar results followed NBM lesions in a DCD tested on a radial arm maze (Bartus et al., 1985b). The maze had 8 arms extending from a central platform. At the beginning of each trial, one pellet of food was placed at the end of each arm. Consequently, the optimal strategy for the rat was to enter each arm once, obtain the food there, and not return to that arm during the rest of the test session. The delay interval between the fourth and fifth choice varied from a few seconds to 24 hours. During initial postoperative testing, the magnitude of the impairment produced by the NBM lesions was greater with longer delays than with shorter delays.

BF lesions consistently produce an impairment in all types of DCDs (for reviews, see Olton and Wenk, 1987; Wenk and Olton, 1987). The delay-related increase in the magnitude of the impairment suggests that these lesions disrupt recent memory.

The cognitive impairments produced by BF lesions include cognitive abilities other than recent memory. Long-term spatial reference memory is also disrupted by these lesions (for a review, see Olton and Wenk, 1987).

In summary, then, BF lesions produce substantial and consistent impairments in both recent memory and other types of memory. These impairments are similar to those produced by lesions of the H and FC.

NBM AND MSA LESIONS PRODUCE DIFFERENT BEHAVIORAL EFFECTS

Determining if NBM and MSA lesions produce different behavioral effects in rats is complicated by the fact that lesions of the FC and H, the target sites of these two BF areas respectively, produce similar changes in many different behavioral tasks (Olton et al., 1979; Kolb, 1984).

Thus, the absence of a dissociation between the effects of NBM and MSA lesions in a task showing no dissociations after F and HC lesions is not informative. Consequently, the most relevant data come from the few tasks in which lesions of the H and FC did produce dissociations. In these tasks, lesions of the MSA and NBM produced similar dissociations.

Three dissociations occurred in tests of timing: reference memory for the expected time of reinforcement (MSA lesions, too short; NBM lesions, too long); working memory for the duration of a previous stimulus following a gap in the stimulus (MSA lesions, impaired; NBM lesions, no effect); divided attention for timing two stimuli simultaneously (MSA lesions, no effect; NBM lesions, impaired). These dissociations were identical to those produced by lesions of the fimbria-fornix (FF), one of the major extrinsic fiber connections of the H, and the FC (Meck et al., 1984; Meck et al., 1987; Olton et al., 1987; Olton et al., 1988).

All three measures of performance were obtained from variations of a fixed interval (FI) schedule of reinforcement. Each rat was first trained with two discriminative stimuli, each one indicating a different FI schedule. For each training trial, one stimulus was turned on. After the appropriate FI interval, the first lever press by the rat produced reinforcement. The *short stimulus* indicated an FI-10-second schedule, with food available for the first lever press 10 seconds after the onset of the stimulus. The *long stimulus* indicated an FI schedule longer than 10 seconds, ranging from 20 seconds to 40 seconds in different experiments.

The optimal strategy for the rat during each of these training trials was to wait until the appropriate FI interval had been completed, and then press the lever. The rats did not perform optimally, but they did develop the usual scalloped response rate function. The response rate was low at the beginning of the trial, and gradually increased until reinforcement was received (when it went to zero because the rat stopped pressing the bar and ate the food).

Probe trials assessed the reference memory for the expected time of reinforcement. For each *probe trial*, the stimulus was turned on as for the training trial. However, it remained on for an extended period of time, and no reinforcement was given for any response. Control (CON) rats had a peak in the response rate at the time when food was available during the training trials. Prior to the time when food had been delivered in the training trials, the response rate function showed the usual positively accelerated increase. After the time when reinforcement had been available, the response rate function had a symmetrical decrease. The *peak time* was the time at which the response rate reached its peak. For CON rats, the peak time was at the time when food had been delivered in the FI training trials. For MSA rats, the peak time was too early. For NBM rats, the peak time was too late. This pattern of results indicates that both the MSA and the NBM are involved in accurate recall of the expected time of reinforcement, but in complementary ways.

Working memory for the duration of a previously presented stimulus was assessed by performance during gap trials. During each *gap trial*, the stimulus was turned on for a brief period (shorter than the FI interval associated with that stimulus), turned off for a short delay (the gap), and turned back on. During training trials, food was delivered for the first bar press after the appropriate duration of the stimulus. Consequently, the optimal strategy for the rat was the following: when the gap occurred, remember the duration of the stimulus prior to the gap; when the gap ended, add that value to the duration of the stimulus that was presented after the gap. The ability to perform this task was assessed in probe trials as described above. In each probe trial, the stimulus after the gap was turned on for an extended period of time, and no reinforcement was given for any bar press.

CON rats had a peak time at the time when reinforcement had been delivered during the training trials; the peak time was shifted to the right by an amount equal to the gap as compared to the standard reference memory trials with no gap. This shift to the right of the peak time by an amount equal to the gap indicated that CON rats remembered the duration of the stimulus prior to the gap when the gap occurred, and added that value to the duration of the stimulus after the gap when the stimulus resumed. NBM rats performed equivalently to CON rats, indicating that they also had an accurate working memory. MSA rats had an additional rightward shift of the peak time, a shift equal to the duration of the gap plus the duration of the stimulus prior to the gap. These data indicate that when the gap occurred, MSA rats forgot the duration of the stimulus prior to the gap, and began timing again from the beginning when the stimulus was turned back on. Thus, MSA lesions impaired working memory for the duration of the stimulus prior to the gap and produced resetting, while NBM lesions had no effect.

Divided attention for timing two stimuli simultaneously was assessed in compound trials. In each *compound trial*, the long stimulus was turned on. Following a brief and variable delay, the short stimulus was turned on. Food was available after the appropriate interval of time from the onset of each stimulus. The optimal strategy for the rat during these compound trials was to time each stimulus simultaneously, which required divided attention.

Compound probe trials, similar to the ones described previously, assessed each rat's ability to perform this divided attention task. For each compound probe trial, the long stimulus was turned on, after a brief and variable delay the short stimulus was turned on, both stimuli remained on for an extended period of time, and no reinforcement was given for any lever press. CON rats had two peak times, one at each of the appropriate intervals following the onset of the stimulus; the peak times for both the short stimulus and the long stimulus in compound probe trials were the same as the peak times for each of those stimuli when presented alone in the reference memory trials. FF rats performed similarly. NBM rats had a rightward shift in the peak time for the long stimulus that was equal to the duration of the short stimulus, and a peak time for the short stimulus that was similar to the peak time in the reference memory probe test when only one stimulus was presented at a time. This selective rightward shift of the peak time for the long stimulus by an interval equal to the duration of the short stimulus indicates that NBM rats were unable to time both stimuli simultaneously. At the beginning of the compound probe trial, when only the long stimulus was present, they timed it. When the short stimulus was subsequently presented, they stopped timing the long stimulus and timed only the short stimulus. At the end of the 10-second FI associated with the short stimulus, when food had been delivered in the training trials, the rats returned to timing the long stimulus. Consequently, the peak time for the long stimulus was offset to the right by a value equal to the duration of the short stimulus. These results indicate that NBM lesions, but not MSA lesions, interfere with the processes of divided attention.

Primacy and recency effects also show dissociations following small MSA and NBM lesions (Kesner et al., 1987; Kesner, 1988; Kesner et al., 1988). The apparatus was a radial arm maze as described previously, with 8 arms extending from a central choice point. At the beginning of each test session, one pellet of food was placed on each of the 8 arms. For the *sample phase*, the rat was allowed to choose each of the 8 arms in an order determined by the experimenter. The rat was placed in the center of the maze. The guillotine door to one arm was raised allowing the rat to enter that arm, obtain the reinforcement, and return to the center. The guillotine door to the arm just chosen was lowered, and the door to another arm was raised. This procedure was repeated until the rat had chosen each of the 8 arms.

For the assessment of primacy and recency in the *study phase*, the rat was given a choice between two of the arms previously chosen. Food was available on the arm that had been chosen first during the study phase. Consequently, the optimal strategy for the rat was to remember the order of the arms chosen during the study phase, and return to the one that had been chosen first.

CON rats showed greater choice accuracy during the test phase for the first two arms entered during the study phase (a primacy effect), and the last two arms entered during the study phase (a recency effect) than for the middle two arms entered during the study phase. Partial MSA lesions disrupted the primacy effect but not the recency effect. Partial NBM lesions produced the complementary pattern of results, an impairment of the recency effect but not the primacy effect.

These results indicate that both the MSA and NBM are involved in remembering serial order, but in complementary ways. The MSA is primarily required for the cognitive processes associated with the primacy effect, while the NBM is primarily associated with the cognitive processes responsible for the recency effect.

Together, these patterns of results clearly demonstrate that functional dissociations can be produced by MSA and NBM lesions. These dissociations follow logically from two other observations. First, lesions of the two BF regions produce behavioral effects similar to those following lesions of their target sites in the H and FC, respectively. Second, lesions of these target sites produce behavioral dissociations in some tasks.

At a behavioral level of analysis, these data indicate that the NBM and MSA must have different functions, as assessed by the effects of lesions in them. At a more molecular level of analysis, of course, these two brain areas may have similar functions. Thus, the projections from both BF nuclei may facilitate individual neurons at the target sites through the same neuronal mechanisms. However, because these neurons process different types of information, the effects of lesions in the NBM and MSA are different. Alternatively, the BF projections to the FC and H may have different functions at a molecular level as well as a behavioral level. More detailed analyses of the neural interactions of basal forebrain neurons with their target neurons are necessary to determine at what level the functional differences arise.

NONCHOLINERGIC SYSTEMS IN THE BASAL FOREBRAIN MAY CONTRIBUTE TO THE COGNITIVE IMPAIRMENTS PRODUCED BY NEUROTOXIC LESIONS

Ibotenic (IBO) acid has been the neurotoxin most often used to produce lesions in the BF. It destroys cells at the site of the injection, and reduces choline acetyltransferase (ChAT) activity at the site normally innervated by the damaged cells. Thus, IBO clearly destroys cholinergic cell bodies in the BF, and the fact that many of the behavioral impairments following BF lesions are similar to those produced by anticholinergic drugs such as scopolamine suggests that cholinergic pathology may be responsible for the resulting cognitive impairments.

However, a comparison of the neurochemical and behavioral effects produced by IBO with those produced by another neurotoxin, quisqualic (QUIS) acid, indicates that destruction of noncholinergic systems may also contribute to the cognitive impairments following neurotoxic lesions of the NBM. The general pattern of the results is as follows. QUIS, as compared to IBO, produces a greater decrease of ChAT in the FC and a greater loss of cholinergic cell bodies in the NBM, indicating that it produces a greater pathological insult to the cholinergic basal forebrain system. Behaviorally, however, the opposite pattern of results occurs. QUIS, as compared to IBO, produces much less of a behavioral impairment. This dissociation of the neural and cognitive effects of these two neurotoxins suggests that noncholinergic damage produced by IBO may contribute to the cognitive impairments following these NBM lesions.

Tests of recent memory in a nonspatial and spatial DCD in a T-maze showed this kind of dissociation following neurotoxic lesions of the NBM by IBO and QUIS (Markowska et al., 1990). IBO reduced ChAT activity by 45%, while QUIS reduced it even further, by 74%. The DCD was a continuous cued delayed nonmatch-to-sample discrimination. The discriminative stimuli were two goal boxes, each with a distinctive visual and tactual pattern. At the beginning of each trial, for the *forced run*, only one goal was available. The rat entered that goal box and obtained reinforcement. For the subsequent *choice run*, which followed the delay, both goal boxes were available. However, reinforcement was available only in the goal box not entered during the forced run prior to the delay.

At the beginning of testing, IBO and QUIS rats showed a substantial and equivalent impairment. After 150 trials, CON rats reached asymptotic performance, about 88% correct responses on the choice trials. Both IBO and QUIS rats had choice accuracy only slightly greater than chance after 150 trials, approximately 65%. With continued testing, QUIS rats consistently improved choice accuracy until they reached a level equivalent to that of CON rats. In contrast, IBO rats had only a slight improvement in choice accuracy, and at the end of behavioral testing (more than 500 trials), still remained at approximately 70% correct.

A similar result occurred in a continuous-trial spatial nonmatch-to-sample discrimination in a T-maze. For the first, *forced trial*, in each test session, only one arm was available. The rat entered that arm and obtained food there. All subsequent trials in each test session were choice trials. During each *choice* trial, both arms were available but food was in only the arm not entered during the previous choice trial. Again, both IBO and QUIS rats had a similar and significant impairment at the beginning of behavioral testing. At the end, however, QUIS rats performed as well as CON rats, while IBO rats still had a substantial impairment.

The significant impairment by both IBO and QUIS at the beginning of behavioral testing is consistent with the idea that dysfunction of cholinergic cells in the NBM is responsible for the impairment of recent memory. However, the normal choice accuracy of QUIS rats at the end of behavioral testing is inconsistent with this hypothesis. QUIS rats, as compared to IBO rats, had a greater decrease in ChAT but a smaller behavioral impairment. Consequently, noncholinergic systems must contribute to the behavioral impairments observed following neurotoxic lesions of the BF produced by IBO (Dunnett et al., 1987; Etherington et al., 1987;Wenk et al., 1989; Markowska et al., 1990).

This pattern of neurochemical and behavioral differences produced by QUIS and IBO provides some challenges to interpretations that emphasize the role of the cholinergic system in memory (For example, see review by Bartus et al., 1985). Some clarification of the "cholinergic hypothesis" is important in order to be specific about the idea that is being evaluated. For the present discussion, two possible versions of the cholinergic hypothesis are not being considered, because these are already proven to be incorrect.

(1) Only the BF cholinergic system is involved in memory.
(2) The BF cholinergic system is involved only in memory.

Rather, the hypothesis being considered is that the BF cholinergic system is involved in memory. The results from the comparison of QUIS and IBO are consistent with this hypothesis, and certainly do not refute it. Thus, the fundamental version of the cholinergic hypothesis clearly remains intact. However, a more inclusive analysis of the neurotransmitter systems involved in memory indicates that some additional mechanisms must be involved in modulating memory function. This section considers some alternative mechanisms that might be responsible for the differences produced by QUIS and IBO.

The measurement of ChAT may not be the optimal measurement for assessing the effects of these two neurotoxins on cholinergic function. ChAT is not rate limiting in the synthesis of acetylcholine. Although it is often useful to determine whether or not an intervention has killed cholinergic cells, it may not accurately assess the extent to which the remaining cholinergic system is functioning effectively. Microdialysis of acetylcholine in the FC, and dynamic measures of acetylcholine release to stimulation of the NBM can help resolve this issue. If QUIS not only destroys more cells but also reduces the effectiveness of the remaining cells, then it should reduce these other measures of cholinergic function. The likelihood of this hypothesis being confirmed is influenced by information about the number of cholinergic cells remaining after QUIS lesions. Because QUIS destroys almost all cholinergic cells, the ability of the remaining few to influence target neurons may be severely limited. However, this hypothesis is consistent with the currently available data, and should be carefully evaluated.

Most interpretations of the neural mechanisms responsible for the different effects of IBO and QUIS suggest that IBO destroys something in addition to that destroyed by QUIS. IBO produced changes in the number of cortical neurotensin receptors while QUIS did not (Wenk et al., 1989), and IBO induced a local inflammatory response (Coffey et al., 1988). Additional analyses are desirable. If IBO does destroy some neural component that is not affected by QUIS, and if this neural component can be manipulated independently of the cholinergic system, then the role of this component in memory functions can be examined. For example, if this additional component is responsible for the prolonged impairments produced by IBO but not by QUIS, then the addition of this component to a lesion produced by QUIS should produce the same kinds of behavioral impairments that follow IBO.

Alternatively, QUIS may be destroying something more than IBO, and that extra destruction compensates for the cholinergic disruption. This compensation might take place either within the cholinergic system, or in some other system. Thus, recovery of function following QUIS might be more effective than that following IBO because changes in the cholinergic cells that survive QUIS may help to compensate for the loss of the cells produced by QUIS (if a sufficient number of cholinergic cells remain after a QUIS lesion to produce compensation). Alternatively, the recovery of function might be mediated by changes in another transmitter system that helps to restore balance between the cholinergic system and some other transmitter system.

Finally, of course, the mechanisms responsible for the behavioral impairments following both IBO and QUIS may not depend upon alterations in the FC, but may be due to changes in other areas of the brain (Dunnett, in press). A thorough search of electrophysiological and neurochemical changes in many different brain areas may help to identify pathological alterations that are more strongly correlated with the magnitude of the behavioral deficit in individual animals than is the change in ChAT activity in the FC.

In summary, then, the pattern of neurochemical and behavioral changes following lesions produced by IBO and QUIS provides an opportunity to investigate the way in which the cholinergic system interacts with other neurotransmitter systems to influence memory processing. All of the ideas discussed above are testable, and a reasonable argument can be made to support each of them. The experimental data obtained from these analyses should help us to gain further information about the role of the basal forebrain system in cognitive processes, and the ways in which cholinergic and noncholinergic systems interact with each other.

FUTURE DIRECTIONS

The use of neurotoxic lesions, rather than physical (electrolytic or radio frequency) lesions, has significantly increased the specificity of the neuropathology. Unlike physical lesions, which destroy fibers of passage as well as cell bodies, these neurotoxic lesions can destroy only cell bodies, sparing fibers of passage. Thus, the behavioral consequences can be attributed to selective damage of the cell bodies in the area of the lesion.

As indicated in the discussion of IBO and QUIS, further increases in specificity are desirable. Microinfusions offer substantial promise. For example, consider the results of an experiment examining the role of GABAergic and cholinergic neurotransmission in the MSA (Givens and Olton, in press). Cholinergic cells in the MSA have both excitatory cholinergic and inhibitory GABAergic synapses on them. If the activity of these cells is important for normal hippocampal function, which is in turn necessary for normal recent memory, then alterations in the activity of these cells should alter hippocampal function and impair recent memory. Hippocampal function was assessed by measuring the theta rhythm, a characteristic slow wave of 7-8 Hz. Recent memory was assessed by measuring choice accuracy in a spatial alternation task in a T-maze. A reduction in the power of hippocampal theta and a decrease in choice accuracy followed microinfusion of scopolamine, a cholinergic antagonist, and muscimol, a GABAergic agonist, into the MSA. These effects were reversible, occurring 10 minutes after the injection, but disappearing by 90 minutes after the injection. These data provide strong support for the conclusion that both cholinergic and GABAergic mechanisms in the MSA portion of the BF have significant effects on neuronal activity in the hippocampus, which in turn affects recent memory.

Microinfusions, as compared to neurotoxic lesions, provide several important advantages. They are reversible, more specific for neurotransmitter systems, and permit both excitation and inhibition of neuronal activity. Consequently, the use of microinfusions, rather than neurotoxic lesions, should provide the opportunity to obtain more detailed information about the functions of different components of the BF system.

Measurements of cholinergic activity at the terminals of the BF neurons should also provide a significant increase in the specificity of information about BF function. High affinity choline uptake (HACU), a measure of the level of the activity of cholinergic neurons, can be altered by behavior (Wenk et al., 1984). HACU can provide significant anatomical and neurochemical specificity to assess the ways in which different types of behavioral experiences and psychological demands engage the cholinergic system. An unfortunate characteristic of HACU is that it can be measured only once in a given animal. In contrast, *in vivo* microdialysis of acetylcholine provides the opportunity for repeated measurements, time locked to different behavioral events. Although this technique is still being developed, its promise is substantial, and should provide an important advance over HACU.

Predicting the future is always difficult. However, given the previous success of the analysis of basal forebrain function with neurotoxic lesions, and the significant improvements offered by microinfusions and *in vivo* microdialysis, these latter two techniques are likely to become predominant in behavioral and psychological investigations of BF function (Olton et al., in press).

CONCLUSIONS

These experiments demonstrate that pathological changes in the cells of the BF can disrupt many different cognitive functions, especially those involved in recent memory. More generally, the cholinergic projections from the NBM to the FC, and from the MSA to the H, are both necessary for normal function of the respective target sites. Thus, any theory that attempts to explain the neural bases of functions related to the FC or H must consider the important involvement of projections from the BF to these areas.

The data summarized here clearly indicate an important role of the BF cells in supporting normal cognitive functions. Future research should focus on the neural mechanisms by which the BF cells mediate these functions. Neural manipulations that are selective for specific types of cells should be an important tool in this endeavor.

REFERENCES

Bartus, R.T., Dean, R.L., Pontecorvo, M.J., and Lippa, A.S. (1985a): The cholinergic hypothesis: an historical overview, current perspective, and future directions. In: *Memory Dysfunctions: An Integration of Animal and Human Research from Preclinical and Clinical Perspectives.* Olton, D., Gamzu, E., Corkin, S., eds. New York: The New York Academy of Sciences Press. pp. 332-358

Bartus, R.T., Flicker, C., Dean R.L., Pontecorvo, M., Figueiredo, J.C., and Fisher, S.K. (1985b): Selective memory loss following nucleus basalis lesions: long term behavioral recovery despite persistent cholinergic deficiencies. *Pharmacol. Biochem. Behav.* 23:125-135

Coffey, P.J., Perry, V.H., Allen, Y., Sinden, J., and Rawlins, J.N.P. (1988): Ibotenic acid induced demyelination in the central nervous system: a consequence of a local inflammatory response. *Neurosci. Lett.* 84:171-184

Dunnett, S.B. (in press): *Symposium Medicum Hoechst.*, 23

Dunnett, S.B., Whishaw, I.Q., Jones, G.H., and Bunch, S.T. (1987): Behavioral, biochemical and histochemical effects of different neurotoxic amino acids injected into nucleus basalis magnocellularis of rats. *Neurosci.* 20:653-669

Etherington, R., Mittleman, G., and Robbins, T.W. (1987): Comparative effects of nucleus basalis and fimbria-fornix lesions on delayed matching and alternation tests of memory. *Neurosci. Res. Commun.* 1:135-143

Fibiger, H.C. (1982): The organization and some projections of cholinergic neurons of the mammalian forebrain. *Brain Res. Rev.* 4:327-328

Fibiger, H.C. (in press): Central cholinergic systems and memory. *Symposium Medicum Hoechst*, 23.

Fuster, J.M. (1989): *The Prefrontal Cortex: Anatomy, Physiology, and Neuropsychology of the Frontal Lobe.* (2nd ed.). New York: Raven Press

Givens, B. and Olton, D. (in press): Cholinergic and GABAergic modulation of medial septal area: effect on working memory. *Behav. Neurosci.*

Hepler, D.J., Olton, D.S., Wenk, G.L. and Coyle, J.T. (1985): Lesions in nucleus basalis magnocellularis and media septal area of rats produce qualitatively similar memory impairments. *J. Neurosci.* 5:866-873

Johnston, M.V., Michael McKinney, and Citke, H.T. (1979): Evidence for a cholinergic projection to neocortex from neurons in basal forebrain. *Neurobiol.* 76 (10): 5392-5396

Kesner, R.P. (1988): Reevaluation of the contribution of the basal forebrain cholinergic system to memory. *Neurobiol. Aging* 9:609–616

Kesner, R.P., Adelstein T., and Crutcher, K.A. (1987): Rats with nucleus basalis magnocellularis lesions mimic mnemonic symptomatology observed in patient with dementia of the Alzheimer's type. *Behav. Neurosci.* 101(4):451-456

Kesner, R.P., Crutcher, K. and Beers, D.R. (1988) : Serial position curves for item (spatial location) information: role of the dorsal hippocampal formation and medial septum. *Brain Res.* 454:219–226.

Kolb, B. (1984): Functions of the frontal cortex of the rat: a comparative review. *Brain Res. Rev.* 8:65-98

Markowska, A.L., Wenk, G. and Olton, D. (1990): Nucleus basalis magnocellularis and memory: differential effects of two neurotoxins. *Behav. Neural Biol.* 54:13-26

Meck, W.H., Church, R.M. and Olton, D.S. (1984): Hippocampus, time, and memory. *Behav. Neurosci.* 98:3-22

Meck, W.H., Church, R.M., Wenk, G.L. and Olton, D.S. (1987) : Nucleus basalis magnocellularis and media septal area lesions differentially impair temporal memory. *J. Neurosci.* 7 (11):3505-3511

Olton, D.S. (1989a): Frontal cortex, timing, and memory. *Neuropsychologia* 27:

121-130.

Olton, D.S. (1989b): Mnemonic functions of the hippocampus: Single unit analyses in rats. In: *The hippocampus: New Vistas*. Chan-Palay, V., ed. New York: Alan R. Liss, pp. 411-424

Olton, D.S., Becker, J.T. and Handelmann, G.E. (1979): Hippocampus, space and memory. *Behav. Br. Sci.* 2:313-322

Olton, D., Markowska, A., Voytko, M.L., Givens, B., Gorman, L., and Wenk, G. (in press): Basal forebrain cholinergic system: a functional analysis. In: *The Basal Forebrain: Anatomy to Function*. Napier, T.C., Kalivas, P., Hanin, I., eds. New York: Plenum Press

Olton, D.S. and Wenk, G.L. (1987): Animal models of the cognitive impairments produced by degeneration of the basal forebrain cholinergic system. In: *Psychopharmacology: A Third Generation of Progress*. Meltzer, H.Y., ed. New York: Raven Press, pp. 941-953

Olton, D.S., Meck, W.H. and Church, R.M. (1987): Separation of hippocampal and amygdaloid involvement in temporal memory dysfunctions. *Brain Res.* 404:180-188

Olton, D.S., Wenk, G.L., Church, R.M. and Meck, W.H. (1988): Attention and the frontal cortex as examined by simultaneous temporal processing and lesions of the basal forebrain cholinergic system. *Neuropsychologia* 26:307-318

Schacter, D.L. (1987): Memory, amnesia, frontal lobe dysfunction. *Psychobiol.* 15(1):21-36

Squire, L.R. (1987): *Memory and Brain*. New York: Oxford University Press

Wenk, H., Bigl, V. and Meyer, U. (1980): Cholinergic projections from magnocellular nuclei of the basal forebrain to cortical areas in rats. *Brain Res. Rev.* 2:295-316

Wenk, G.L., Hepler, D. and Olton, D. (1984): Behavior alters the uptake of [^{3}H]choline into acetylcholinergic neurons of the nucleus basalis magnocellularis and medial septal area. *Behav. Brain Res.*, 13:129-138

Wenk, G.L. and Olton, D.S. (1987): Basal forebrain cholinergic neurons and Alzheimer's disease. In: *Experimental Models of Dementing Disorders: A Synaptic Neurochemical Perspective*. Coyle, J., ed. New York: Alan R. Liss, Inc. pp 81-101

Wenk, G.L., Markowska, A.L. and Olton, D.S. (1989): Basal forebrain lesions and memory: alteration in neurotensin, not acetylcholine, may cause amnesia. *Behav. Neurosci.* 103:1624-1628

An Analysis of the Basal Forebrain Contribution to Learning and Memory

Raymond P. Kesner and Debra L. Johnson

INTRODUCTION

In the last thirty years a large number of neural regions (e.g., hippocampus, amygdala, neocortex) have been identified as playing important roles in mediating memory. More recently, a new neural region has been discovered as a potentially important new area subserving memory function. This neural region is known as the basal forebrain area. It has gained prominence because dysfunction (cell loss) of this area may be associated with dementia of the Alzheimer's type.

In Alzheimer's disease not only is there a cell loss in the basal forebrain area, but there are also reduced levels of cortical and limbic cholinergic activity as well as the formation of neurofibrillary tangles and senile plaques in neocortex, amygdala and hippocampal formation (Tomlinson and Kitchener, 1972; Bowen et al., 1976; Ball, 1977; Tomlinson, 1977; Bird et al., 1983; Kemper, 1983; Hyman et al., 1984; Price, 1986; Van Hoesen et al., 1986). These latter neural regions represent target areas for cholinergic neurons of the basal forebrain areas (Coyle et al., 1983; McKinney et al. 1983; Carlsen et al., 1985; Butcher and Woolf, 1986) and these areas have also been implicated in memory function (Corkin, 1982; Mishkin, 1982; Olton, 1983; Kesner and DiMattia, 1987).

Further evidence that the cholinergic basal forebrain system might indeed play a critical role in mnemonic function comes from studies with humans that have sustained damage to the basal forebrain due to rupture of anterior cerebral or anterior communicating aneurysms or war wounds. The general findings are a deficit in episodic coding of contextual information and the inability to code temporal information (Salazar et al.,

1981; Alexander and Freedman, 1983; Volpe and Hirst, 1983; Damasio et al., 1985).

Even though the data are suggestive that the basal forebrain contributes to memory function, the progressive nature of Alzheimer's disease, the inability to clearly determine the extent of cell loss until autopsy, and the variability in memory dysfunction have made it difficult to ascertain the strength of the neuroanatomy-memory relationship. In order to test further the exact role of the cholinergic basal forebrain system in mediating memory, a number of investigators have used animal models, for which the rodent has been used extensively. In these models the basal forebrain cholinergic system or its cholinergic targets is damaged and behavioral tests are performed to determine mnemonic function. It is assumed that anatomically the basal forebrain cholinergic system and its targets in the rat are homologous to humans.

In this chapter an attempt will be made to clarify further the relationship between the basal forebrain cholinergic system and mnemonic function by addressing two specific issues. First, does the cholinergic basal forebrain system play a role in mediating memory, and does this system act as a single unit or do the different components (e.g., medial septum (MS), vertical nucleus of diagonal band (VNDB), horizontal nucleus of the diagonal band (HNDB), and nucleus basalis magnocellularis (NBM)) have different or similar functions? Second, to what extent are the deficits observed in the basal forebrain system due to interference with its cholinergic projection? In order to answer this second question, a number of strategies have been used. The first involves the determination of whether the basal forebrain cholinergic system mediation of memory function is paralleled by its specific cholinergic target(s), which would be the hippocampus in the case of MS and VNDB, the medial prefrontal cortex, orbital frontal cortex, visual cortex, entorhinal cortex, and olfactory bulb in the case of the HNDB and the dorsolateral frontal cortex, parietal cortex and basolateral amygdala in the case of the NBM.

The second strategy involves the determination of whether specific relationships exist between degree of damage to the cholinergic system and behavioral performance. The third strategy involves the use of pharmacological manipulations of the cholinergic system aimed at potentially reversing basal forebrain damage-induced memory deficits. The fourth strategy involves an analysis of different potential neural transmitters affected by basal forebrain damage as well as an analysis of the role of afferent inputs into the basal forebrain area from the neocortex and limbic system. In order to address specifically these two issues, this review will be somewhat limited with a primary emphasis on lesion research in rats.

MEDIAL SEPTUM, NUCLEUS BASALIS MAGNOCELLULARIS, HORIZONTAL NUCLEUS OF THE DIAGONAL BAND AND MEMORY

A number of neuroanatomists have suggested that the cholinergic basal forebrain system can on the basis of its projections be divided into at least three systems, namely, the MS and VNDB with its primary cholinergic projection to the hippocampus, the HNDB with its primary cholinergic projection to the olfactory bulbs, medial prefrontal, orbital frontal, insular, visual and entorhinal cortex and NBM with its primary cholinergic projection to dorsolateral frontal and parietal cortex as well as basolateral amygdala (Bigl et al., 1982; Woolf and Butcher 1982; McKinney et al., 1983; Mesulam et al., 1983; Carlsen et al., 1985; Záborszky et al., 1986).

Since very little work has been done with damage to the HNDB systems, most of the comparisons will be made between MS and NBM. It should be noted that caution is necessary whenever one compares the behavioral (memory) consequences of lesions in these two brain areas. First, there are only a few studies in which both MS and NBM lesions are made using the same paradigm and procedures to test memory function. Second, it is relatively easier to deplete the target of most of its cholinergic input with MS in comparison with NBM lesions. Third, within the NBM there are more cholinergic efferents projections (80-90%) than within the MS (30-35%). Fourth, the number of cholinergic cells that need to be destroyed to produce an observable behavioral impairment might vary between the two regions. Fifth, it is difficult to assess the contribution of damage to non-cholinergic cells within the two regions. Sixth, possible dissociations of function between MS and NBM might be dependent on the ability to dissociate the functional contribution to memory of its separate target structures. Even though these problems exist, there are two specific outcomes that are somewhat easier to interpret. In the first case, one can conclude that MS and NBM share a similar mnemonic function when the same effects (deficits or facilitation) occur on one or more behavioral tasks following MS and NBM lesions, even though it is always possible that alterations in mnemonic function could be due to different mechanisms. In the second case one can conclude that MS and NBM have an independent or parallel mnemonic function, when animals with MS lesions affect memory on Task A but not Task B, while animals with NBM lesions affect memory on Task B but not Task A. In general, the data indicate that MS and NBM share some mnemonic functions, but mediate independently other mnemonic functions.

Passive and Active Avoidance Tasks

It is clear that both NBM and MS lesions impair acquisition and retention of passive avoidance (Flicker et al., 1983; Altman et al., 1985; Hepler et al., 1985; Lerer et al., 1985; Miyamoto et al., 1985; Dunnett et al.,1987; Berman et al., 1988). In contrast, the majority of MS lesion studies show facilitation of two-way active avoidance learning (Gray and McNaughton, 1983), while NBM lesions either impair or facilitate two-way active avoidance learning (LoConte et al., 1982; Hepler et al.,1985; Miyamoto et al, 1985; Kessler et al., 1986).

Win-Shift Tasks

With respect to acquisition on tasks requiring a win-shift rule for lists of spatial locations, Hepler et al. (1985) reported a deficit for both NBM or MS lesions for 8 spatial locations. Similar deficits were reported by Beninger et al. (1986) with NBM lesioned animals for 4 spatial locations. However, Murray and Fibiger (1985) did not find a deficit with NBM lesioned animals for 9 spatial locations. With respect to performance on win-shift tasks, after extensive pretraining, both MS and NBM lesions resulted in a deficit followed by recovery on a 2 arm task, but performance on the win-shift component of an 8 arm task was impaired following MS, but not NBM lesions (Olton, et al., 1978; Crutcher et al., 1983; Bartus et al., 1985; Hepler et al. 1985). Thus, both similarities and differences can be found between MS and NBM on tasks requiring a win-shift rule for spatial information depending to some extent on task difficulty and extent of preoperative training.

Time Estimation Task

With respect to time estimation, it appears that animals with MS lesions overestimate the duration of a stimulus, while animals with NBM lesions underestimate the duration of a stimulus (Meck et al., 1984; Wenk and Olton, 1987).

Water Maze Task

Hagan et al. (1988) have shown that animals with MS/VNDB lesions are impaired in a place navigation learning task in a water maze, but animals with NBM lesions are not impaired. It should be noted, however, that others (Whishaw et al., 1985; Dunnett et al., 1987; Mandel et al., 1989) have shown that NBM lesions can impair the learning of a place navigation task, but in these studies a group with MS/VNDB lesions was not included.

Item-Order List Tasks

In our laboratory we have selected to study the contribution of MS and NBM in two complex item and order list learning tasks in which both rats and humans display serial position curves (better memory for the first and last events compared to the middle events within the list) for the occurrence of specific events (spatial locations) labelled *item* recognition memory or the *sequential* occurrence of specific events labelled *order* recognition memory.

Details of the procedures used to assess item and order recognition memory can be found in DiMattia and Kesner (1984) and Kesner et al. (1984). Briefly, for the *item* memory task each animal was allowed to visit a sequence of five arms on each trial (one per day), which was selected on a pseudo-random basis. This constituted the study phase. Immediately after the animal had received reinforcement from the last of the five arms, the test phase began. Only one test was given for each trial and consisted of opening two doors simultaneously, with one door representing an arm previously visited for that trial and the other door representing a novel arm for that trial. The rule to be learned leading to an additional reinforcement was to choose the arm that had been previously visited during the study phase of the trial (win-stay).

For the *order* memory task, each animal was allowed on each trial (one per day) to visit all eight arms in an order that was randomly selected for that trial. This constituted the study phase. Immediately after the animal had received reinforcement from the last of the eight arms, the test phase began. Only one test was given for each trial and consisted of opening two doors simultaneously. On a random basis either the

1st and 2nd, 4th and 5th, or 7th and 8th doors that occurred in the sequence were selected for the test. The rule to be learned leading to an additional reinforcement was to choose the arm that occurred earlier in the sequence. After extensive training and reaching criterion performance animals received lesions of specific neural regions followed by a new set of trials.

Results indicated that animals with large MS or NBM lesions had a deficit for all choice orders in the order memory task (see Table 1). However, with small (asymetric or unilateral) MS or NBM lesions, there was a double dissociation effect with MS lesions producing an impairment only for the first choice order without altering performance for the last choice order and NBM lesions producing an impairment only for the last choice order without altering performance for the first choice order (Kesner et al., 1986). Furthermore, animals with large MS lesions were impaired for most serial positions in the item memory task, while animals with large NBM lesions showed no impairment (Kesner et al., 1988). In addition, preliminary data indicate that HNDB lesions result in a deficit for item memory, but not order memory. Thus, there appears to be a double dissociation between NBM and HNDB in terms of differential mediation of item and order recognition memory. In general, the MS and NBM systems have a few shared, but mostly separate and independent functions. On the basis of the above mentioned studies, it is difficult to assign a specific mnemonic function to either MS or NBM, but it appears that the NBM region is very sensitive to coding of temporal information, while MS is critical for coding of temporal-spatial (contextual) information.

Table 1. Memory for spatial location information following medial septum, nucleus basalis magnocellularis or horizontal nucleus of the diagonal band lesions.

	Order		Item	
	Sequential Position		Sequential Position	
	Early	Late	Early	Late
Small MS	Deficit	Intact	Deficit	Intact
Small NBM	Intact	Deficit	Intact	Intact
Large MS	Deficit	Deficit	Deficit	Deficit
Large NBM	Deficit	Deficit	Intact	Intact
Large HNDB	Intact	Intact	Deficit	Deficit

Medial Septum and Hippocampus

Whenever one compares the behavioral (memory) consequences of lesions of the cholinergic basal forebrain system with lesions of its target systems (e.g., neocortex, hippocampus, amygdala), one needs to take into account a number of methodological problems. First, lesions of the cholinergic basal forebrain system are rarely complete, leaving the target with significant levels of residual cholinergic activity. In contrast, it is easier to damage all the tissue associated with a specific target, especially a neocortical one. Any differences in behavioral recovery could be due to remaining functional activity. Second, many subregions of the cholinergic basal forebrain system have distributions to multiple target areas. Thus, lesion of one target area, like dorsolateral frontal cortex for the NBM projection, might not be representative of the total projection system of the NBM. Third, different lesion techniques are often used in removing neocortex (e.g., aspiration) vs. basal forebrain systems (e.g., ibotenic acid injections). Furthermore, lesion size is often not varied in a systematic fashion. In the case of our own studies, a "small" lesion of the MS or NBM is characterized by unilateral or minimal bilateral cell loss in MS or NBM in conjunction with asymmetrical or minimal symmetrical depletion of the cholinergic target areas. A "large" lesion of MS or NBM is characterized by extensive bilateral cell loss in MS or NBM in conjunction with extensive bilateral depletion of cholinergic target areas. Fourth, because of the likelihood of reciprocal connections between the cholinergic basal forebrain system and its targets, there is always the possibility that some of the behavioral effects of a lesion in the basal forebrain are due to retrograde degeneration of the target (e.g., neocortex). Conversely, a lesion of the target (e.g., neocortex) might produce behavioral effects that are due to retrograde degeneration of the basal forebrain.

Even though these methodological problems need to be addressed, the hypothesis that a cholinergic input to a particular target plays an important role in mediating a given mnemonic function is supported when parallel effects upon that memory function are produced by lesions in both the cholinergic basal forebrain system and its targets. However, to the extent that there is a double dissociation of memory function between a region of the cholinergic basal forebrain system and its target, then the cholinergic input to its target probably does not play an important role in mediating mnemonic functions.

A great deal of systematic research has been carried out in comparing the MS and its cholinergic target, the hippocampus. In general, there is a consensus that the cholinergic input to the hippocampus is critical for a variety of mnemonic functions associated with the hippocampus. For example, both MS and hippocampal or fimbria-fornix lesions impair passive avoidance learning and retention, impair acquisition or retention on an 8 arm win-shift task, produce an overestimation of duration of a stimulus in a time estimation task (Olton et al., 1978; Crutcher et al., 1983; Gray and McNaughton, 1983; Olton et al., 1987; Wenk and Olton 1987). However, these animals also show an improvement in the acquisition of two-way avoidance learning (Gray and McNaughton, 1983). With respect to taste aversion learning, both septal and hippocampal lesions disrupt development of taste aversion learning with small doses of LiCl, but do not affect the acquisition of taste aversion learning with large doses of LiCl (Nonneman and Curtis, 1978). In a place navigation learning task both septal and hippocampal lesions impair acquisition of the task (Morris, et al., 1982; Hagan et al, 1988). In the case of order and item recognition memory, small MS or hippocampal lesions produce an impairment for the early spatial locations, while memory for the last spatial location within the list remains intact (see Table 2). Large MS or hippocampal lesions produce an impairment for all spatial locations for order or item recognition memory (see Table 2) (Kesner et al., 1988). Thus, there is an impressive set of data that suggests that the MS mediated cholinergic input into the hippocampus might be of critical importance for mnemonic activity associated with hippocampal function.

Table 2. Memory for spatial location information following medial septum or hippocampus lesions.

	Order		Item	
	Sequential Position		Sequential Position	
	Early	Late	Early	Late
Small MS	Deficit	Intact	Deficit	Intact
Small Hippocampus	Deficit	Intact	Deficit	Intact
Large MS	Deficit	Deficit	Deficit	Deficit
Large Hippocampus	Deficit	Deficit	Deficit	Deficit

Nucleus Basalis Magnocellularis and Dorsolateral Frontal Cortex

It has been shown that animals with dorsolateral frontal cortex lesions underestimate time duration in a timing task (Meck et al., 1987). Similar results were found for animals with NBM lesions (Meck et al., 1987) It should be noted that animals with basolateral amygdala lesions show normal time estimation (Olton et al., 1987). Thus, in this situation the dorsolateral frontal cortex rather than the amygdala cholinergic target appears to be of importance.

In the order recognition memory task for spatial location information there are no deficits in animals with dorsolateral frontal cortex lesions (see Table 3). However, there are deficits in animals with NBM lesions. In a somewhat different task, it has been shown that animals will switch to a non-preferred hand in a hand reaching task with lesions of the dorsolateral frontal cortex contralateral to the preferred hand (Castro, 1972). Preliminary data in our laboratory indicate that NBM lesions ipsilateral to the preferred hand do not alter hand preference in the same hand reaching task.

There are other tasks (e.g., taste aversion learning) in which neither dorsolateral frontal cortex nor NBM lesions produce deficits (Kesner et al., unpublished observations).

Table 3. Memory for spatial location information following dorsolateral frontal cortex, parietal cortex or nucleus basalis magnocellularis lesions.

	Order		Item	
	Sequential Position		Sequential Position	
	Early	Late	Early	Late
Dorsolateral Frontal Cortex	Intact	Intact	—	—
Large NBM	Deficit	Deficit	Intact	Intact
Parietal Cortex	—	—	Deficit	Deficit

In summary, it appears, thus far, that cholinergic projections from NBM to dorsolateral frontal cortex play a role in only a limited set of tasks. In some tasks there is a clear dissociation between lesion effects of NBM compared to the dorsolateral frontal cortex.

Nucleus Basalis Magnocellularis and Parietal Cortex

It has been shown that animals with lesions of the parietal cortex have deficits in acquisition of a place navigation task in a water maze and a dry land version of the water maze (a cheese board task) (DiMattia and Kesner, 1988a; Kesner et al., 1989). Similar deficits have been described for animals with NBM lesions in both the water maze and the dry land version (Whishaw et al., 1985; Dunnett et al., 1987; Mandel et al., 1989). It should be noted, however, that in at least one study NBM lesions do not impair acquisition of the place navigation task in the water maze (Hagan et al., 1988).

In another study it was found that parietal cortex lesions impaired tactile discrimination learning, but not black-white discrimination learning, in a T maze. Comparable deficits in tactile, but not brightness, discrimination learning were reported for NMDA-induced lesions of NBM (Wozniak et al. 1989; Wozniak et al., in press).

In an 8-arm task in which 4 spatial locations were never rewarded (reference memory) and 4 spatial locations were rewarded only for the first visit (working memory), both NBM lesions and parietal cortex lesions produced a deficit in reference, but not working memory (Kesner et al., 1987).

In the item recognition memory task for eight spatial locations there are deficits in animals with parietal cortex lesions, but no deficits in animals with NBM lesions (See Table 3) (DiMattia and Kesner, 1988b; Kesner, 1988).

In summary, it appears that cholinergic projections from NBM to parietal cortex play a role in most of the tasks studied thus far. However, in at least one task (item recognition), there is a dissociation between NBM and parietal cortex, suggesting that cholinergic input from NBM to parietal cortex might not always be of importance.

Nucleus Basalis Magnocellularis and Amygdala

With respect to passive and active avoidance learning and retention, there are comparable deficits for animals with NBM and basolateral amygdala lesions (Altman et al., 1985; Lerer et al., 1985; Miyamoto et al., 1985; Sarter and Markowitsch, 1985; Berman et al., 1988; Dunnett et al., 1987).

In the item and order recognition memory for spatial location tasks, animals with either NBM or basolateral amygdala lesions display a total deficit for order memory, but display normal performance for item memory (see Table 4) (Kesner et al., 1989; Kesner et al., 1990).

Table 4. Memory for spatial location information following amygdala or nucleus basalis magnocellularis lesions.

	Order		Item	
	Sequential Position		Sequential Position	
	Early	Late	Early	Late
Amygdala	Deficit	Deficit	Intact	Intact
Large NBM	Deficit	Deficit	Intact	Intact

Animals with amygdala lesions are profoundly impaired in acquiring taste aversion, but in this case animals with NBM lesions do not show a deficit in taste aversion learning (McGowan et al. 1972; Everitt et al., 1987).

In summary, it appears that for some learning situations the cholinergic projection from NBM to amygdala might play an important role, but not in other learning tasks. Thus, for the NBM the role of the cholinergic projection system is of importance in a few, but certainly not all learning and memory situations.

Horizontal Nucleus of Diagonal Band and Medial Prefrontal, Entorhinal Cortex

As a relatively obscure component of the basal forebrain, the HNDB and its functions have not been widely studied. Mayo et al. (1988) reported deficits in acquiring a spatial navigation task in the Morris water maze and a spontaneous alternation task following ibotenate lesions of the HNDB (based on reported coordinates of the lesions). With respect to performance in these tasks, comparable deficits have been reported for animals with medial prefrontal cortex or entorhinal cortex lesions (Loesche and Steward, 1977; Kolb, 1984; Schenk and Morris, 1985; Kesner et al., 1989), suggesting that there might be an important cholinergic contribution from HNDB to the medial prefrontal and entorhinal cortex.

Preliminary results in our laboratory indicate that ibotenate lesions of the HNDB disrupt item recognition memory for spatial location information, but do not affect order recognition memory for spatial location information (Table 5). Animals with medial prefrontal cortex lesions are impaired for order recognition memory for all items within a list whereas on item recognition memory they are impaired on only the last items within the list (Table 5) (Kesner and Holbrook, 1987). This pattern of results is not consistent with observation of deficits with HNDB lesions. Thus far, animals with entorhinal cortex lesions have not been tested for item or order recognition memory for a list of spatial locations, but animals with entorhinal cortex lesions are impaired in remembering a single spatial location (Evans and Kesner, unpublished observations). Thus, it is likely that animals with entorhinal cortex lesions will, like animals with HNDB lesions, show impairment on the item recognition task. Clearly, more research needs to be done in order to evaluate more precisely the cholinergic contribution of the HNDB to the medial prefrontal and entorhinal cortex.

Thus far, only the cholinergic contribution of the MS appears to be of importance in almost all the tasks that have been shown to be sensitive to its target, namely the hippocampus.

Table 5. Memory for spatial location information following medial prefrontal cortex or horizontal nucleus of diagonal band lesions.

	Order Sequential Position		Item Sequential Position	
	Early	Late	Early	Late
Medial Prefrontal Cortex	Deficit	Deficit	Intact	Deficit
HNDB	Intact	Intact	Deficit	Deficit

BASAL FOREBRAIN LESIONS: DEGREE OF RELATIONSHIP BETWEEN THE CHOLINERGIC SYSTEM AND MEMORY FUNCTION

There are at least three methods that have been used to assess the degree of relationship of the cholinergic system with memory function. The first method involves manipulation of lesion size of the basal forebrain. Based on the observation of level of AChE depletion of the hippocampus following MS lesions, it has been shown that on the item recognition task a small amount of AChE depletion only impairs memory for the early items within the list, whereas an extensive AChE depletion produces a total deficit (Table 1). In a 1-trial delayed-matching-to-sample task for spatial location, a small amount of AChE depletion of the dorsal hippocampus following MS lesions only produces a transient memory deficit, whereas extensive AChE depletion of the dorsal hippocampus following MS lesions produces a permanent memory deficit (Kesner, unpublished observations). Based on the observation of the level of AChE depletion in dorsolateral frontal cortex following NBM lesions, it has been shown that in the order recognition memory task a small amount of AChE depletion results only in a memory impairment for the later items within the list, whereas an extensive AChE depletion produces a total deficit (Table 1). Thus, with the use of AChE histochemistry the more extensive the depletion in the target the greater the memory deficit.

With the use of a different, more quantitative method, a positive relationship between cholinergic dysfunction and deficits in memory performance has not been observed. In this second method, ibotenic or quisqualic acid is injected into NBM with subsequent higher ChAT depletion in frontal cortex for quisqualate compared to ibotenate injections. On a number of behavioral tasks, namely place navigation in a water maze, recent memory in a T maze, and delayed matching and delayed alternation in an operant chamber (Etherington et al., 1987; Wenk et al.,1989; Dunnett et al., in press), there was a greater behavioral deficit for the ibotenate injected group. Thus, there appears to be a negative relationship between degree of cholinergic depletion in frontal cortex and memory performance. It should be noted that the dorsolateral cortex may not play a very important role in the tasks that were employed so that a relationship between ChAT levels and memory performance might not be expected. Since ChAT levels were not measured in the parietal cortex or basolateral amygdala, it is always a possibility that in those two areas quisqualic acid might not produce a greater ChAT depletion compared to ibotenic acid. Also, it will be necessary to compare memory function following ibotenic acid and quisqualic acid injections into MS or HNDB.

A third method is to correlate memory performance with depletion of ChAT in the target structure. In a number of studies the level of frontal ChAT depletion following NBM lesions has been correlated with memory deficits in a variety of tasks (see Table 6). Unfortunately, in the majority of studies the relationship between the observed behavioral deficits and ChAT depletion within the target structures has not been reported. In those studies that do report this relationship, the correlations are in most studies low and nonsignificant. These data imply that there might not be a major cholinergic contribution of the NBM to memory function.

PHARMACOLOGIC REVERSAL OF BASAL FOREBRAIN INDUCED DEFICITS

Another strategy that can be used to determine whether the cholinergic basal forebrain system does indeed play a role in memory is to attempt to reverse NBM lesion-induced deficits with either cholinergic agonists or AChE inhibitors.

In an early study Murray and Fibiger (1985) demonstrated improvements for NBM lesioned animals in both working and reference memory in a 16-arm radial maze following high doses (0.5 mg/kg, i.p.) of physostigmine. It is difficult to interpret these results, because control animals were immobilized by this high dose and no tests were given after cessation of physostigmine treatments so that a return to baseline level could not be measured.

In a subsequent study, animals with NBM lesions were impaired in the retention of spatial memory in a food searching task as well as acquisition of spontaneous and reinforced alternation in a T maze (Murray and Fibiger, 1986). Injections of pilocarpine nitrate reversed the spatial memory deficit. The animals returned to an impaired performance baseline following the cessation of pilocarpine treatments. Injections of pilocarpine or physostigmine reversed the spatial alternation deficits, but it should be noted that pilocarpine disrupted performance of the control

Table 6. Correlations between ChAT level in target structures following basal forebrain lesions and memory.

Lesion structure	Target structure	Learning and memory test	Correlation	Reference
NBM	Frontal Cortex	retention passive avoidance	.19	Berman et al. (1988)
NBM	Frontal Cortex	retention passive avoidance	.64°	Santucchi et al. (1989)
NBM	Frontal Cortex	retention passive avoidance	.03	Mandel et al. (1989)
NBM	Dorsolateral Frontal Cortex	passive avoidance acquisition	.11	Dunnett et al. (1989)
NBM	Dorsolateral Frontal Cortex	passive avoidance retention	.03	Dunnett et al. (1989)
NBM	Frontal Cortex	water maze acquisition (latency)	.88*	Mandel et al. (1989)
NBM	Frontal Cortex	visual discrimination	–.19	Thompson et al. (1986)
	Parietal Cortex	visual discrimination	–.15	
NBM	Parietal Cortex	cheese board acquisition (latency)	.59°	Kesner et al. (unpublished observations)
NBM	Amygdala	cheese board acquisition (latency)	.06	Kesner et al. (unpublished observations)
NBM	Parietal Cortex	taste aversion learning	–.50	Kesner et al. (unpublished observations)
	Amygdala	taste aversion learning	–.59	
MS/VNDB	Posterior Hippocampus	water maze acquisition	.61°	Hagan et al. (1988)

* significant $P < .05$

°Approach significance $P < .10$ – $P < .05$

subjects, whereas physostigmine (0.5 mg/kg) in this experiment did not affect performance of the control subjects. Following cessation of treatment, the lesioned animals again displayed spatial alternation deficits.

In additional studies, it has been shown that relative to controls a 0.06 mg/kg dose of physostigmine improves performance in a water maze navigation task in rats with NBM lesions, but a dose of .32 mg/kg physostigmine disrupts performance in the water maze task. It should be noted, however, that this improvement was small and certainly not complete (Mandel and Thal, 1988). In a somewhat different study, Santucci et al., 1989 demonstrated that 0.03 mg/ kg dose of physostigmine facilitated memory in a passive avoidance task for both sham and NBM lesioned rats, but there was a greater increase in NBM lesioned animals. Higher doses (0.06 mg/kg) did not produce facilitatory effects.

Finally, Tilson et al. (1988) demonstrated that in a standard 8-arm radial maze test, colchicine-induced lesions in the NBM were attenuated with a .24 mg/kg, but not a .12 mg/kg, dose of physostigmine, 1.0 mg/kg dose of RS-86, or a 1.5 mg/kg dose of nicotine.

In general, it appears that physostigmine, a cholinergic agent, can at specific dose levels for each task reverse to some extent an NBM induced memory deficit. Thus, the pharmacological reversal data suggest a possible role for the cholinergic NBM system in mediating memory function.

NONCHOLINERGIC EFFECTS OF BASAL FOREBRAIN LESIONS

Within each component of the basal forebrain, there are cells that contain neurotransmitters and neuropeptides other than acetylcholine. For example, within the medial septum one finds cells containing GABA, galanin, CCK, dynorphin and substance P (Senut, et al., 1989). Only 30-35% of MS cells contain acetylcholine (Alonso and Kohler, 1984). Within the HNDB there are cells that contain neuropeptide Y, GABA, CCK, neurotensin and somatostatin (Senut et al., 1989). Within the NBM the great majority of cells (90-95%) are cholinergic, but there are probably other cells within the NBM that contain neurotensin. In addition, many fibers of passage course through the basal forebrain containing norepinephrine, dopamine, serotonin and glutamate (Sofroniew et al., 1983; Arrendash et al., 1987; Wenk et al., 1987). Thus, one would expect that following lesions of the basal forebrain, especially with toxins that alter cell activity, that other neurotransmitters or neuropeptides could also play a role in affecting memory function. One example is provided by Wenk et al. (1989). They injected either ibotenic or quisqualic acid into the NBM and tested rats in an alternation task in a T-maze. Animals with ibotenic acid injections were more impaired than animals with quisqualic acid injections. Furthermore, ChAT activity in frontal cortex was reduced less for animals with ibotenic acid compared to quisqualic acid injections, suggesting that cholinergic activity is not likely to mediate alternation performance in the T maze. However, neurotensin levels were reduced more in frontal cortex with ibotenic acid compared to quisqualic acid, suggesting a possibility that T maze alternation performance might be mediated by changes in neurotensin levels.

Another possibility is that lesions of the basal forebrain may affect memory, because of subsequent degeneration of descending afferent inputs, especially from neocortex and limbic system. It is likely that glutamate might be the critical neurotransmitter that is altered after basal forebrain lesions.

In the case of the medial septum, descending projections from the hippocampus synapse in the lateral septum; the lateral septal neurons, in turn, project to the medial septum (Swanson and Cowan, 1977). Thus, there is not a direct reciprocal projection between the MS and the hippocampus. In the case of the NBM and HNDB there is not much known about the neocortical descending projections. Saper (1984) and Lemann and Saper (1985) based on HRP and electron microscope studies suggested that there were reciprocal connections between NBM and neocortex. In a recent study Beers and Kesner (1988) have studied the descending projections of the dorsolateral frontal and medial prefrontal cortex (anterior cingulate and limbic cortex) to the basal forebrain region with the use of a retrograde transported fluorescent tracer (bis-Benzimide) and an anterograde tracer (PHA-L). They found that there were indeed reciprocal connections between dorsolateral frontal cortex and NBM, but even though the HNDB projects to the cingulate cortex and prelimbic cortex, the cingulate cortex does not project back to the HNDB, rather it projects to NBM. The prelimbic cortex, however, does project back to the HNDB (Sesack et al., 1989). Reciprocal connections also exist for NBM and basolateral amygdala (Woolf and Butcher, 1982; Krettek and Price, 1978) as well as HNDB and lateral entorhinal cortex (Witter et al., 1989).

Thus, lesions of the basal forebrain (especially NBM, but also to some extent the HNDB) could affect memory, because of a direct disruption of descending systems making the interpretation of a cholinergic effect following basal forebrain lesions more difficult. It should be noted, however, that there have not been any published reports of neocortical or limbic degeneration following NBM or HNDB lesions. In summary, it is likely that other neurotransmitters that are manufactured in basal forebrain cells or influence the operation of basal forebrain neurons also play a role in mediating memory functions.

SUMMARY

The aim of this chapter was to address the question of whether the cholinergic basal forebrain system plays a role in mediating and/or modulating memory. Before one can answer this question, it is necessary to recognize that the basal forebrain is a complex neural entity that can be divided into at least three major regions (MS and VNDB, HNDB, and NBM) with differential cholinergic projections to limbic and neocortical targets.

The best support, thus far, for a strong cholinergic influence on memory function is for the MS and VNDB and their projections to the hippocampal formation. This is primarily based on the observation of parallel patterns of memory impairments in animals with MS or hippocampus lesions and a positive relationship between lesion size of MS with degree of memory impairment. However, it should be noted that other neurotransmitters (e.g., GABA) might also contribute to memory function. If one assumes that the hippocampus plays a critical role in mediating spatial and temporal information within a data-based or working memory system (Kesner and DiMattia, 1987), then it is possible that the MS and VNDB as a critical component of the cholinergic basal forebrain system, modulate spatial and temporal information within the data-based or working memory system.

Support for a strong cholinergic influence of the NBM on memory function is mixed. With respect to the NBM projection to dorsolateral frontal cortex there are parallel patterns of deficits for NBM and dorsolateral frontal cortex lesions for a duration timing task, but there is a dissociation between the two areas in an order recognition memory task. Furthermore, with the exception of one study, there are usually no significant correlations or at times negative correlations between depletion of ChAT in cortex following NBM lesions and memory performance. It is, thus, likely that other neural transmitters within the NBM might also play an important role in mediating memory function. With respect to the NBM projection to parietal cortex and amygdala, there are again some parallel patterns of deficits between NBM and parietal cortex in the acquisition of spatial navigation and tactile discrimination learning, and between NBM and amygdala in passive and active avoidance learning as well as order recognition memory. But there are also dissociations between NBM and parietal cortex on item recognition memory and NBM and amygdala on taste aversion learning. Some support for a cholinergic role of NBM in modulating memory comes from the findings that it has been possible to reverse an NBM lesion-induced memory deficit with physostigmine.

In general, there is some support for a cholinergic role of the NBM, as a critical component of the cholinergic basal forebrain system, in mediating memory, but at best it appears to be task specific. Because of the NBM's varied cholinergic projection system and the uncertainty of its cholinergic contribution, it is very difficult at present to assign any specific memory function to the NBM.

It is not yet possible at present to assess the cholinergic contribution of the HNDB component of the basal forebrain area because not enough data have been reported on the role of the HNDB in mediating memory. It appears that the cholinergic projection of HNDB to entorhinal cortex might be of importance in modulating memory function.

In general, the cholinergic basal forebrain system is not likely to mediate or modulate a single memory function, because of its multiple projections to a variety of limbic and neocortical targets and because of the observation of double dissociation effects among the specific subcomponents of the basal forebrain on specific tasks measuring memory.

ACKNOWLEDGMENTS

Support for this research was provided by NIH Grant NS19406-03 and NIH Grant R01NS20771-04.

REFERENCES

Alexander, M. P. and Freedman, M. (1983): Amnesia after anterior communicating artery aneurysm rupture. *Neurol.* 33:104

Alonso, A. and Kohler, C. (1984): A study of the reciprocal connections between septum and the entorhinal area using anterograde and retrograde axonal transport methods in the rat brain. *J. Comp. Neurol.* 225:327-343

Altman, H.J., Crosland, R.D., Jenden, D.J. and Berman, R.F. (1985): Further characterizations of the nature of the behavioral and neurochemical effects of lesions to the nucleus basalis of Meynert in the rat. *Neurobiol. Aging* 6:125-130

Arrendash, G.W., Millard, W.J., Dunn, A.J. and Meyer, E.M. (1987): Long term neuropathological and neurochemical effects of nucleus basalis lesions in the rat. *Science* 238:952-956

Ball, M.J. (1977): Neuronal loss, neurofibrillary tangle and granulovacuolar degeneration in the hippocampus with aging and dementia. *Acta Neuropathol.* 37:111-118

Bartus, R.T., Flicker, C., Dean, R.L., Pontecorvo, M., Figueiredo, J.C. and Fisher, S.K. (1985): Selective memory loss following nucleus basalis lesions: long term behavioral recovery despite persistent cholinergic deficiencies. *Pharmacol. Biochem. Behav.* 23:125-135

Beers, D.R. and Kesner, R.P. (1988): Differential anatomical projections between frontal cortices and the basal forebrain in the rat. *Soc. Neurosci. Abst.* 14:12-25

Beninger, R.J. Wirsching, B.A., Jhamandas, K., Boegman, R.J. and El-Defrawy, S.R. (1986): Effects of altered cholinergic function on working and reference memory in the rat. *Can. J. Physiol. Pharmacol.* 64:376-382

Berman, R.F., Crosland, R.D., Jenden, D.J. and Altman, H.J. (1988): Persisting behavioral and neurochemical deficits in rats following lesions of the basal forebrain. *Pharmacol. Biochem. Behav.* 29:581-586

Bigl, B., Woolf, N.J. and Butcher, L.L. (1982): Cholinergic projections from the basal forebrain to frontal, parietal, temporal, occipital, and cingulate cortices: a combined fluorescent tracer and acetylcholinesterase analysis. *Brain. Res. Bull.* 8:727-749

Bird, T.D., Stranahan, S.M., Sumi, S.M. and Raskind, M. (1983): Alzheimer's disease: choline acetyltransferase activity in brain tissue from clinical and pathological subgroups. *Ann. Neurol.* 14:284

Bowen, D.M., Smith, C.B., White, P. and Davison, A.N. (1976): Neurotransmitter-related enzymes and indices of hypoxia in senile dementia and other abiotrophies. *Brain* 99:459-469

Butcher, L.L. and Woolf, N.T. (1986): Central cholinergic systems: Synopsis of anatomy and overview of physiology and pathology. In: *The Biological substrates of Alzheimer's disease.* Scheibel, A.B., Wechsler, A.F., Brazier, M.A.B., eds. New York: Academic Press

Carlsen, J.L., Záborszky, L. and Heimer, L. (1985): Cholinergic projections from the basal forebrain to the basolateral amygdaloid complex: a combined retrograde fluorescent and immunohistochemical study. *J. Comp. Neurol.* 234:155-165

Castro, A.J. (1972): The effects of cortical ablations on digital usage in the rat. *Brain Res.* 44:313-323

Corkin, S. (1982): Some relationships between global amnesias and the memory impairments in Alzheimer's disease. In: *Alzheimer's Disease: A Report of Progress, Vol. 19, Aging.* Corkin, S., Davis, K.L., Growdon, J.H., Usdin, E. and Wurtman, P.J., eds. New York: Raven Press

Coyle, J.T., Price, D.L., and DeLong, R. (1983): Alzheimer's disease: a disorder of cortical cholinergic innervation. *Science* 219:1184-1190

Crutcher, K.A., Kesner, R.P., and Novak, J.M. (1983): Medial septal lesions, radial arm maze performance, and sympathetic sprouting: a study of recovery of function. *Brain Res.* 262:91-98

Damasio, A.R., Graff-Radford, N.R., Eslinger, P.J., Damasio, H. and Kassell, N. (1985): Amnesia following basal forebrain lesions. *Arch. Neurol.* 42:263-271

DiMattia, B.V. and Kesner, R.P. (1984): Serial position curves in rats: automatic vs. effortful information processing. *J. Exp. Psy: An. Behav. Proc.* 10:557-563

DiMattia, B.V. and Kesner, R.P. (1988a): Spatial cognitive maps: differential role of parietal cortex and hippocampal formation. *Behav. Neurosci.* 102:471-480

DiMattia, B.V. and Kesner, R.P. (1988b): The role of the posterior parietal association cortex in the processing of spatial event information. *Behav. Neurosci.* 102:397-403

Dunnett, S.B., Rogers, D.C. and Jones, G.H. (in press): Effects of nucleus basalis magnocellularis lesions on delayed matching and non-matching to position tasks: disruption of conditional discrimination learning but not of short-term memory. *Europ. J. of Neurosci.*

Dunnett, S.B., Whishaw, I.Q., Jones, G.H. and Bunch, S.T. (1987): Behavioural, biochemical and histochemical effects of different neurotoxic amino acids injected into nucleus basalis magnocellularis of rats. *Neurosci.* 20:653-699

Etherington, R., Mittleman, G. and Robbins, T.W. (1987): Comparative effects of nucleus basalis and fimbria-fornix lesions on delayed matching and alternation tests of memory. *Neurosci. Res. Commu.* 3:135-143

Everitt, B.T., Robbins, T.W., Evenden, J.L., Marston, H.M., Jones, G.H., Sirkia, T.E. (1987) The effects of excitotoxic lesions of the substantia innominata, ventral and dorsal globus pallidus on the acquisition and retention of a conditional visual discrimination: implications for cholinergic hypotheses of learning and memory. *Neurosci.* 22:441-469

Flicker, C., Dean, R.L., Watkins, D.L., Fisher, S.K. and Bartus, R.T. (1983): Behavioral and neurochemical effects following neurotoxic lesions of a major cholinergic input to the cerebral cortex in the rat. *Pharmacol. Biochem. Behav.* 18:973-981

Gray, J.A. and McNaughton, N. (1983): Comparison between the behavioural effects of septal and hippocampal lesions: a review. *Neurosci. and Biobeh. Rev.* 7:119-188

Hagan, J.J., Salamone, J.D., Simpson, J., Iversen, S.D. and Morris, R.G.M. (1988): Place navigation in rats is impaired by lesions of medial septum and diagonal band but not nucleus basalis magnocellularis. *Behav. Brain Res.* 27:9-20

Hepler, D.J., Wenk, G.L., Cribbs, B.L., Olton, D.S. and Coyle, J.T. (1985): Memory impairments following basal forebrain lesions. *Brain Res.* 346:8-14

Hepler, D.J., Olton, D.S., Wenk, G.L. and Coyle, J.T. (1985): Lesions in nucleus basalis magnocellularis and medial septal area of rats produce qualitatively similar memory impairments. *J. Neurosci.* 5:866-873

Hyman, B.T., Van Hoesen, G.W., Damasio, A.R. and Barnes, C.L. (1984): Alzheimer's disease: cell-specific pathology isolates the hippocampal formation. *Science* 225:1168-1170

Kemper, T.L. (1983): Organization of the neuropathology of the amygdala in Alzheimer's disease. Biological Aspects of Alzheimer's Disease. *Banbury Rep.* 15:31-35

Kesner, R.P. (1988): Reevaluation of the contribution of the basal forebrain cholinergic system to memory. *Neurobiol. Aging* 9:609-616

Kesner, R.P., Crutcher, K.A. and Beers, D.R. (1988): Serial position curves for item (spatial location) information: role of the dorsal hippocampal formation and medial septum. *Brain Res.* 454:219-226

Kesner, R.P., Crutcher, K.A. and Measom, M.O. (1986): Medial septal and nucleus basalis magnocellularis lesions produce order memory deficits in rats which mimic symptomatology of Alzheimer's disease. *Neurobiol. Aging* 7:287-295

Kesner, R.P., Crutcher, K.A. and Omana, H. (1990): Memory deficits following nucleus basalis magnocellularis lesions may be mediated through limbic but not neocortical targets. *Neurosci.* 38:93-102

Kesner R.P, DiMattia, B.V. and Crutcher, K.A. (1987): Evidence for neocortical involvement in reference memory. *Behav. Neurol. Biol.* 47:40-53

Kesner, R.P. and DiMattia, B.V. (1987): Neurobiology of an attribute model of memory. In: *Progress in Psychobiology and Physiological Psychology*. Epstein, A.N., Morrison, A., eds. New York: Academic Press

Kesner, R.P., Farnsworth, G. and DiMattia, B.V. (1989): Double dissociation of egocentric and allocentric space following medial prefrontal and parietal cortex lesions in the rat. *Behav. Neurosci.* 103: 956-961

Kesner, R.P. and Holbrook, T. (1987): Dissociation of item and order spatial memory in rats following medial prefrontal cortex lesions. *Neuropsychol.* 25:653-664

Kesner, R.P., Measom, M.O., Forsman, S.L. and Holbrook, T.H. (1984): Serial position curves in rats: order memory for episodic spatial events. *Animal Learn. and Behav.* 12:378-382

Kessler, J., Markowitsch, H.J. and Sigg, G. (1986): Memory related role of the posterior cholinergic system. *Intern. J. Neurosci.* 30:101-119

Krettek, J.E. and Price, J.L. (1978): Amygdaloid projections to subcortical structures within the basal forebrain and brainstem in the rat and cat. *J. Comp. Neurol.* 178:225-280

Kolb, B. (1984): Functions of the frontal cortex of the rat: a comparative review. *Brain Res. Rev.* 8:65-98

Lemann, W. and Saper, C.B. (1985): Evidence for a cortical projection to the magnocellular basal nucleus in the rat: an electron microscopic axonal transport study. *Brain Res.* 334:339-343

Lerer, B., Warner, J., Friedman, E., Vincent, G. and Gamzu, E. (1985): Cortical cholinergic impairment and behavioral deficits produced by kainic acid lesions of rat magnocellular basal forebrain. *Beh. Neurosci.* 99:661-677

LoConte, G., Bartolini, L., Casamenti, F., Marconcini-Pepeu, I. and Pepeu, G. (1982): Lesions of cholinergic forebrain nuclei: changes in avoidance behavior and scopolamine actions. *Pharmacol. Biochem. and Beh.* 17:933-937

Loesche, J. and Steward, O. (1977): Behavioral correlates of denervation and reinnervation of the hippocampal formation of the hippocampal formation of the rat: recovery of alternation performance following unilateral entorhinal cortex lesions. *Brain Res. Bull.* 2:31-39

Mandel, R.J., Gage, F.H. and Thal, L.J. (1989): Spatial learing in rats: correlation with cortical choline acetyltransferase and improvement with NGF following NBM damage. *Exper. Neurol.* 104:208-217

Mandel, R. J., Thal, L. T. (1988): Physostigmine improves water maze performance following nucleus basalis magnocellularis lesions in rats. *Psychopharm.* 96: 421- 425

Mayo, W., Kharouby, M., Le Moal, M. and Simon, H. (1988): Memory disturbances following ibotenic acid injections in the nucleus basalis magnocellularis of the rat. *Brain Res.* 455: 213-222

McGowan, B.K., Hankins, W.G. and Garcia, J. (1972): Limbic lesions and control of the internal and external environment. *Behav. Biol.* 7:841-852

McKinney, M., Coyle, J.T. and Hedreen, J.C. (1983): Topographic analysis of the innervation of the rat neocortex and hippocampus by the basal forebrain cholinergic system. *J. Comp. Neurol.* 217:103-121

Meck, W.H., Church, R.M. and Olton, D.S. (1984): Hippocampus, time and memory. *Beh. Neurosci.* 98:3-22

Meck, W.H., Russell, M.C., Wenk, G.L. and Olton, D.S. (1987): Nucleus basalis magnocellularis and medial septal area lesions differentially impair temporal memory. *J. Neurosci.* 11:3505-3511

Mesulam, E., Mufson, J., Wainer, B.H. and Levey, A.I. (1983): Central cholinergic pathways in the rat: an overview based on an alternative nomenclature (Chl-Ch6). *Neurosci.* 10:1185-1201

Mishkin, M. (1982): A memory system in the monkey. *Phil. Trans. Royal Soc. London Series* B 298:85-95

Miyamoto, M., Shintani, M., Nagaoka, A. and Nagawa, Y. (1985): Lesioning of the rat basal forebrain leads to memory impairments in passive and active avoidance tasks. *Brain Res.* 328:97-104

Morris, R.G.M. Garrud, P., Rawlins, J.N.P. and O'Keefe, J. (1982): Place navigation impaired in rats with hippocampal lesions. *Nature* 297:681-683

Murray, C.L. and Fibiger, H.C. (1985): Learning and memory deficits after lesions of the nucleus basalis magnocellularis: reversal by physostigmine. *Neurosci.* 14:1025-1032

Murray, C.L. and Fibiger, H.C. (1986): Pilocarpine and physostigmine attenuate spatial memory impairments produced by lesions of the nucleus basalis magnocellularis. *Behav. Neurosci.* 100:23-32

Nonneman, A.J. and Curtis, S.D. (1978): Strength of conditioning determines the effects of septo-hippocampal lesions on tastaversion learning. *Physiol. Psychol.* 6:249-254

Olton, D.S. (1983): Memory functions and the hippocampus. In: *Neurobiology of the Hippocampus*. Seifert, W. ed. New York: Academic Press

Olton, D.S., Meck, W.H. and Church, R.M. (1987): Separation of hippocampal and amygdaloid involvement in temporal memory dysfunctions. *Brain Res.* 404:180-188

Olton, D.S., Walker, J.A. and Gage, F.H. (1978): Hippocampal connections and spatial discrimination. *Brain Res.* 139:295-308

Price, D.L. (1986): New perspectives on Alzheimer's disease. *Ann. Rev. Neurosci.* 9:489-512

Salazar, A.H., Grafman, J., Schlesselman, S., Vance, S.C., Mohr, M., Carpenter, M., Pevsner, P., Ludlow, C. and Weingartner, H. (1981): Penetrating war injuries of the basal forebrain: neurology and cognition. *Neurol.* 36:459-465

Saper, C. (1984): Organization of cerebral cortical afferent systems in the rat. I. Magnocellular basal nucleus. *J. Comp. Neurol.* 222:313-342

Santucci, A.C., Kanof, P.D. and Haroutunian, V. (1989): Effect of physostigmine on memory consolidation and retrieval processes in intact and nucleus basalis-lesioned rats. *Psychopharm.* 99:70-74

Sarter, M. and Markowitsch, H. T. (1985): Involvement of the amygdala in learning and memory: a critical review, with emphasis on anatomical relations. *Beh. Neurosci.* 99: 342-380

Schenk, F. and Morris, R.G.M. (1985): Dissociation between components of spatial memory in rats after recovery from the effects of retrohippocampal lesions. *Exper. Brain Res.* 58:11-28

Sesack, S.R., Deutch, A.Y., Roth, R.H. and Bunney, B.S. (1989): Topographical organization of the efferent projections of the medial prefrontal cortex in the rat: an anterograde tract-tracing study with *Phaseolus vulgaris* leucoagglutinin. *Comp. Neurol.* 290:213-242

Senut, M., Menetrey, C. and Lamour, V. (1989): Cholinergic and peptidergic projection from the medial septum and nucleus of the diagonal band of broca to dorsal hippocampus, cingulate cortex, and olfactory bulb: a combined wheatgerm agglutinin-apohorseradish peroxidase-gold immunohistochemical study. *Neurosci.* 30:385-403

Sofroniew, M.V., Pearson, R.C.A., Eckenstein, F., Cuello, A.C. and Powell, T.P.S. (1983): Retrograde changes in cholinergic neurons in the basal nucleus of the forebrain of the rat following cortical damage. *Brain Res.* 289:370-374

Swanson, L.W. and Cowan, W.M. (1977): An autoradiographic study of the organization of the efferent connections of the hippocampal formation in the rat. *J. Comp. Neurol.* 172:49-84

Thompson, R., Gibbs, R.B., Ristic, G.A., Cotman, C.W. and Yu, J. (1986): Lack of correlation between cortical levels of choline acetyltransferase and learning scores in rats with globus pallidus lesions. *Brain Res.* 367:402-404

Tilson, H.A., McLamb, R.L. Shaw, S., Rogers, B.C., Pediaditakis, P. and Cook, L. (1988): Radial-arm maze deficits produced by colchicine administered into the area of the nucleus basalis are ameliorated by cholinergic agents. *Brain Res.* 438:83-94

Tomlinson, B.E. (1977): Morphological changes and dementia in old age. In: *Aging and Dementia.* Smith, W.L., Kinsbourne, M. eds. New York: Spectrum Publications, Inc.

Tomlinson, B.E. and Kitchener, D. (1972): Granulovacuolar degeneration of hippocampal pyramidal cells. *J. Pathol.* 106:165

Van Hoesen, G.W., Hyman, B.T. and Damasio, A.R. (1986): Cell specific pathology in neural systems of the temporal lobe in Alzheimer's disease. In: *Progress in Brain Research.* Swaab, D., ed. Amsterdam: Elsevier

Volpe, B.T. and Hirst, W. (1983): Amnesia following the rupture and repair of an anterior communicating artery aneurysm. *J. Neurol. Neurosurg. Psych.* 46:704-709

Wenk, G.L., Hughey, D., Boundy, V., Kim, A., Walker, L. and Olton, D.S. (1987): Neurotransmitters and memory: role of cholinergic, serotonergic, and noradrenergic systems. *Behav. Neurosci.* 101:325-332

Wenk, G. L., Markowska, A. L., Olton, D. S. (1989): Basal forebrain lesions and memory: alterations in neurotensin, not acetylcholine, may cause amnesia. *Behav. Neurosci.* 103:765-769

Wenk, G.L. and Olton, D.S. (1987): Basal forebrain cholinergic neurons and Alzheimer's disease. In: *Animal models of dementia: a synaptic neurochemical perspective.* Coyle, J.T., ed. New York: Alan Liss, Inc.

Whishaw, I.Q., O'Connor, W.T. and Dunnett, S.T. (1985): Disruption of central cholinergic systems in the rat by basal forebrain lesions: effects on feeding, sensorimotor behaviour, locomotor activity and spatial navigation. *Brain Res.* 17:103-115

Witter, M.P., Groenewegen, H.J., Lopes Da Silva, F.H. and Lohman, A.H. (1989):

Functional organization of the extrinsic and intrinsic circuitry of the parahippocampal region. *Neurobiol.* 33 :161-253

Woolf, N.J. and Butcher, L.L. (1982): Cholinergic projections to the basolateral amygdala: a combined Evans Blue and acetylcholinesterase analysis. *Brain Res. Bull.* 8:751-763

Wozniak, D.F., Stewart, G.R., Finger, S. and Olney, T.W. (in press): Comparison of behavioral effects of nucleus basalis magnocellularis lesions and somatosensory cortex ablation in the rat. *Neurosci.*

Wozniak, D.F., Stewart, G.R., Finger, S., Olney, J.W. and Cozzari, C. (1989): Basal forebrain lesions impair tactile discrimination and working memory. *Neurobiol. Aging* 10:173-179

Záborszky, L., Carlsen, J., Brastear, H.R. and Heimer, L. (1986): Cholinergic and GABAergic afferents to the olfactory bulb in the rat with special emphasis on the projection neurons in the nucleus of the horizontal limb of the diagonal band. *J. Comp. Neurol.* 243:488-509

Ocular Dominance Plasticity in Kitten Visual Cortex: Integration of Noradrenergic and Cholinergic Regulation

Takuji Kasamatsu and Kazuyuki Imamura

INTRODUCTION

Sensory cortex is a part of various ascending fiber projection systems, each of which originates from a relatively small number of chemically identified cells in the basal forebrain, brainstem or medulla. Catecholamine (CA) histochemistry, invented by the Swedish school in the early 1960's, indeed opened up a new possibility of identifying each neuron based on its chemical signature or transmitter phenotype. The recent advent in development of specific immunological probes has further led to the explosion of detailed cytochemical mapping on the ascending fiber projection systems. Noradrenaline (NA) fibers, originating from the locus coeruleus (LC) in the dorsal tegmentum, mesocortical dopamine (DA) fibers from the mesencephalon, serotonin (5-HT) fibers from the raphe groups in the pons, and the basal forebrain acetylcholine (ACh) system, are among the best characterized ascending projection systems. They consist of slow-conducting, non-myelinated or poorly myelinated axons.

Giving off many branches along respective long ascending paths, these monosynaptic projection fibers eventually innervate visual cortex as their last target area. In keeping with the above anatomical organization, endogenous molecules in neocortex related to the ascending projections typically show the lowest content in the occipital area. The low endogenous content, as usually expressed per unit weight of tissue or protein, of neurotransmitters/neuromodulators, however, does not mean that the molecules lack *biological significance* in visual cortex. Rather, because of accumulated knowledge about basic single-cell physiology and connectivity among functionally characterized cells, visual cortex has been a favorite test ground for proposed functions of selected molecules released from the ascending projection systems.

In the present review, we are going to focus our attention on function of the NA and the ACh system because: (i) both NA and ACh are known to modulate neural excitability of cortical cells, (ii) their ionic mechanisms have been worked out in detail, and (iii) the two systems seem to participate in the regulation of *visual cortical plasticity,* a type of synaptic plasticity which is typically expressed by visuocortical cells in the developing brain. The review consists of three parts. First, we will briefly introduce our paradigm in studying visual cortical plasticity, followed by a concise synopsis of topics on the NA-regulated plasticity. We next review new evidence for interactions of the NA and the ACh system in visuocortical plasticity, preceded by comments on ACh actions in cortical physiology. Finally, an integrated view on neurochemical control of visuocortical plasticity will be presented. Further reference to neural mechanisms underlying visuocortical plasticity, especially "activity-dependent processes," was not included here, but left for a future review.

VISUAL CORTICAL PLASTICITY: THE NEW PARADIGM

Cat visual cortex has provided us with an unique opportunity to explore *developmental plasticity,* one of the central questions in modern neuroscience ever since the days of Ramón-y-Cajal. In the early '60's, new paradigms were devised to study "experience-dependent modification" of neuronal connections in immature visual cortex of kittens (Wiesel and Hubel, 1963; Hubel and Wiesel, 1965). For example, when a kitten is subjected to monocular vision as briefly as a few days, the majority of neurons in kitten visual cortex lose their functional connections with the closed eye, leaving only a small fraction of the cells excitable by stimulation of the closed eye (*ocular dominance plasticity*). Because of *apparent* simplicity in designing physiological experiments, their execution and interpretations of results, monocular deprivation has quickly become the paradigm in this newly created research interest. However, despite the vast amount of information accumulated over the last 25 years, molecular and cellular bases of this unique susceptibility of the developing neocortex to experience have not yet been revealed (Movshon and Van Sluyters, 1981; Sherman and Spear, 1982; Wiesel, 1982; Frégnac and Imbert, 1984; Hirsch and Tieman, 1987). Neurochemical or theoretical aspects of regulatory mechanisms of visuocortical plasticity have been reviewed (Kasamatsu 1982, 1983, 1986b, 1987, 1989; Kasamatsu et al., 1984, 1989; Kasamatsu and Shirokawa, 1988; Singer, 1984; Cooper, 1987; Frégnac, 1987; Bear et al., 1987; Rauschecker, 1987; Stryker, 1989; Zahs, 1989).

Noradrenergic Control of Cortical Plasticity: A Thesis

A few chemically defined signaling systems within visual cortex have been implied as plausible carriers of cellular mechanisms of ocular dominance plasticity. Earlier, we proposed that the CA-containing system, especially NA-containing one, in the brain may play a crucial regulatory role in ocular dominance plasticity (Kasamatsu and Pettigrew, 1976, 1979; Pettigrew and Kasamatsu, 1978; Kasamatsu et al., 1979, 1981b; Kasamatsu, 1982, 1983; Kasamatsu et al., 1984). The thesis was based on the following three points: (i) the plasticity was not detectable in kitten visual cortex in which the release of endogenous NA was *maximally* suppressed by destruction of CA terminals with a CA-related neurotoxin, 6-hydroxydopamine (6-OHDA); (ii) a direct infusion of exogenous NA *restored the plasticity* to the cortex which had been rendered aplastic due to the preceding 6-OHDA treatment; and (iii) cortical recovery from the effects of monocular deprivation was suppressed by directly infused 6-OHDA, while enhanced by directly infused NA. The critical importance of the *maximal suppression* of NA release (point (i), above) is well illustrated recently. The endogenous level of NA in hippocampal dialysates was unaffected by a lesion with 6-OHDA unless the tissue NA content became less than 50% of control. If the NA depletion remained modest, tail shock or local infusion of excess K^+ increased NA in dialysates as seen in control animals (Abercrombie and Zigmond, 1989).

Extension of the NA Hypothesis: β Adrenoreceptors

Our early work suggested that β adrenoreceptors (Kasamatsu, 1979) and a second messenger (Kasamatsu, 1980; 1986a) are indeed involved in the maintenance of visuocortical plasticity. Subsequently, we biochemically studied ontogeny of the central NA-β adrenoreceptor system in cat visual cortex. Endogenous NA was measured by a high-pressure liquid chromatography and β adrenoreceptors by *in vitro* binding of a radiolabelled antagonist (Jonsson and Kasamatsu, 1983). The number of specific β adrenoreceptor binding sites was very low at birth and became larger than the adult value between the 5th and 13th week of age. Endogenous NA increased more or less continuously toward adulthood. The results suggested that the ontogeny of β adrenoreceptors, rather than endogenous NA, might be a better indicator of the duration as well as the strength of ocular dominance plasticity in the postnatal susceptible period. Recently, this proposal was tested directly. We found that a continuous infusion with a β-adrenoreceptor antagonist, propranolol, of kitten visual cortex suppressed in a concentration-dependent manner the expected shift of ocular dominance in monocularly deprived kittens (Kasamatsu and Shirokawa, 1985; Shirokawa and Kasamatsu, 1986).

The above finding is significant since the disappearance of ocular dominance plasticity from kitten visual cortex, the original finding, was replicated by means other than using 6-OHDA. These new results with propranolol thus provided a practical answer to the skepticism that ocular dominance plasticity stayed unimpaired despite *significant* decreases in endogenous NA within kitten visual cortex (Bear and Daniels, 1983; Bear et al., 1983; Daw et al., 1984; 1985ab, Adrien et al., 1985; Trombley et al., 1986). Another "6-OHDA-free" test was carried out by using clonidine, an α_2-adrenergic agonist, which was thought to decrease the release of NA from the NA-containing nerve terminals within visual cortex (Nelson et al., 1985).

Subsequently, a converse experiment was carried out to substantiate a causal link between β adrenoreceptors and cortical plasticity; the plasticity increased in kitten visual cortex when *in vivo* availability for endogenous NA of unoccupied β adrenoreceptors was expected to increase some time after the termination of a continuous infusion with propranolol (Shirokawa and Kasamatsu, 1987). In the same study, naturally occurring recovery of the plasticity was accelerated by a cortical infusion of (–)-NA and suppressed by that of tunicamycin, an inhibitor of protein glycosylation. Glycosylation is a key step in the biosynthesis of β adrenoreceptors and other glycoproteins.

Antithesis and Synthesis

As mentioned earlier, several investigators obtained a usual shift of ocular dominance in monocularly deprived kittens whose NA content in visual cortex had been significantly reduced by various means except for a continuous cortical infusion of 6-OHDA. Some common problems in designing these studies are: (i) induced changes in the NA system are obviously *not* confined to visual cortex; (ii) physiological recordings were made to assess changes in the level of plasticity a few weeks to months after placing lesions aimed at the NA system; (iii) reported depletion of endogenous NA in visual cortex was not complete but at the 75-90% level; (iv) it has not been addressed where the remaining NA molecules are localized in visual cortex and how they behave; and (v) induced changes in function of NA-related receptors were totally ignored.

There is little disagreement between results obtained by other investigators (Bear et al., 1983; Daw et al., 1983; Paradiso et al., 1983) and our results (Kasamatsu et al., 1979, 1981b), regarding the plasticity-suppressing effects of cortically infused 6-OHDA. However, there were significant differences in their interpretations. Some suggested the involvement of unspecified "compensatory" processes which counteract with plasticity-suppressing effects of 6-OHDA outside the NA system (Bear and Daniels, 1983; Bear et al., 1983). Others further argued that "non-specific" effects of 6-OHDA might account for our early findings of lowered plasticity (Daw et al., 1984, 1985a,b,c; Trombley et al., 1986; Gordon et al., 1988).

However, an obvious possibility that has not been considered by other investigators is "compensation for NA depletion within the NA system" through either an increase in the density of NA-related receptors (up-regulation) or reinnervation of the visual cortex in which NA-containing terminals have been destroyed by a preceding 6-OHDA treatment (regenerative NA fibers). Previous authors showed in rat neocortex the presence of compensation mechanisms for the NA depletion within the central NA system through either up-regulation of β adrenoreceptors, an increase in turnover of NA and reinnervation by NA fibers of the neocortex which has suffered from 6-OHDA-caused denervation (Kostrzewa and Jacobowitz, 1974; Harden et al., 1977; Jonsson et al., 1979; Jonsson, 1980). Similarly, pre- and postsynaptic compensatory changes occur in remaining DA neurons after electrolytic lesions or lesions with 6-OHDA of the nigrostriatal system (Stricker and Zigmond, 1986).

To substantiate these possibilities, we studied the time course of various changes caused in the 6-OHDA-infused visual cortex by utilizing biochemical, pharmacological, histochemical and electron microscopic methods. We showed that compensatory processes were indeed set in action at both pre- and postsynaptic sites after NA afferents had been impaired by cortically infused 6-OHDA. We first established the presence of *specific degeneration* of CA terminals in the 6-OHDA-infused cortex and estimated the spatial extent of such an effect. We next elucidated processes of reinnervation by NA terminals of the 6-OHDA-affected cortex (Nakai et al., 1987). Within 2 weeks after stopping the continuous infusion of 6-OHDA, the size of the CA terminal-denervated area was substantially smaller than before. In 4 weeks, the cortical area, devoid of fluorescent CA fibers and terminals, was no longer found histochemically. The 6-OHDA-affected area was almost totally reinnervated in 24 weeks or earlier. The similar recovery trend was also obtained in the spatial distribution of endogenous NA and DA, and *in vitro* uptake of ^{3}H-NA by cortical slices. Electron microscopic demonstration of the presence of CA terminal boutons in the 6-OHDA-affected area strongly indicated that these reemerged CA boutons were indeed regenerative (Nakai, 1987). A sign of the postsynaptic compensation of the lack of NA afferents was also shown by light microscopic autoradiography with a radiolabelled β-adrenoreceptor antagonist. In one week after the end of a cortical 6-OHDA infusion, there was noted a ~50% increase of β-adrenoreceptor binding sites in the 6-OHDA-affected cortical area (Nakai et al., 1987). This is consistent with previous findings obtained from the hippocampus treated by DSP4, another type of NA-related neurotoxin (Dunwiddie et al., 1983).

ACh ACTIONS IN CORTICAL PHYSIOLOGY

Laminar Pattern

The majority of ACh afferents, if not all, to neocortex was visualized by the presence of immunoreactive choline acetyltransferase (ChAT)-positive fibers and varicosities which originate from the basal forebrain (Kimura et al., 1981; Houser et al., 1983; Mesulam et al., 1983; de Lima and Singer, 1986). In cat visual cortex ChAT immunoreactivity was found in all 6 layers, showing the highest density in layer I and a sharp drop in layers II and III followed by a gradual decrease toward deep layers (Stichel and Singer, 1987a). This laminar distribution is to be compared to that of muscarinic ACh receptors measured by quinuclidinyl benzilate (QNB) binding. The highest density of QNB binding was seen in supragranular three layers and the lowest in layer IV, showing an intermediate level in infragranular two layers (Shaw et al., 1986). NA afferents and β adrenoreceptors are also present throughout the 6 layers in cat visual cortex. The laminar correspondence between the density of afferent terminals and postsynaptic binding sites seems to be better in the NA-β adrenoreceptor system (Itakura et al., 1981; Nakai et al., 1987) than the ACh-muscarinic receptor system.

Ionic Mechanisms in Neocortex

Long before neuromodulator roles have been assigned to endogenous ACh in the brain, modulation of neural excitability by iontophoretically injected ACh and related drugs was studied by early investigators in mammalian neocortex (Rinaldi and Himwich, 1955; Krnjević and Phillis, 1963; Spehlmann, 1963; Shute and Lewis, 1967; Krnjević et al., 1971; Woody et al., 1978). An early study showed that ACh iontophoreses to cells in neocortex *in vivo* produced a brief decrease in spontaneous discharges followed by an increase (Krnjević, 1974). Recording mostly from layer V pyramidal cells in the anterior cingulate (and less frequently from layers II, III and V in the sensorimotor or visual cortex) of guinea pigs *in vitro*, McCormick and Prince (1985, 1986) examined in detail a sequence of short-latency hyperpolarization followed by long-lasting depolarization and action potentials in response to local application of ACh. The sequence was evident at the membrane potential just below firing threshold and not seen at the resting level, indicating that this effect of ACh is due to voltage-dependent conductances which are most active at depolarized membrane potentials. Both hyperpolarization and slow depolarization were blocked by muscarinic antagonists. Detailed analyses of the spatial distribution of the two responses and their pharmacology strongly suggested that the hyperpolarization is Ca^{++}-dependent and caused by synaptic activation of γ-amino butyric acid (GABA) cells in the vicinity. In some cases, ACh also caused short-latency excitatory responses of action potentials with unusually fast repolarizing phases. This characteristic response was recorded from anatomically identified aspiny, multipolar cells, most likely GABAergic interneurons. McCormick and Prince (1986) also showed that pressure-injected ACh facilitated layer V pyramidal cells' responses by reducing the amplitude and duration of afterhyperpolarization (AHP). This is possibly through muscarinic *slow* EPSP which effectively reduces both voltage-dependent (Ca^{++}-

independent) K^+ current (M-current, for review, see Brown, 1983) and Ca^{++}-dependent (voltage-independent) K^+ current. Essentially the same ionic mechanisms have been proposed earlier for the facilitatory effect of ACh on CA1 pyramidal cells in hippocampus (Benardo and Prince, 1982; Halliwell and Adams, 1982; Krnjević and Ropert, 1982). The mode of excitatory effects of ACh on hippocampal pyramidal cells is similar to that reported on NA's action, although a likely ionic mechanism of the latter is due mainly to reduction of β adrenoreceptor-mediated, Ca^{++}-dependent K^+ current, decreasing in effect the amplitude and duration of AHP, rather than voltage-dependent K^+ current (Madison and Nicoll, 1986). Constanti and Sim (1987) recorded from the pyramidal cell layers (II-IV) of the guinea pig olfactory cortex *in vitro*. In response to a brief depolarizing current pulse under current/voltage clamp, they obtained slow AHPs with an increase in input resistance at the membrane potential between -70 and -45 mV. Muscarine at low concentrations (1-2 μM) were found to reduce, probably via activation of M_2 receptors, the slow AHP current, most of which was Ca^{++}-sensitive. When the concentration was high ($>10\mu$M), however, muscarine reduced the voltage-dependent, Ca^{++}-independent M-current. It was noted that slow AHP currents mediated through the Ca^{++}- dependent K^+ current was also significantly reduced by NA, tetraethylammonium and tetrodotoxin. It is a distinct possibility that NA and ACh facilitate neural excitability in neocortex, thus reducing the same K^+ current synergistically under certain conditions.

ACh Effects on Visual Receptive Fields

While respective receptive fields were stimulated by optimal stimuli, modulatory roles of exogenous ACh were studied in some detail in cat visual cortex (Sillito and Kemp, 1983) and in somatosensory cortex (Metherate et al., 1988). In most cortical cells, visually evoked responses were augmented by iontophoreses of ACh. Both facilitatory (majority) and suppressive (minority) effects of ACh were blocked by iontophoresis of atropine (Sato et al., 1987a). In visual cortex ipsilateral to kainate lesions of the basal forebrain, half the recorded cells from area 17 lost visual responsiveness, which seemed to be restored by ACh iontophoreses (Sato et al., 1987b).

CONTRIBUTION OF ACh AFFERENTS TO CORTICAL PLASTICITY

Our studies in the last 14 years indicate strongly that activation of the NA-β adrenoreceptor system is sufficient, though not necessarily excluding contribution of other factors under usual conditions, in enhancing visuocortical plasticity.

Why ACh Afferents?

Bear and Singer (1986) reported that ocular dominance plasticity was substantially reduced in kitten visual cortex only when its noradrenergic and cholinergic afferents had been impaired concurrently. The impairment of NA fibers was made at the ascending dorsal bundle and that of ACh afferents at the basal forebrain. Based on these results and others, they argued that a cortical 6-OHDA infusion might have disrupted the plasticity by simultaneously interfering with both the NA and ACh transmission within the 6-OHDA-affected cortex. As will be discussed in some detail below, interpretations of their findings are not as straightforward as they were presented and turned out to be highly problematic. Nevertheless, we took their suggestion as a *testable* hypothesis and examined further the involvement of ACh-related receptors and especially their interaction with the NA system in the regulation of ocular dominance plasticity.

Our own reasoning behind this new direction was as follows: (i) Neocortex is an ultimate target area of many projection systems which have long ascending axons originating from a limited number of cells in the basal forebrain, the brainstem and the medulla. The cortical NA system, working together with specific receptors, is merely one of such projection systems. It is thus quite conceivable that multilayered regulatory mechanisms normally responsible for ocular dominance plasticity may shift their mode of operation from the NA system to others as a consequence of "heterologous" compensation for the severely impaired NA system. (ii) Among various ways we had tried to reduce ocular dominance plasticity, we obtained so far the best effect with a cortical infusion of propranolol. Yet, the proportion of binocular cells (binocularity, B) preserved in monocularly deprived kittens was maximally B = 0.67 (Shirokawa and Kasamatsu, 1986). Though this value is certainly above the lower end of 5% rejection intervals of normal binocularity (B $\geq$ 0.53), it is below that of 95% confidence intervals (B $\geq$ 0.69) (mean binocularity, B = 0.75) (Kasamatsu et al., 1985). (iii) No molecules have been identified yet in mammalian neocortex which uniquely appear at the beginning of the physiologically defined postnatal susceptible period and disappear toward its end. The time course of the susceptible period varies, depending on physiological parameters of cortical cells under study and their laminar location. For example, the susceptibility profile of modifiability of directional selectivity (Daw and Wyatt, 1976) rises and ends earlier than that of ocular dominance (Hubel and Wiesel, 1970; Olson and Freeman, 1980). (iv) Rather, it seems likely that the difference among immature and mature cortex is quantitative but not qualitative, the former showing larger values in accumulation of a few yet-to-be-identified molecules than the latter during the envelope of the susceptibility profile defined physiologically. (v) Based on the above premise, we tried to restore cortical plasticity to the mature cortex by activation of the central NA system (including electric stimulation of NA-containing somata in the LC), and cortical infusions of NA (for up to 3 weeks), stimulants of adenylate cyclase (AC), and dibutyryl 3′,5′-adenosine cyclic monophosphate (dibutyryl cAMP). Results remain *partially satisfactory.* We have not yet succeeded in recreating kitten cortex in the adult brain; ocular dominance distribution was U- or W-shaped in response to monocular deprivation, dominated by two types of monocular cells (group−1 and −7 cells of Hubel and Wiesel, 1962), and the average binocularity was lowered to about B = 0.4, still higher than that seen in kittens under comparable conditions. Taken together, a logical conclusion is that a few regulatory mechanisms including the NA-β adrenoreceptor system may work in concert.

A contribution of ACh afferents thus became our immediate concern. We devised a series of experiments to test it, especially in relation to interactions with the NA system (Imamura and Kasamatsu, 1989). We addressed the following two main questions: (i) Can activation of ACh receptors by a muscarinic agonist, bethanechol, restore the plasticity, as shown by an NA infusion, to kitten visual cortex rendered to be aplastic due to a preceding infusion of 6-OHDA or propranolol, and, (ii) conversely, how much can the plasticity be suppressed by an infusion of a muscarinic ACh antagonist, scopolamine, into kitten visual cortex?

Muscarinic ACh Agonist Restored Cortical Plasticity

First, the overwhelming majority of recorded cells showed normal responsiveness as well as receptive-field properties. The proportion of visually unresponsive cells and those with abnormal properties along a given recording track stayed within the usual range. Thus, under the present design of experiments (Fig. 1), there were no discernible side effects of directly infused chemical agents used here [6-OHDA, (±)-propranolol, (–)-NA, bethanechol chloride, and 0.4% ascorbate saline].

Effects of directly infused bethanechol (1 or 5mM) into the 6-OHDA-pretreated cortex was clear-cut: there was a shift in ocular dominance to the open eye (Fig. 2A), while the shift was not seen in the control,

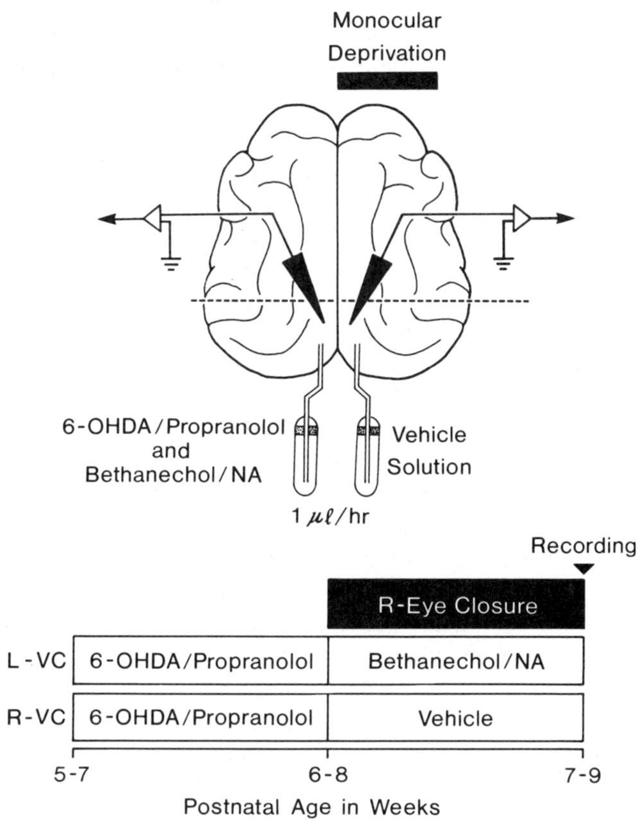

Figure 1. The upper drawing shows schematically relations among placement of recording microelectrodes, monocular lid suture of the right eye, and implantation of cannulae for a continuous cortical infusion (Kasamatsu et al., 1979; 1981a) of four drugs; i.e., 6-hydroydopamine (6-OHDA), propranolol, bethanechol and noradrenaline (NA). Timing of the various treatments is indicated below in terms of the postnatal age of kittens.

vehicle-infused hemisphere of the same animals (Fig. 2B). Accordingly, binocularity in the bethanechol-infused hemisphere (B = 0.27) was significantly smaller than that in control (B = 0.60). A direct infusion of kitten visual cortex with 4mM 6-OHDA, due to a significant reduction in cortical plasticity, blocks the expected shift in ocular dominance following brief monocular deprivation (Kasamatsu et al., 1979; Bear et al., 1983; Daw et al., 1983; Paradiso et al., 1983). Furthermore, the plasticity-suppressing effects of 6-OHDA are sustained, with slightly reduced strength, through at least a week after the end of the 6-OHDA infusion (Kasamatsu and Heggelund, unpublished observation). Therefore, the clear-cut shift in ocular dominance observed here was interpreted to be due to the "plasticity-enhancing" effects of bethanechol.

Figure 2. Effects of cortical infusion with bethanechol chloride and monocular deprivation for the second week of ocular dominance in kitten visual cortex which was pretreated with either 6-OHDA(A,B) or propranolol (C,D) for the first week. **A**: Composite ocular dominance histogram which comprised 5 original histograms (N = 5) based on 150 visually active cells (n = 150) recorded from the bethanechol-infused, left hemisphere (L-VC). **B**: Composite histogram which comprised 3 original histograms (N = 3) based on 90 visual cells (n = 90) obtained in the control, right hemisphere (R-VC) which was infused with the vehicle solution (ascorbate saline) alone. **C**: Composite histogram which comprised 3 original histograms based on 90 visually active cells recorded from the bethanechol-infused, left hemisphere. **D**: Composite histogram comprised 2 original histograms based on 60 visually active cells recorded from the control, right hemisphere. Note that a clear shift in ocular dominance was obtained in A but *not* in C, despite the same bethanechol infusion for both experiments. Each original histogram contained 30 visually active cells which were recorded along mostly one (occasionally two) electrode track. Ocular dominance of each cell was based on Hubel and Wiesel's 7-group scheme (1962). GL and U indicate unit activity of lateral geniculate axons and visually unresponsive units, respectively. Binocularity (B) was initially calculated for each original histogram as the ratio of cells in groups 2-6 to the total number of visually responsive cells and then its mean was calculated for a composite histogram by averaging the individual B values. Vertical thin bars at the top of columns refer to a standard deviation of means in each group. Adapted with permission of Elsevier Science Publishers BV, Amsterdam from Imamura and Kasamatsu (1989): Interaction of noradrenergic and cholinergic systems in regulation of ocular dominance plasticity, *Neuroscience Research* 6: 519-536.

See Figure 2 on next page

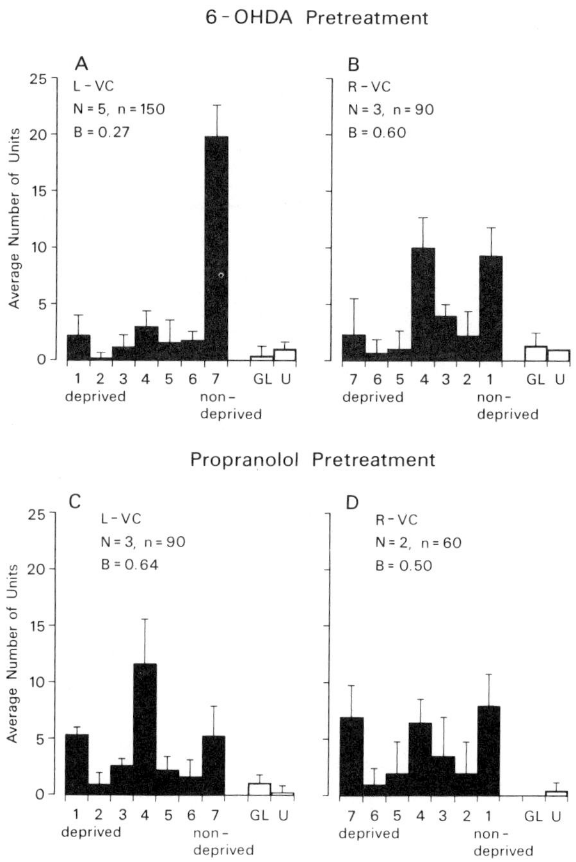

Figure 2.

Relative Strength of "Plasticity-enhancing" Effects of Bethanechol

To have a clue to the strength of the bethanechol infusion in restoring the plasticity, we compared a concentration-effect relationship for bethanechol with that for (–)-NA. The results are summarized in Fig. 3. First, we found that a shift in ocular dominance became less obvious and binocularity stayed higher when concentrations of bethanechol were lowered from 5mM, the highest tested here, to 10μM, the lowest. The results suggested to us that there is a positive correlation between concentrations of bethanechol infused into aplastic cortex and the plasticity-enhancing effect restored by such an infusion. Second, under the comparative condition, we found almost always a clear shift in ocular dominance in the visual cortex which had been infused with 1-100μM NA. Thus, it is evident that the bethanechol infusion was at least 100-fold less effective than that of (–)-NA in restoring the plasticity to the aplastic kitten cortex priorly infused with 6-OHDA.

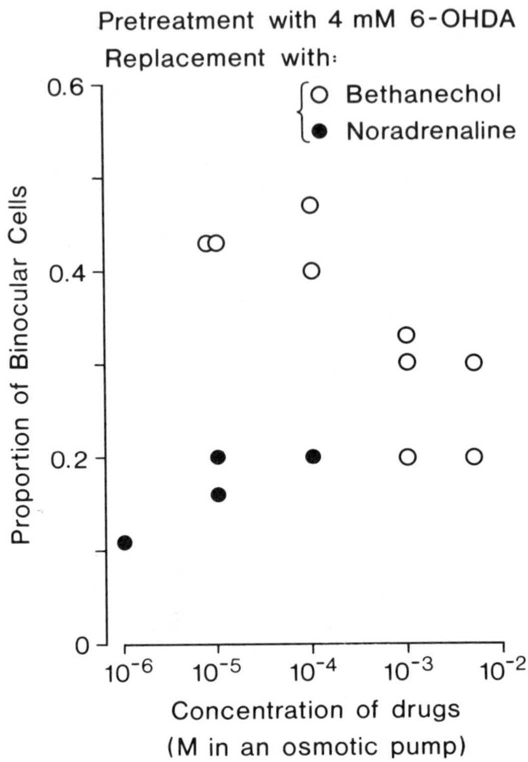

Figure 3. Relationships between a logarithmic concentration of drugs in an osmotic minipump (abscissa) and binocularity (ordinate). Visual cortex of 13 kittens was bilaterally infused with 4 mM 6-OHDA for the first week and with either bethanechol chloride (N = 9) or (–)-noradrenaline (N = 4) for the second week, through the same cannula chronically implanted in the left hemisphere. Note that strength of bethanechol in reversing the plasticity-suppressing effect of 6-OHDA is concentration-dependent and that bethanechol is at least 100-fold less effective than (–)-NA when the concentrations of the two drugs necessary for the maximal effect were compared. Reprinted with permission of Elsevier Science Publishers BV, Amsterdam from Imamura and Kasamatsu (1989): Interaction of noradrenergic and cholinergic systems in regulation of ocular dominance plasticity. *Neuroscience Research* 6:519-536.

Weak Suppression of Plasticity by Scopolamine

The above results with a bethanechol infusion into the 6-OHDA pre-infused cortex definitely indicated that muscarinic ACh receptors are involved in the regulation of cortical plasticity, though their activation is far less effective than that of β adrenoreceptors. An obvious question then is how the two receptor systems possibly work in this matter.

As a first step to address the above question, we carried out a converse experiment using scopolamine, a muscarinic antagonist. Scopolamine at concentrations higher than 100mM (in an osmotic minipump) prevented us from carrying out "clean" physiological recordings due to strong non-specific tissue damage left in a wide cortical area. Within a concentration limit thus imposed ($\leq$100mM), the expected shift in ocular dominance to the nondeprived eye appeared to be *partially* suppressed in the scopolamine-infused hemisphere. Scopolamine at 1mM was totally ineffective. With 10 or 100mM scopolamine, ocular dominance distribution became U-shaped. This was so far the strongest effect we obtained in the present study. Average binocularity values of B = 0.43 (with 100mM) and B = 0.42 (with 10mM) were significantly larger than the control from the opposite, drug-free hemisphere (B = 0.22 and 0.30), though still smaller than the lower end of 5% rejection intervals of normal binocularity (B = 0.53) (Kasamatsu et al., 1985). We are inclined to conclude that functional blockade of muscarinic receptors by scopolamine exerts a very *modest* action in reducing ocular dominance plasticity. We compared a concentration-effect curve obtained for scopolamine in this study (Fig. 4) with a similar curve obtained for ($\pm$)-propranolol in the previous study (Shirokawa and Kasamatsu, 1986). By comparing a pair of drug concentrations for the half-maximal effect, we concluded that a scopolamine infusion was at least 172-fold less effective than a ($\pm$)-propranolol infusion under comparable conditions.

Bethanechol Infusion Does Not Always Restore Plasticity

According to Bear and Singer's understanding of how cortically infused 6-OHDA reduces cortical plasticity (1986), the plasticity-restoring effect of bethanechol shown here in the 6-OHDA-infused cortex might be explained as follows: bethanechol in 10mM or more restored the plasticity by simply activating muscarinic ACh receptors, thus compensating for the lack of ACh impulse transmission which had been caused by a preceding 6-OHDA infusion. At the same time the NA-β adrenoreceptor system remained dysfunctional throughout the period of a bethanechol infusion due to "residual" effects of 6-OHDA which was discontinued earlier. There are some factual and conceptual problems in their explanation.

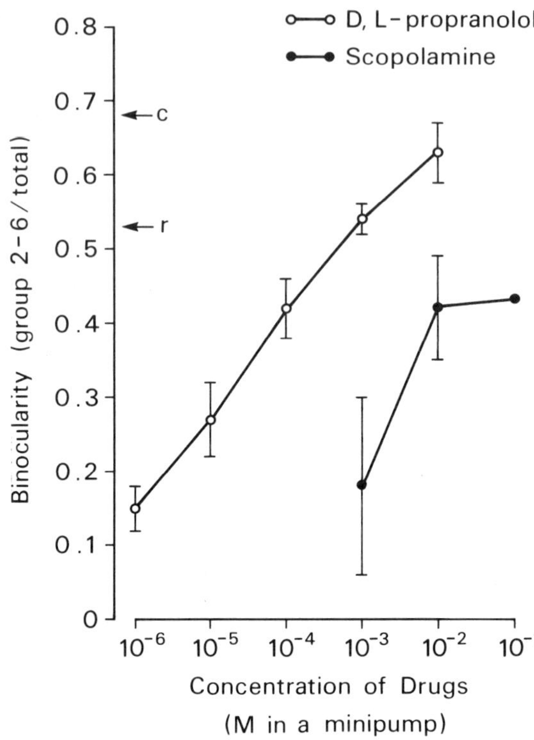

Figure 4. Relationship between a logarithmic concentration of drugs in an osmotic minipump (abscissa) and binocularity (ordinate). Three filled circles refer to binocularity obtained in the scopolamine-infused visual cortex of 8 kittens. Five open circles refer to binocularity previously obtained in the propranolol-infused visual cortex of 19 kittens (Shirokawa and Kasamatsu, 1986). Each circle with vertical bars shows the mean binocularity and its standard deviation at a given concentration. No vertical bar was shown at 10^{-1} M scopolamine, since two animals had an identical binocularity value by chance. The two curves are distinctly different from each other. c and r are the lower end of the 95% confidence intervals ($B \geq 0.69$) and the 5% rejection intervals ($B \geq 0.53$) of normal binocularity (Kasamatsu et al., 1985). Reprinted with permission of Elsevier Science Publishers BV, Amsterdam from Imamura and Kasamatsu (1989): Interaction of noradrenergic and cholinergic systems in regulation of ocular dominance plasticity. *Neuroscience Research* 6:519-536.

First, there is no independent evidence for the proposed effects of 6-OHDA on ACh transmission, especially for its long-lasting effects in a micromolar range at the site of physiological recordings. Second, the proposed scheme works only on the premise that both the NA-β adrenoreceptor system and the ACh-muscarinic receptor system contribute equally to the regulation of plasticity. Is this really so?

Using the paradigm exemplified in Fig. 1, we first infused kitten visual cortex for a week with 10mM ($\pm$)-propranolol, in place of 4mM 6-OHDA. We asked if a subsequent cortical infusion of 1,5 or 10mM bethanechol for the second week restored the plasticity. We knew that as an initial treatment, a cortical infusion of 4mM 6-OHDA and 10mM ($\pm$)- propranolol are equally effective in suppressing ocular dominance plasticity (Shirokawa and Kasamatsu, 1986). We later learned that the suppression of plasticity by propranolol remained for a week after the end of its infusion and that a cortical infusion of 50μM (–)-NA restored the plasticity to such a cortex (Shirokawa and Kasamatsu, 1987).

We encountered an intriguing result. The "expected" shift in ocular dominance due to monocular deprivation failed this time to reveal itself in the bethanechol-infused cortex (Fig. 2C). There was no significant difference in binocularity between the bethanechol-infused (B = 0.64) and the control (B = 0.50) hemisphere. The resulting ocular dominance histograms from the two hemispheres (Fig. 2C,D) differ neither from each other nor from the control histogram obtained in the vehicle-infused hemisphere of 6-OHDA-pretreated kittens (Fig. 2B).

Taken together, the present results indicate that the "plasticity-enhancing" effect of bethanechol is not expressed when β adrenoreceptors have been functionally blocked by propranolol. In other words, the availability of β adrenoreceptors seems to be a prerequisite for integrating the NA and muscarinic components in the regulation of ocular dominance plasticity. We conclude that the contribution of the ACh system is secondary to the plasticity-enhancing mechanisms maintained through activation of the NA-β adrenoreceptor system.

NEUROCHEMICAL BASES OF CORTICAL PLASTICITY: A DISCUSSION

Ontogeny of ACh and NA Systems in Cat Visual Cortex

We described effects of activation and inactivation of the muscarinic ACh system on ocular dominance plasticity in kitten visual cortex (Table 1). Ocular dominance plasticity is typically expressed in immature kitten visual cortex. One of a few strategies to analyze neurochemical bases of developmental plasticity is to examine, biochemically, histologically or autoradiographically, the normal ontogeny of "targeted" molecules in an effort to detect their accumulation in early postnatal life above the level which is eventually attained in adulthood. If a profile of this maturation curve changes in parallel to the electrophysiologically determined time course of the plasticity, one tentatively takes this parallelism as a piece of evidence for the involvement of "targeted" molecules in the plasticity.

Bear et al. (1985) histochemically examined postnatal changes in acetylcholinesterase (AChE) staining in cat visual cortex. They found that by 4 weeks of age the number of AChE-positive fibers in layer IVc to VI exceeded the adult value, remained high through 8 weeks, and decreased to the adult value by 13 weeks. AChE-positive fibers in layer II, III and IVab, especially at the bottom of layer III, increased gradually to reach the mature laminar pattern at about 6 weeks of age. Earlier, Potempska et al. (1979) showed biochemically that AChE activity in cat visual cortex was relatively high already at 1 week of age and dropped to 65% of the adult value during the second postnatal week, remaining so throughout the end of 2 months before showing a gradual increase in later months. This trend was basically shared by a profile of ChAT activity, except for its peaking at 3 months followed by a gradual decline to adulthood. Muscarinic receptor binding with QNB, already as high as the adult level at birth, showed an early peak at 5 weeks of age, remained high over 14 weeks of age, and thereafter appeared to gradually decline to adulthood (Shaw et al., 1984).

Taken together, Bear et al. (1985) then argued that "the levels of this cholinergic marker (i.e., AChE staining) correlate with synaptic plasticity in both the spatial and temporal domains." It is, however, not immediately clear how they reached this conclusion from the material they took into consideration. In addition, there is doubt of the usefulness of AChE staining as a marker of ontogeny of the ACh system because of its low specificity, as evidenced by the transient nature of staining patterns under certain conditions, e.g., AChE-containing non-cholinergic fibers (Butcher et al., 1975; Robertson et al., 1989).

Later, an immunostaining study in cat visual cortex showed that by 4 weeks of age the density of ChAT-positive fibers and varicosities reached the adult level in layer V and VI, and the maturation in layer I-IV lagged behind by 9 weeks. They thus concluded that there was *no* evidence for a particular narrow correlation between the density of the ACh innervation and modifiability of neural connections during the postnatal susceptible period (Stichel and Singer, 1987b). This conclusion is further corroborated by a recent biochemical study which showed a "biphasic" time course of ChAT activity throughout the susceptible period in area 17 and 18 (a first peak at the second week followed by a very slow maturation process), (Fosse et al., 1989). In short, the two reliable markers of ACh maturation, ChAT activity and muscarinic receptor binding, showed a maturation profile quite different from that of ocular dominance plasticity, which is defined physiologically (Hubel and Wiesel, 1970; Olson and Freeman, 1980). Thus, the ACh system cannot be a main carrier of ocular dominance plasticity in cat visual cortex. Rather, it is intriguing that ontogeny curves of other molecules such as β adrenoreceptor (Jonsson and Kasamatsu, 1983), phosphatidyl inositol (PI) turnover induced by ibotenate (Dudek and Bear, 1989), and protein kinase C (PKC), (Sheu et al., 1990) in cat visual cortex are comparable to those of the plasticity defined physiologically.

Second Messengers

Activation of β adrenoreceptors causes AC-dependent accumulation of cAMP, involving an excitatory type of guanosine triphosphate (GTP)-binding transducer protein, termed G_s. Muscarinic activation of ACh receptors is known to lead to various biochemical changes in cells such as a decrease in cAMP and an increase in PI turnover (Fisher and Bartus, 1985). In the former, the decrease is caused by inhibition of a key enzyme, AC, the inhibition being mediated by inhibitory G proteins, G_i or G_o (Watanabe et al., 1978; Jakobs et al., 1979). In the latter, the muscarinic activation causes first activation of phospholipase C, which metabolizes PI to produce two second messengers, inositol 1,4,5-triphosphate (IP_3) and diacylglycerol (DAG). IP_3 is thought to be responsible for release of Ca^{++} from the intracellular pool (Berridge and Irvine, 1984; 1989), and DAG works as an endogenous activator of PKC (Nishizuka,

Table 1. Summary of changes in cortical plasticity by various drug treatments given to kitten visual cortex, individually or in pairs, following the matrix shown below. A few null hypotheses are proposed and rejected as follows:

(i) Both NA and ACh terminals are *equally* destroyed by a cortical 6-OHDA infustion; not rejected by finding (1), but rejected by comparison of findings (4) and (6).

(ii) Both β-adrenergic and muscarinic receptors are *equally* blocked by a cortical infusion of propranolol; not rejected by finding (2), but rejected by comparison of findings (5) and (7).

(iii) Both NA-β adrenoreceptors and ACh-muscarinic receptors are *equally* needed for cortical plasticity; not rejected by findings (1) and (2), but rejected by combination of findings (2) and (3), (4) and (6), and (5) and (7).

(↑, weak increase; ↑↑, strong increase; ↓, weak decrease; ↓↓, strong decrease; ∼, no change).

Pretreatment (first week)

Replacement (second week)	6-OHDA 4mM	Propranolol 10mM	Scopolamine 10-100mM	lesion of ACh terminals
none	(1) ↓↓	(2) ↓↓	(3) ↓	not tested
Bethanechol 1-5mM	(4) ↑	(5) ∼	not tested	
(−)-NA 1-100μM	(6) ↑↑	(7) ↑ (see ref.*)	not tested	

* Shirokawa and Kasamatsu, 1987

1986; 1988). It is interesting that a family of phorbol esters, potent activators of PKC, was found to block slow AHP in hippocampal pyramidal cells (Malenka et al., 1986; Baraban, 1987).

Currently, five molecularly distinct subtypes of muscarinic ACh receptors (m_1-m_5) are known. Some of these subtypes are also functionally different from each other; activation of m_2 or m_3 inhibits effectively AC without having facilitatory effects on PI turnover in non-neural cell lines, and the reverse is the case for m_1 and m_4 activation (Fukuda et al., 1988; Peralta et al., 1988). It is intriguing if the 5 subtypes are also assigned to various consequences of ACh applications mentioned above. Neocortex and hippocampus (CA1) are known for their rich presence of PKC activity (Worley et al., 1986; Saito et al., 1988). A crucial role of PKC in memory and neural plasticity (long-term potentiation, LTP) has been implied (Akers et al., 1986; for review see Benowitz and Routtenberg, 1987). PKC is also known to inactivate G_i through its phosphorylation, thus enhancing AC activity (Katada et al., 1985). Likewise, PKC potentiates agonist-induced accumulation of cAMP (Sugden et al., 1985).

Central Core Control

Singer and associates have recognized, as we did, the necessity of "non-retinal" afferents besides Hebb synapses in maintenance of ocular dominance plasticity in immature visual cortex. In two kittens *under anesthesia and paralysis*, monocular exposure for 15-18 hrs to a rotating black/white grating conditioned with electric stimulation of the thalamic nuclei or mesencephalic reticular formation (MRF) caused a change in ocular dominance toward the stimulated eye or augmentation of visual cortical potentials evoked by electric stimulation of the optic nerve (Singer, 1979). Taken together with an accompanying result from kittens which received unilateral lesions at the mediodorsal nucleus of the thalamus (Singer, 1982), Singer and Rauschecker (1982) suggested that the MRF/nonspecific thalamic nuclei is the site of "gating" function which regulates experience-dependent modifications of neural connections in kitten visual cortex. There are, however, serious difficulties in the interpretations of their results. For example, the majority of single cells recorded in the above stimulation study remained binocular ($B = 0.67$), though the ocular dominance distribution was dominated by cells receiving stronger inputs from the exposed eye. One would *not* call this distribution shifted. Furthermore, an unusually high proportion (43%) of cells had receptive-field properties described as outside the normal range (e.g., sluggish responses and broad orientation tuning).

It is thought that electric stimulation of the MRF induces release of ACh in neocortex (Szerb, 1967), probably together with simultaneous release of other substances. Therefore, the proposed role of the MRF in enhancement of cortical plasticity appears to be mediated, at least in part, by activation of the ACh system. However, there is a conceptual difficulty left unsolved before the Singer's proposal is evaluated properly. On the one hand, in reference to his study of cats that experienced surgical strabismus (Singer et al., 1979a) or a combined manipulation of intraorbital rotation of one eye and monocular lid suture of the other eye (Singer et al., 1979b), Singer claims that "visual attention" plays a vital role in gating experience-dependent modification of neural connections. On the other hand, activation of the MRF, which is supposed to enhance "visual attention" through the ACh system, significantly *reduces* specificity of visuocortical cells such as orientation tuning and direction selectivity (Singer et al., 1976). Later studies by other authors on cortical effects of iontophoretically injected ACh were inconsistent; Sillito and Kemp (1983) reported an increase in cortical cells' specificity and Sato et al. (1987a) obtained the opposite results. Thus, it is fair to say that neurochemical consequences of MRF stimulation *in vivo* are much more complicated than originally imagined by Singer and associates. For example, the MRF is rich of NA terminals beside other types of terminals.

Furthermore, we recently showed that distinct changes in ocular dominance can be induced under general anesthesia and paralysis. In NA-infused, otherwise normal visual cortex of acutely prepared *adult* cats, the proportion of binocular cells decreased significantly in response to the divergence of the visual axes and binocularity returned normal when they were realigned by placing prism(s) in front of the eye (Heggelund et al., 1987). The experimental condition was typical of receptive-field recordings; the cat was anesthetized with $N_2O/O_2/CO_2$ (75/22.5/2.5) supplemented by $\sim$2 mg/kg/h of Surital, and paralysis was maintained by a continuous infusion of Flaxedil at $\sim$10 mg/kg/hr. The maximal change was obtained, regardless of the direction in changes, in about 22 hrs of the combined manipulations. We subsequently found that a shift in ocular dominance takes place in kittens under anesthesia and paralysis when a NA infusion is combined with pattern vision through one eye (Imamura and Kasamatsu, 1988). Taken together, we conclude that activation by NA of β adrenoreceptors is *sufficient* to restore plasticity at least partly in anesthetized and paralyzed preparations.

Therefore, if some mental process called "visual attention" is an indispensable part of regulatory mechanisms of cortical plasticity operative in freely behaving animals such that the attentional process may well be expressed through activation of the NA-β adrenoreceptor-cAMP system in the brain.

Interaction Between NA and ACh Systems

It was suggested that the ACh and NA afferents independently promote ocular dominance plasticity working through a common molecular mechanism in an additive manner (Bear and Singer, 1986). As discussed above, however, the ACh system is not equipped with molecular machinery which is capable to execute its plasticity-enhancing action independent of functional states of the NA system. Then, how and what kind of interaction is possible among the two neuromodulator systems in promotion of the cortical plasticity?

Recently, Nicoll (1988) raised a possibility that a Ca^{++}-activated K^+ channel responsible for slow AHP is under dual control of cAMP and DAG-activated PKC through phosphorylation of the same K^+ channel protein, which has yet to be identified structurally. In the other system, the presence of a similar phosphorylation scheme was also noted (Takai et al., 1984). Despite these possibilities, it is *not* immediately clear if NA-activated and ACh-activated blockade of slow AHP are equally responsible for the enhancement of visually evoked responses *in vivo*. Rather, it is our common knowledge that effects on cortical excitability of iontophoretically injected ACh (Sillito and Kemp, 1983; Sato et al., 1987a) are far stronger than those of NA (Kasamatsu and Heggelund, 1982; Videen et al., 1984) when individual visual-receptive fields are stimulated with optimal visual stimuli.

Presynaptic ACh receptors are generally thought to decrease transmitter release (Yamamoto and Kawai, 1967). An inhibitory effect of ACh on NA release was shown in cerebellar slices (Westfall, 1974) and the peripheral NA system (Kadlec et al., 1986). In freshly dissociated gastric smooth muscles, a β-adrenergic agonist and an analog of cAMP induced the M-current (Brown, 1983), while a muscarinic agonist suppressed this current (Sims et al., 1988). Strong light flash or electric stimulation of the forelimb was found to decrease "nonspecifically" the release of NA into cortical perfusate and increase the ACh release in cat visual cortex, the changes being counteracted by atropine or nicotine (Reader et al., 1976). These inhibitory effects of ACh on NA release are due presumably to ACh afferents terminating presynaptically on NA boutons, and activating the M_2 subtype of muscarinic receptors (Meyer and Otero, 1985). Obviously, however, these effects would not explain "the plasticity-enhancing effect" of bethanechol shown in our study.

A family of G proteins may be involved in the NA and ACh interaction in the regulation of ocular dominance plasticity. G proteins are indeed a molecular entity which is responsible for modulatory interaction among various ion channels, transmitter receptors and hormone receptors (Cerione et al., 1983; Gilman, 1984; Andrade et al., 1986; Sasakai and Sato, 1987; Nicoll, 1988). For example, Watanabe et al. (1978) reported in membrane preparation of dog myocardium that a muscarinic agonist, methacholine, increased β-adrenergic agonist (isoprenaline) binding up to 3-fold by blocking GTP's inhibitory action on the apparent affinity of isoprenaline for cardiac β receptors. Conversely, Rosenberger et al. (1980) found that isoprenaline decreased the apparent affinity of a muscarinic agonist (oxotremoline) for cardiac muscarinic receptors. In the cat submandibular salivary gland, vasoactive intestine peptide (VIP) increased carbachol binding to muscarinic receptors by 10^5-fold (Lundberg et al., 1982). Both VIP and NA are thought to facilitate synergistically glycogenolysis in cerebral cortex by α_1-adrenoreceptor-mediated potentiation of VIP effects on accumulation of cAMP (Magistretti and Schorderet, 1984). Co-localization of VIP-and ChAT-immunoreactivity was shown in rat cerebral cortex (Eckenstein and Baughman, 1984). Ontogeny of VIP-immunoreactive cells was described in cat visual cortex (Wahle and Meyer, 1989).

Integration of NA and ACh Effects on Plasticity

We hypothesize as follows: while NA-initiated, β adrenoreceptor-mediated and G_s protein-enhanced accumulation of cAMP plays a primary role in the regulation of ocular dominance plasticity, ACh afferents may exert a secondary, yet important regulatory control in this matter (Table 2).

Our preliminary results showed that ocular dominance plasticity was substantially decreased in visual cortex of kittens which had been intraperitoneally injected with a lithium salt (Li_2CO_3) for some time (Ohashi et al., 1988; Ohashi and Kasamatsu, 1989). Recent *in vitro* and *ex vivo* studies in rat neocortex showed that lithium at therapeutic concentrations blocked both NA-agonist (isoprenaline)- and ACh-agonist (carbachol)-induced increases in GTP binding to membrane preparations (Avissar et al., 1988). Berridge and Irvine (1989) favored an idea that lithium reduces more PI turnover rather than dually blocks binding of G_s and G_i/G_o proteins. Taken together, the plasticity-enhancing effect of ACh may be mediated by activated M_2/M_3 receptors, causing G_i/G_o protein-dependent inhibition of ACh activity (and thus a decrease in desensitization of β adrenoreceptors, (Cerione et al., 1983; Sibley and Lefkowitz, 1985), or activation of m_1/m_4 receptors (further leading to activation of IP_3 and PKC) or both.

Table 2. Contribution of a few receptor systems to modulation of visually evoked responses and regulation of ocular dominance plasticity.

	Modulation of visual response	**Regulation of cortical plasticity**
Acetylcholine — muscarinic receptor	++	+
Noradrenaline — β adrenoreceptor	+	+++
Glutamate — NMDA receptor	+++	(+)
GABA– $GABA_A$ receptor	+++	+

(+, weak; ++ moderate, +++ strong; (+) in question)

CONCLUSION

We presented a unified view, including both the NA-β adrenoreceptor and the ACh-muscarinic receptor systems, of the regulation of visual cortical plasticity in immature visual cortex. We found: (i) within concentration limits imposed by recordability of visually evoked activity, there was *no* discernible effects on visual responsiveness and receptive field properties of individual cells by a direct infusion of drugs used here (6-OHDA, propranolol, NA, bethanechol, scopolamine, and 0.4% ascorbate saline); (ii) activation of ACh receptors by bethanechol indeed restored cortical susceptibility to brief monocular deprivation of kitten visual cortex rendered aplastic due to a preceding direct infusion of 6-OHDA; (iii) there was a positive correlation between concentrations of bethanechol infused into aplastic cortex and the extent of cortical susceptibility thus restored. The bethanechol infusion was at least 100-fold *less* effective than NA infusion in this matter; (iv) functional blockade of muscarinic receptors by scopolamine at high concentrations resulted in a *modest* reduction of cortical susceptibility to monocular deprivation (no shift in the U-shaped distribution of ocular dominance); (v) finally, the bethanechol infusion *failed* to restore the cortical susceptibility to kitten visual cortex pretreated with propranolol in place of 6-OHDA.

Taken together, the presence of β adrenoreceptors seems to be a pivot in integrating the NA and ACh components in the regulation of ocular dominance plasticity, the former playing a primary role and helped by the latter. Yet, as the current state of the affair dictates, it seems almost inevitable to widen our search for contributing neurochemical factors in this matter. They may include various ascending fiber projections, slow heterosynaptic release or co-release of modulator substances, or an age-dependent expression of receptor subtypes and second messengers. Especially urgent is the integration of the two separately pursued avenues of research in the regulation of cortical plasticity: activity dependency within the visual pathway on the one hand, and global neurochemical factors, such as the NA and ACh system, on the other. In normally developing visual cortex, all these factors can be brought into action synergistically in an overlapping mosaic fashion, each uniquely contributing to the maintenance of cortical plasticity.

ACKNOWLEDGMENTS

We are grateful to Mr. J. Brodale and Ms. R. Smith for their art work. Supported by USPHS Grants EY06733 (to T.K.), Core Grant EY06883 and BRSG RR05981. K. Imamura was a recipient of the R.C. Atkinson Fellowship.

REFERENCES

Abercrombie, E.D. and Zigmond, M.J. (1989): Partial injury to central noradrenergic neurons: reduction of tissue norepinephrine content is greater than reduction of extracellular norepinephrine measured by microdialysis. *J. Neurosci.* 9:4062-4067

Adrien, J., Blanc, G., Buisseret, P., Frégnac, Y., Gary-Bobo, E., Imbert, M., Tassin, J.-P. and Trotter, Y. (1985): Noradrenaline and functional plasticity in kitten visual cortex: a re-examination. *J. Physiol.* (Lond.) 367:73-98

Akers, R.F., Lovinger, D.M., Colley, P., Linden, D. and Routtenberg, A. (1986): Translocation of protein kinase C activity may mediate hippocampal long-term potentiation. *Science* 231:587-589

Andrade, R., Malenka, R.C. and Nicoll, R.A. (1986): A G protein couples serotonin and GABA receptors to the same channels in hippocampus. *Science* 234:1261-1265

Avissar, S., Schreiber, G., Danon, A. and Belmaker, R.Hh (1988): Lithium inhibits adrenergic and cholinergic increases in GTP binding in rat cortex. *Nature* (Lond.) 331:440-442

Baraban, J.M. (1987): Phorbol esters: probes of protein kinase C function in the brain. *Trends Neurosci.* 10:57-58

Bear, M.F., Carnes, K.M. and Ebner, F.F. (1985): Postnatal changes in the distribution of acetylcholinesterase in kitten visual cortex. *J. Comp. Neurol.* 237:519-532

Bear, M.F., Cooper, L.N. and Ebner, F.F. (1987): A physiological basis for a theory of synaptic modification. *Science* 237:42-48

Bear, M.F. and Daniels, J.D. (1983): The plastic response to monocular deprivation persists in kitten visual cortex after chronic depletion of norepinephrine. *J. Neurosci.* 3:407-416

Bear, M.F., Paradiso, M.A., Schwartz, M., Nelson, S.B., Carnes, K.M. and Daniels, J.D. (1983): Two methods of catecholamine depletion in kitten visual cortex yield different effects on plasticity. *Nature* (Lond.) 302:245-247

Bear, M.F. and Singer, W. (1986): Modulation of visual cortical plasticity by acetylcholine and noradrenaline. *Nature* (Lond.) 320:172-176

Benardo , L.S. and Prince, D.A. (1982): Ionic mechanisms of cholinergic excitation in mammalian hippocampal pyramidal cells. *Brain Res.* 249:333-344

Benowitz, L.I. and Routtenberg, A. (1987): A membrane phosphoprotein associated with neural development, axonal regeneration, phospholipid metabolism, and synaptic plasticity. *Trends Neurosci.* 10:527-532

Berridge, M.J. and Irvine, R.F. (1984): Inositol triphosphate, a novel second messenger in cellular signal transduction. *Nature* (Lond.) 312:315-321

Berridge, M.J. and Irvine, R.F. (1989): Inositol phosphates and cell signalling. *Nature* (Lond.) 341:197-205

Brown, D.A. (1983): Slow cholinergic excitation-a mechanism for increasing neuronal excitability. *Trends Neurosci.* 6:302-307

Butcher, L.L., Talbot, K. and Bilezikijan, L. (1975): Acetylcholinesterase neurons in dopamine-containing regions of the brain. *J. Neurol. Trans.* 37:127-153

Cerione, R.A., Staniszewski, C., Caron, M.G., Lefkowitz, R.J., Codina, J. and Birnbaumer, L. (1983): A role for Ni in the hormonal stimulation of adenylate cyclase. *Nature* (Lond.) 318:293-295

Constanti, A. and Sim, J.A. (1987): Calcium-dependent potassium conductance in guinea-pig olfactory cortex neurones *in vitro*. *J. Physiol.* (Lond.) 387:173-194

Cooper, L.N. (1987): Cortical plasticity: theoretical analysis, experimental results. In: *Imprinting and Cortical Plasticity, Comparative Aspects of Sensitive Periods*. Rauschecker, J.P., Marler, P.R., eds. New York: John Wiley & Son, pp 177-192

Daw, N.W., Rader, R.K., Robertson, T.W. and Ariel, M. (1983): Effects of 6-hydroxydopamine on visual deprivation in kitten striate cortex. *J. Neurosci.* 3:907-914

Daw, N.W., Robertson, T.W., Rader, R.K., Videen, T.O. and Coscia, C.J. (1984): Substantial reduction of cortical noradrenaline by lesions of adrenergic pathway does not prevent effects of monocular deprivation. *J. Neurosci.* 4:1354-1360

Daw, N.W., Videen, T.O., Parkinson, D. and Rader, R.K. (1985a) DSP-4 (N-(2-chloroethyl)-N-ethyl-2-bromobenzylamine) depletes noradrenaline in kitten visual cortex without altering the effects of monocular deprivation. *J. Neurosci.* 5:1925-1933

Daw, N.W., Videen, T.O., Rader, R.K., Robertson, T.W. and Coscia, C.J. (1985b): Substantial reduction of noradrenaline in kitten visual cortex by intraventricular injections of 6-hydroxydopamine does not always prevent ocular dominance shifts after monocular deprivation. *Exp. Brain Res.* 59:30-35

Daw, N.W., Videen, T.O., Robertson, T. and Rader, R.K. (1985c): An evaluation of the hypothesis that noradrenaline affects plasticity in the developing visual cortex. In: *The Visual System.* Fein, A., ed. New York: Alan R. Liss, Inc. pp 133-144

Daw, N.W. and Wyatt, H.J. (1976): Kittens reared in a unidirectional environment: evidence for a critical period. *J. Physiol.* (Lond.) 257:155-170

de Lima, A.D. and Singer, W. (1986): Cholinergic innervation of cat striate cortex: a choline acetyltransferase immunocytochemical analysis. *J. Comp. Neurol.* 250:324-338

Dunwiddie, T.V., Mueller, A.L., Bickford, P.C. and Zahniser, N.R. (1983): Electrophysiological and biochemical sequelae of the destruction of hippocampal noradrenergic afferents by DSP4. *Brain Res.* 269:311-317

Dudek, S.M. and Bear, M.F. (1989): A biochemical correlate of the critical period for synaptic modification in the visual cortex. *Science* 246:673-675

Eckenstein, F. and Baughman, R.W. (1984): Two types of cholinergic innervation in cortex, one co-localized with vasoactive intestinal polypeptide. *Nature* (Lond.) 309:152-155

Fisher, S.K. and Bartus, R.T. (1985): Regional differences in the coupling of muscarinic receptors to inositol phospholipid hydrolysis in guinea pig brain. *J. Neurochem.* 45:1085-1095

Fosse, V.M., Heggelund, P. and Fonnum, F. (1989): Postnatal development of glutamatergic, GABAergic, and cholinergic neurotransmitter phenotypes in the visual cortex, lateral geniculate nucleus, pulvinar, and superior colliculus in cats. *J. Neurosci.* 9:426-435

Frégnac, Y. (1987): Cellular mechanisms of epigenesis in cat visual cortex. In: *Imprinting and Cortical Plasticity.* Rauschecker, J.P., Marler, P., eds. New York: John Wiley & Sons, pp 221-266

Frégnac, Y. and Imbert, M. (1984): Development of neuronal selectivity in primary visual cortex of cat. *Physiol. Rev.* 64:325-434

Fukuda, K., Higashida, H., Kubo, T., Maeda, A., Akiba, I., Bujo, H., Mishina, M. and Numa, S. (1988): Selective coupling with K^+ currents of muscarinic acetylcholine receptor subtypes in NG 108-15 cells. *Nature* (Lond.) 335:355-358

Gilman, A.G. (1984): G proteins and dual control of adenylate cyclase. *Cell* 36:577-579

Gordon, B., Allen, E.E. and Trombley, P.Q. (1988): The role of norepinephrine in plasticity of visual cortex. *Prog. Neurobiol.* 30:171-191

Halliwell, J.V. and Adams, P.R. (1982): Voltage-clamp analysis of muscarinic excitation in hippocampal neurons. *Brain Res.* 250:71-92

Harden, T.K., Wolfe, B.B., Sporn, J.R., Poulos, J.R. and Molinoff, P.B. (1977): Effects of 6-hydroxydopamine on the development of the beta adrenergic receptor/adenylate cyclase system in rat cerebral cortex. *J. Pharmacol. Exp. Ther.* 203:132-143

Heggelund, P., Imamura, K. and Kasamatsu, T. (1987): Reduced binocularity in the noradrenaline-infused striate cortex of acutely anesthetized and paralyzed, otherwise normal cats. *Exp. Brain Res.* 68:593-605

Hirsch, H.V.B. and Tieman, S.B. (1987): Perceptual development and experience-dependent changes in cat visual cortex. In: *Sensitive Periods in Development: Interdisciplinary Perspectives.* Bornstein, M., ed. Hillsdale, NJ: Lawrence Erlbaum Assoc., pp 39-79

Houser, C.R., Crawford, G.D., Barber, R.P., Salvaterra, P.M. and Vaughn, J.E. (1983): Organization and morphological characteristics of cholinergic neurons: an immunocytochemical study with a monoclonal antibody to choline acetyltransferase. *Brain Res.* 266:97-119

Hubel, D.H. and Wiesel, T.N. (1962): Receptive fields, binocular interaction and functional architecture in the cat's visual cortex. *J. Physiol.* (Lond.) 160:106-154

Hubel, D.H. and Wiesel, T.N. (1965): Binocular interaction in striate cortex of kittens reared with artificial squint. *J. Neurophysiol.* 28:1041-1059

Hubel, D.H. and Wiesel, T.N. (1970): The period of susceptibility to the physiological effects of unilateral eye closure in kittens. *J. Physiol.* (Lond.) 206:419-436

Imamura, K. and Kasamatsu, T. (1988): Acutely induced shift in ocular dominance during brief monocular exposure: effects of cortical noradrenaline infusion. *Neurosci. Lett.* 88:57-62

Imamura, K. and Kasamatsu, T. (1989): Interaction of noradrenergic and cholinergic systems in regulation of ocular dominance plasticity. *Neurosci. Res.* 6:519-536

Itakura, T., Kasamatsu, T. and Pettigrew, J.D. (1981): Norepinephrine-containing terminals in kitten visual cortex: laminar distribution and ultrastructure. *Neurosci.* 6:159-175

Jakobs, K.H., Aktories, K. and Schulz, G. (1979): GTP-dependent inhibition of cardiac adenylate cyclase by muscarinic cholinergic agonists. *Naunyn-Schmiedeberg's Arch. Pharmacol.* 310:113-119

Jonsson, G. (1980): Chemical neurotoxins as denervation tools in neurobiology. *Ann. Rev. Neurosci.* 3:169-187

Jonsson, G. and Kasamatsu, T. (1983): Maturation of monoamine neurotransmitters and receptors in cat occipital cortex during postnatal critical period. *Exp. Brain Res.* 50:449-458

Jonsson, G., Wiesel F.-A. and Hallman, H. (1979): Developmental plasticity of central noradrenaline neurons after neonatal damage–changes in transmitter functions. *J. Neurobiol.* 10:337-353

Kadlec, O., Somogyi, G.T., Seferna, I., Masek, K. and Vizi, E.S. (1986): Interactions between the duration of stimulation and noradrenaline on cholinergic transmission in the myenteric plexus-smooth muscle preparation. *Brain Res. Bull.* 16:171-178

Kasamatsu, T. (1979): Involvement of the β-adrenergic receptor in cortical plasticity. *ARVO Abstr. Suppl. Invest. Ophthalmol. Vis. Sci.* 18:135

Kasamatsu, T. (1980): A possible role for cyclic nucleotides in plasticity of visual cortex. *Soc. Neurosci. Abstr.* 6:494

Kasamatsu, T. (1982): A role of the central norepinephrine system in regulation of neuronal plasticity in cat visual cortex. In: *Neurotransmitters in the Retina and the Visual Centers*, Kaneko, A., Tsukahara, N., Uchizono, R., eds. Tokyo: Biomed. Res. Suppl. 3, Biomed. Res. Foundation, pp 87-93

Kasamatsu, T. (1983): Neuronal plasticity maintained by the central norepinephrine system in the cat visual cortex. In: *Progr. Psychobiol. Physiol. Psych., Vol. 10*. New York: Academic Press, pp 1-112

Kasamatsu, T. (1986a): Changes in ocular dominance of adult cats following monocular lid suture: the effect of directly infused forskolin. *ARVO Abstr. Suppl. Invest. Ophthalmol. Vis. Sci.* 27:153

Kasamatsu, T. (1986b): A regulatory mechanism of changes in ocular dominance. In: *Adaptive Processes in Visual and Oculomotor Systems*. Keller, E.L., Zee, D.S., eds. Oxford: Pergamon Press, pp 71-78

Kasamatsu, T. (1987): Norepinephrine hypothesis for visual cortical plasticity: thesis, antithesis, and recent development. In: *Current Topics in Developmental Biology, Vol. 21*. New York: Academic Press, pp 367-389

Kasamatsu, T. (1989): Experimental amblyopia ex anopsia in kittens: neuropharmacological approach. In: *Problems and Concepts in Developmental Neurophysiology.* Kellaway, P., Noebels, J.L., eds. Baltimore: The Johns Hopkins Univ. Press, pp 75-91

Kasamatsu, T. and Heggelund, P. (1982): Single cell responses in cat visual cortex to visual stimulation during iontophoresis of noradrenaline. *Exp. Brain Res.* 45:317-327

Kasamatsu, T., Itakura, T. and Jonsson, G. (1981a): Intracortical spread of exogenous catecholamines: effective concentration for modifying cortical plasticity. *J. Pharmacol. Exp. Ther.* 217:841-850

Kasamatsu, T., Itakura, T., Jonsson, G., Heggelund, P., Pettigrew, J.D., Nakai, K., Watabe, K., Kuppermann, B.D. and Ary, M. (1984): Neuronal plasticity in cat visual cortex: a proposed role for the central noradrenaline system. In: *Monoamine Innervation of Cerebral Cortex.* Descarries, L., Reader, T., Jasper, H.H., eds. New York: Alan R. Liss, Inc., pp 301-319

Kasamatsu, T., Ohashi, T. and Imamura, K. (1989a): Integration of adrenergic and cholinergic regulation in ocular dominance plasticity. *Biomed. Res. 10 Suppl.* 2:43-53. The Proceedings of the 14th Seiriken Conference on "The Neural Basis of Cortical Plasticity."

Kasamatsu, T. and Pettigrew, J.D. (1976): Depletion of brain catecholamines: failure of ocular dominance shift after monocular occlusion in kittens. *Science* 194:206-209

Kasamatsu, T. and Pettigrew, J.D. (1979): Preservation of binocularity after monocular deprivation in the striate cortex of kittens treated with 6-hydroxydopamine. *J. Comp. Neurol.* 185:139-162

Kasamatsu, T., Pettigrew, J.D, and Ary, M. (1979): Restoration of visual cortical plasticity by local microperfusion of norepinephrince. *J. Comp. Neurol.* 185:163-182

Kasamatsu, T., Pettigrew, J.D. and Ary, M.. (1981b): Cortical recovery from effects of monocular deprivation: acceleration with norepinephrine and suppression with 6-hydroxydopamine. *J. Neurophysiol.* 45:254-266

Kasamatsu, T. and Shirokawa, T. (1985): Involvement of β adrenoreceptors in the shift of ocular dominance after monocular deprivation. *Exp. Brain Res.* 59:507-514

Kasamatsu, T. and Shirokawa, T. (1988): Norepinephrine-dependent neuronal plasticity in kitten visual cortex. In: *Cellular Mechanisms of Conditioning and Behavioral Plasticity.* Woody, C.D., Alkon, D.L., McGaugh, J.L., eds. New York, Plenum, pp 437-444

Kasamatsu, T., Watabe, K., Heggelund, P. and Schöller, E. (1985): Plasticity in cat visual cortex restored by electrical stimulation of the locus coeruleus. *Neurosci. Res.* 2:365-386

Katada, T., Gilman, A.G., Watanabe, Y., Bauer, S. and Jakobs, K.H. (1985): Protein kinase C phosphorylates the inhibitory guanine-nucleotide-binding regulatory component and apparently suppresses its function in hormonal inhibition of adenylate cyclase. *Eur. J. Biochem.* 151:431-437

Kimura, H., McGeer, P.L., Peng, J.H and McGeer, E.G. (1981): The central cholinergic system, studied by choline acetyltransferase immunohistochemistry in the cat. *J. Comp. Neurol.* 200:151-201

Kostrzewa, R.M. and Jacobowitz, D.M. (1974): Pharmacological actions of 6-hydroxydopamine. *Pharmac. Rev.* 26:199-288

Krnjević, K. (1974): Chemical nature of synaptic transmission in vertebrates. *Physiol. Rev.* 54:418-540

Krnjević, K. and Phillis, J.W. (1963): Acetylcholine sensitive cells in the cerebral cortex. *J. Physiol.* (Lond.) 166:296-327

Krnjević, K., Pumain, R. and Renaud, L. (1971): The mechanism of excitation by acetylcholine in the cerebral cortex. *J. Physiol.* (Lond.) 215:247-268

Krnjević, K. and Ropert, N. (1982): Electrophysiological and pharmacological characteristics of facilitation of hippocampal population spikes by stimulation of the medial septum. *Neurosci.* 7:2165-2183

Lundberg, J.M., Hedlund, B. and Bartfai, T. (1982): Vasoactive intestinal polypeptide enhances muscarinic ligand binding in cat submandibular salivary gland. *Nature* (Lond.) 295:147-149

Madison, D.V. and Nicoll, R.A. (1986): Actions of noradrenaline recorded intracellularly in rat hippocampal CA1 pyramidal neurones, ***in vitro***. *J. Physiol.* (Lond.) 372:221-244

Magistretti, P.J. and Schorderet, M. (1984): VIP and noradrenaline act synergistically to increase cyclic AMP in cerebral cortex. *Nature (Lond.)* 308:280-282

Malenka, R.C., Madison, D.V., Andrade, R. and Nicoll, R.A. (1986): Phorbol esters minic some cholinergic actions in hippocampal pryamidal neurons. *J. Neurosci.* 6:475-480

McCormick, D.A. and Prince, D.A. (1985): Two types of muscarinic response to acetylcholine in mammalian cortical neurons. *Proc. Natl. Acad. Sci. USA* 82:6344-6348

McCormick, D.A. and Prince, D.A. (1986): Mechanisms of action of acetylcholine in the guinea-pig cerebral cortex ***in vitro***. *J. Physiol.* (Lond.) 375:169-194

Mesulam, M.-M., Mufson, E.J., Levey, A.I. and Wainer, B.H. (1983): Cholinergic innervation of cortex by the basal forebrain: cytochemistry and cortical connections of the septal area, diagonal band nuclei, nucleus basalis (substantia innominata), and hypothalamus in the rhesus monkey. *J. Comp. Neurol.* 214:170-197

Metherate, R., Tremblay, N. and Dykes, R.W. (1988): The effects of acetylcholine on response properties of cat somatosensory cortical neurons. *J. Neurophysiol.* 59:1231-1252

Meyer, E.M. and Otero, D.H. (1985): Pharmacological and ionic characterizations of the muscarinic receptors modulating [^{3}H] acetylcholine release from rat cortical synaptosomes. *J. Neurosci.* 5:1202-1207

Movshon, J.A. and Van Sluyters, R.C. (1981): Visual neural development. *Ann. Rev. Psychol.* 32:477-522

Nakai, K. (1987): Regenerative catecholamine-containing terminals in kitten visual cortex: an ultrastructural study. *Neurosci. Res.* 4:475-485

Nakai, K., Jonsson, G. and Kasamatsu, T. (1987): Norepinephrinergic reinnervation of cat occipital cortex following localized lesions with 6-hydroxydopamine. *Neurosci. Res.*4:433-453

Nelson, S.B., Schwartz, M.A. and Daniels, J.D. (1985): Clonidine and cortical plasticity: possible evidence for noradrenergic involvement. *Dev. Brain Res.* 23:39-50

Nicoll, R.A. (1988): The coupling of neurotransmitter receptors to ion channels in the brain. *Science* 214:545-551

Nishizuka, Y. (1986): Studies and perspectives of protein kinase C. *Science* 233:305-312

Nishizuka, Y. (1988): The molecular heterogeneity of protein kinase C and its possibilities for cellular regulation. *Nature* (Lond.) 334:661-665

Ohashi, T. and Kasamatsu, T. (1989): Concentration-dependent suppression by lithium of effects on monocular deprivation in kittens. *Soc Neurosci. Abstr.* 15:795

Ohashi, T., Imamura, K. and Kasamatsu, T. (1988): Lithium reduces effects of monocular deprivation. *Soc. Neurosci. Abstr.* 14:189

Olson, C.R. and Freeman, R.D. (1980): Profile of the sensitive period for monocular deprivation in kittens. *Exp. Brain Res.* 39:17-21

Paradiso, M.S., Bear, M.F. and Daniels, J.D. (1983): Effects of intracortical infusion of 6-hydroxydopamine on the response of kitten visual cortex to monocular deprivation. *Exp. Brain Res.* 51:413-422

Peralta, E.G., Ashkenazi, A., Winslow, J.W., Ramachandran, J. and Capon, D.J. (1988): Differential regulation of PI hydrolysis and adenylyl cyclase by muscarinic receptor subtypes. *Nature* (Lond.) 334:434-437

Pettigrew, J.D. and Kasamatsu, T. (1978): Local perfusion of noradrenaline maintains visual cortical plasticity. *Nature* (Lond.) 271:761-763

Potempska, A., Skangiel-Kramska, J. and Kossut, M. (1979): Development of cholinergic enzymes and adenosine-triphosphate activity of optic system of cats in normal and restricted visual input conditions. *Dev. Neurosci.* 2:38-45

Rauschecker, J.P. (1987): What signals are responsible for synaptic changes in visual cortical plasticity. In: *Imprinting and Cortical Plasticity, Comparative Aspects of Sensitive Periods*. Rauschecker, J.P., Maler, P., eds. New York: John Wiley & Sons, pp 193-220

Reader, T.A., De Champlain, J. and Jasper, H.H. (1976): Catecholamines released from cerebral cortex in the cat: decrease during sensory stimulation. *Brain Res.* 111:95-108

Rinaldi, F. and Himwich, H. (1955): Alerting responses and actions of atropine and cholinergic drugs. *Arch. Neurol. Psychiatr.* 73:387-395

Robertson, R.T., Ambe, R.K. and Yu, J. (1989): Intraocular injections of tetrodotoxin reduce transiently expressed acetylcholinesterase activity in developing rat visual cortex. *Dev. Brain Res.* 46:69-84

Rosenberger, L.B., Yamamura, H.I. and Roeske, W.R. (1980): The regulation of cardiac muscarinic cholinergic receptors by isoproterenol. *Eur. J. Pharmacol.* 65:129-130

Saito, N., Kikkawa, U., Nishizuka, Y. and Tanaka, C. (1988): Distribution of protein kinase C-like immunoreactive neurons in rat brain. *J. Neurosci.* 8:369-382

Sasaki, K. and Sato, M. (1987): A single GTP-binding protein regulates K^+-channels coupled with dopamine, histamine, and acetylcholine receptors. *Nature* (Lond.) 325:259-262

Sato, H., Hata, Y., Hagihara, K. and Tsumoto, T. (1987a): Effects of cholinergic depletion on neuron activities in the cat visual cortex. *J. Neurophysiol.* 58:781-794

Sato, H., Hata, Y., Masui, H. and Tsumoto, T. (1987b): A functional role of cholinergic innervation to neurons in the cat visual cortex. *J. Neurophysiol.* 58:765-780

Shaw, C., Wilkinson, W., Cynader, M., Needler, M.C., Aoki, C. and Hall, S.E. (1986): The laminar distributions and postnatal development of neurotransmitter and neuromodulator receptors in cat visual cortex. *Brain Res. Bull.* 16:661-671

Shaw, C., Needler, M.C. and Cynader, M. (1984): Ontogenesis of muscarinic acetylcholine binding sites in cat visual cortex: reversal of specific laminar distribution during the critical period. *Dev. Brain Res.* 14:295-299

Sherman, S.M. and Spear, P.D. (1982): Organization of visual pathways in normal and visually deprived cats. *Psychol. Rev.* 62:738-855

Sheu, F.-S., Kasamatsu, T. and Routtenberg, A. (1990): Protein kinase C activity and substrate (FI/GAP-43) phosphorylation in developing cat visual cortex. *Brain Res.* 524:144-148

Shirokawa, T. and Kasamatsu, T. (1986): Concentration-dependent suppression by β-adrenergic antagonists of the shift in ocular dominance following monocular deprivation in kitten visual cortex. *Neurosci.* 18:1035-1046

Shirokawa, T. and Kasamatsu, T. (1987): Reemergence of ocular dominance plasticity during recovery from the effects of propranolol infused in kitten visual cortex. *Exp. Brain Res.* 68:466-476

Shute, C.C.D. and Lewis, P.R. (1967): The ascending cholinergic reticular system: neocortical, olfactory and subcortical projections. *Brain* 90:497-520

Sibley, D.R. and Lefkowitz, R.J. (1985): Molecular mechanisms of receptor desensitization using the B-adrenergic receptor-coupled adenylate cyclase system as a model. *Nature* (Lond.) 317:124-129

Sillito, A.M. and Kemp, J.A. (1983): Cholinergic modulation of the functional organization of the cat visual cortex. *Brain Res.* 289:143-155

Sims, S.M., Singer, J.J. and Walsh, Jr. J.V. (1988): Antagonistic adrenergic- muscarinic regulation of M current in smooth muscle cells. *Science* 239:190-193

Singer, W. (1979): Central-core control of visual-cortex functions. In: *The Neuroscience, Fourth Study Program.* Schmitt, F.O., Worden, F.G., eds. Cambridge, MA: MIT Press, pp 1093-1109

Singer, W. (1982): Central core control of developmental plasticity in the kitten visual cortex: I. Diencephalic lesions. *Exp. Brain Res.* 47:209-222

Singer, W. (1984): Learning to see: mechanisms in experience-dependent development. In: *The Biology of Learning.* Marler, P.R., Terrace, H.S., eds. Dahlem Konferenzen, Berlin, New York: Springer-Verlag, pp 461-477

Singer, W., von Gruenau, M. and Rauschecker, J. (1979a): Requirements for the disruption of binocularity in the visual cortex of strabismic kittens. *Brain Res.* 171:536-540

Singer, W. and Rauschecker, J.P. (1982): Central core control of developmental plasticity in the kitten visual cortex: II. Electrical activation of mesencephalic and diencephalic projections. *Exp. Brain Res.* 47:223-233

Singer, W., Tretter, F. and Cynader, M. (1976): The effect of reticular stimulation in spontaneous and evoked activity in the cat visual cortex. *Brain Res.* 102:71-90

Singer, W., Yinon, U. and Tretter, F. (1979b): Inverted monocular vision prevents ocular dominance shift in kittens and impairs the functional state of visual cortex in adult cats. *Brain Res.* 164:294-299

Spehlmann, R. (1963): Acetylcholine and prostigmine electrophoresis at visual cortex neurons. *J. Neurophysiol.* 26:127-139

Stichel, C.C. and Singer, W. (1987a): Quantitative analysis of the choline acetyltransferase-immunoreactive axonal network in the cat primary visual cortex: I. Adult cats. *J. Comp. Neurol.* 258:91-98

Stichel, C.C. and Singer, W. (1987b): Quantitative analysis of the choline acetyltransferase-immunoreactive axonal network in the cat primary visual cortex: II. Pre- and postnatal development. *J. Comp. Neurol.* 258:99-111

Stricker, E.M. and Zigmond, M.J. (1986): Brain monoamines, homeostasis and adaptive behavior. In: *Handbook of Physiology – The Nervous System IV.* Mountcastle, V.B., Bloom, F.E., Geiger, S.R., eds. Bethesda: Am. Physiol. Soc., pp 677-700

Stryker, M.P. (1989): Evidence for a possible role of spontaneous electrical activity in the development of the mammalian visual cortex. In: *Problems and Concepts in Developmental Neurophysiology.* Kellaway, P., Noebels, J.L., eds. Baltimore: The Johns Hopkins Univ. Press, pp 110-130

Sugden, D., Vanecek, J., Klein, D.C., Thomas, T.P. and Anderson, W.B. (1985): Activation of protein kinase C potentiates isoprenaline-induced cyclic AMP accumulation in rat pinealocytes. *Nature* (Lond.) 314:359- 361

Szerb, J.C. (1967): Cortical acetylcholine release and electroencephalic arousal. *J. Physiol.* (Lond.) 192:329-343

Takai, Y., Kikkawa, U., Kaibuchi, K. and Nishizuka, Y. (1984): Membrane phospholipid metabolism and signal transduction for protein phosphorylation. *Adv. Cyclic Neucleotide Res.* 18:119-154

Trombley, P., Allen, E.E., Soyke, J., Blaha, C.D., Lane, R.F. and Gordon, B. (1986): Doses of 6-hydroxydopamine sufficient to deplete norepinephrine are not sufficient to decrease plasticity in the visual cortex. *J. Neurosci.* 6:266-273

Videen, T.O., Daw, N.W. and Rader, R.K. (1984): The effect of norepinephrine on visual cortical neurons in kitten and adult cats. *J. Neurosci.* 4:1607-1617

Wahle, P. and Meyer, G. (1989): Early postnatal development of vasoactive intestine polypeptide- and peptide histidine isoleucine-immunoreactive structures in the cat visual cortex. *J. Comp. Neurol.* 282:215-248

Watanabe, A.M., McConnaughey, M.M., Strawbridge, R.A., Fleming, J.W., Jones, L.R. and Besch, Jr. H.R. (1978): Muscarinic cholinergic receptor modulation of B-adrenergic receptor affinity for catecholamines. *J. Biol. Chem.* 253:4833-4836

Westfall, T.C. (1974): Effect of nicotine and other drugs on the release of ^{3}H-norepinephrine and ^{3}H-dopamine from rat brain slices. *Neuropharmacol.* 13: 693-700

Wiesel, T.N. (1982): Postnatal development of the visual cortex and the influence of environment. *Nature* (Lond.) 299:583-591

Wiesel, T.N. and Hubel, D.H. (1963): Single-cell responses in striate cortex of kittens deprived of vision in one eye. *J. Neurophysiol.* 26:1003-1017

Woody, C.D., Swartz, B.E. and Gruen, E. (1978): Effects of acetylcholine and cyclic GMP on input resistance of cortical neurons in awake cats. *Brain Res.* 158:373-395

Worley, P.F., Baraban, J.M. and Snyder, S.H. (1986): Heterogeneous localization of protein kinase C in rat brain: autoradiographic analysis of phorbol ester receptor binding. *J. Neurosci.* 6:199-207

Yamamoto, C. and Kawai, N. (1967): Presynaptic action of acetylcholine in thin sections from the guinea pig dentate gyrus in vitro. *Exp. Neurol.* 19:176-187

Zahs, K.R. (1989): Influences of neural activity on the development and plasticity of the cat's visual cortex. In: *The Assembly of the Nervous System.* Liss, A.R., ed. New York, pp 259-278

Cholinergic Modulation of Synaptic Plasticity in Sensory Neocortex

Robert W. Dykes, Nicole Tremblay, Richard A. Warren and Mark F. Bear

INTRODUCTION

Activity-dependent synaptic plasticity occurs in neocortex devoted to each sensory system at all postnatal ages. The process is crucial for the refinement of topographic cortical representations and the development of stimulus selectivity in the neonate, and although the plasticity is more subtle in the adult cortex, it probably forms the basis of dynamic changes in sensory representations and may account for some forms of memory. A question of central importance is whether the fundamental mechanisms of neuronal plasticity are the same at different ages and in different cortical areas.

Modification of cortical circuits by sensory experience must, at some level, involve biochemical mechanisms that are driven by thalamocortical and intracortical synaptic transmission. It is just as clear, however, that synaptic plasticity in the neocortex depends on more than simply the patterns and amount of activity arising at the periphery. Evidence from both adult and developing cortex suggests that an additional requirement for synaptic plasticity is that the animal attend to the sensory stimuli and use them to guide behavior. This requirement has led to the idea that synaptic modification in the neocortex is facilitated or "enabled" by signals arising from central modulatory systems whose activity is linked to a behavioral state (Singer, 1979). Converging lines of evidence suggest that one of these enabling factors is acetylcholine (ACh) released in the neocortex by fibers arising from the basal forebrain. It should be emphasized that, according to this hypothesis, acetylcholine does not cause neuronal plasticity; rather, the release of ACh (and/or other enabling factors such as norepinephrine) is a necessary condition for the cortical modification which will occur if certain other conditions are fulfilled.

In this chapter we review our evidence favoring such a modulatory role for ACh in the experience-dependent synaptic plasticity that has been demonstrated in the adult and juvenile cat cerebral cortex. We begin by briefly summarizing the anatomical organization of the cat cortical cholinergic pathways, and what is known of their synaptic physiology. Next, we review the evidence that the cholinergic projection participates in the control of long-term synaptic plasticity. The specific forms of plasticity considered are ocular dominance modifications in the kitten visual cortex and adjustments of the body representation in the adult somatic sensory cortex. Finally, we suggest a possible common mechanism for ACh modulation of synaptic plasticity in the neocortex at all postnatal ages.

THE ANATOMY OF CHOLINERGIC INPUTS TO SENSORY NEOCORTEX IN THE CAT

In 1967, Shute and Lewis mapped the central cholinergic pathways in the rat by using a histochemical stain for acetylcholinesterase (AChE). The AChE-containing pathways of the forebrain seemed to be derived largely from cells in the reticular formation of the brain-stem and included cell groups in the intralaminar thalamus and basal telencephalon. They called this the "ascending cholinergic reticular activating system" because electrical stimulation of these regions had been shown to desynchronize the cortical EEG (Morrison and Dempsey, 1942; Moruzzi and Magoun, 1949). This idea fits well with the observation that reticular stimulation causes a large increase in ACh release from the cerebral cortex (Szerb, 1967).

With the subsequent elucidation of the monoaminergic pathways of the rat forebrain (Lindvall and Björklund, 1974) came the realization that AChE was often associated with catecholaminergic neurons, and therefore was not a specific marker for cholinergic cells or fibers (Butcher, 1977); strategies other than AChE histochemistry were required to identify the sources of neocortical ACh. However, while not all AChE-positive cells are cholinergic, all cholinergic cells are AChE-positive (Fibiger, 1982). In the rat, Johnston et al. (1981) used this line of reasoning to identify the source of the cholinergic projections to the neocortex. These investigators made excitotoxic lesions of the AChE -positive cell groups that are known to project to the cortex and measured subsequent changes in cortical choline acetyltransferase (ChAT) activity and ACh levels. They reported a 70% drop in ChAT activity after lesions of the basal forebrain (BF). In contrast, lesions in the thalamus or brainstem produced no significant drop in the levels of this cholinergic marker. These results indicate that the extrinsic cholinergic innervation of rat neocortex arises from cells in the basal telencephalon. Importantly, lesions which depleted ChAT also decreased AChE staining in the cortex. That AChE staining in the cortex was only affected by lesions of known cholinergic cells and that the changes in AChE closely paralleled changes in ChAT are strong evidence that AChE in the mature neocortex is a useful cholinergic marker. These findings largely vindicate Shute and Lewis (1967), and generally support the concept of an ascending cholinergic activating system.

In the cat, the anatomical organization of the cortical cholinergic projection has been characterized using AChE histochemistry (Bear et al., 1985a, b) and, more recently, ChAT immunocytochemistry (deLima and Singer, 1986; Stichel and Singer, 1987). Both methods have yielded similar conclusions. This work has shown that all layers of cat neocortex are richly innervated by cholinergic fibers, with the highest density occurring in layer I. The elegant electron microscopic immunocytochemical studies of Houser et al. (1985) in the rat and deLima and Singer (1986) in the cat demonstrate that these fibers form synapses in all layers, with the preferred target being the dendritic shafts of both stellate and pyramidal neurons.

Cortical undercutting eliminates all AChE-stained axons in cat postlateral gyrus, suggesting that the cholinergic innervation of visual cortex arises entirely from an extrinsic source (Bear et al., 1985a). This conclusion is supported by the failure of immunocytochemical studies to detect ChAT-positive neurons in cat neocortex [in contrast to rat; Stichel and Singer (1987)]. Retrograde transport experiments reveal that the large cholinergic neurons of the basal telencephalon project to both visual and somatic sensory cortex (Bear et al., 1985a,b; Bear and Singer, 1986; Barstad and Bear, 1990). It remains possible that direct brainstem projections to cortex may have a cholinergic component; however, unilateral lesions of the midbrain lead to no detectable depletion of AChE-positive axons in visual cortex (Bear et al., 1985 a,b). This contrasts with the severe depletion of acetylcholinesterase-containing axons in both visual and somatic sensory cortex after excitotoxic lesions of the BF (Fig. 1).

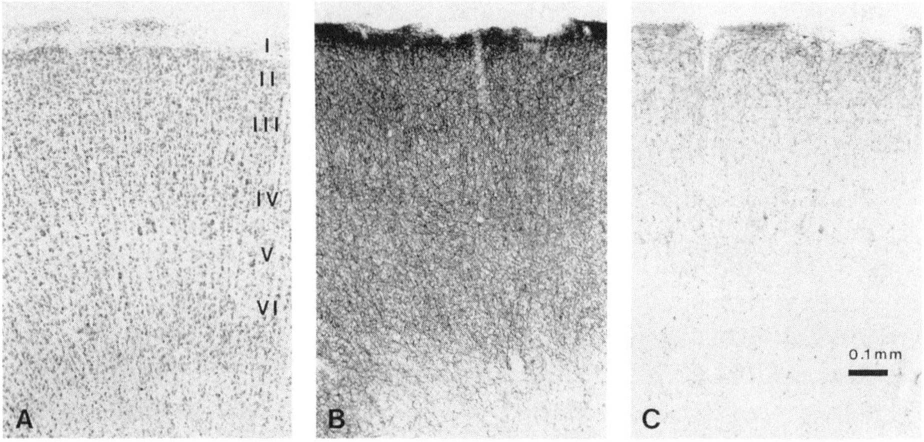

Figure 1. A: Nissl cytoarchitecture of somatic sensory cortex in a normal cat. **B:** Section adjacent to that shown in A stained for acetylcholinesterase to reveal the normal pattern and density of AChE-positive axons. **C:** Section, stained for AChE, through somatic sensory cortex of a cat that received a unilateral lesion of the basal telencephalon 7 days earlier. Note the striking depletion of AChE+ staining. Reproduced with permission from Barstad and Bear (1990).

In order to produce the cholinergic depletion illustrated in Fig. 1, it is necessary to destroy neurons in a considerable volume of the BF. The reason for this is illustrated in Fig. 2, where the distribution of retrogradely-labelled neurons in the basal telencephalon is shown after a discrete injection of horseradish peroxidase in the kitten visual cortex (Bear and Singer, unpublished data). HRP-positive neurons were found scattered within the internal capsule, substantia innominata, and both limbs of the diagonal band of Broca. Hence, cholinergic projections to visual cortex arise from neurons that are scattered widely in the BF. Neurons with projections to somatosensory cortex can also be demonstrated in the diagonal band and internal capsule; however, the major source of cholinergic input to this cortical area appears to be the region immediately ventrolateral to the globus pallidus (Barstad and Bear, 1990). Thus, it appears that a crude topography exists in the neocortical projections of the BF in the cat. This organization is schematically illustrated in Fig. 3.

The wide distribution of cortically projecting BF neurons raises the question of whether different groups of the cholinergic neurons in the BF have different patterns of afferent connectivity. It remains an intrigu-

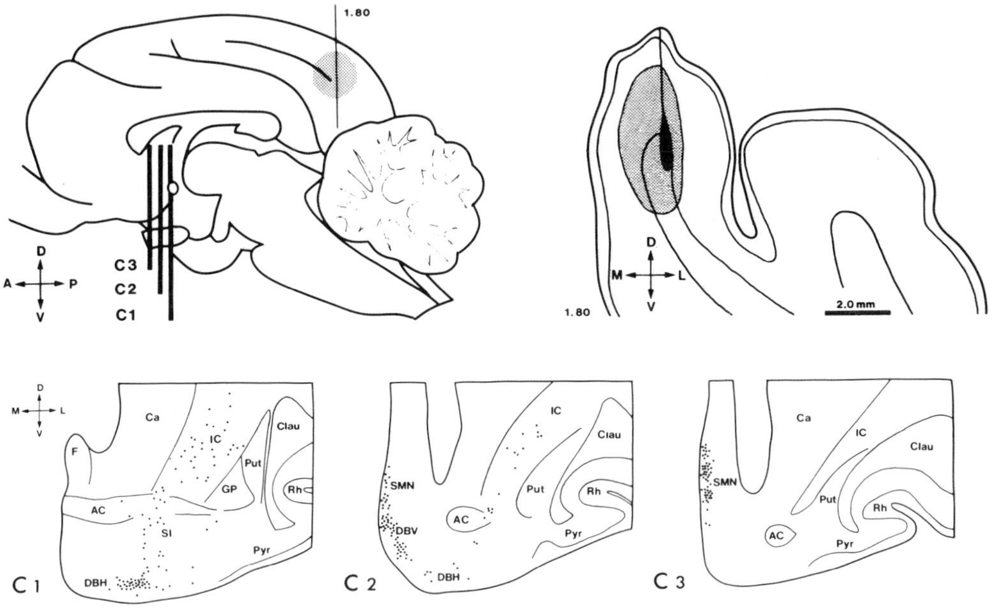

Figure 2. At the top left is a schematic midsagittal view of a cat brain to illustrate the location of an HRP injection (lightly shaded) into visual cortex. A drawing of a coronal section through this injection is shown at the top right. C1, 2 and 3 are plots of the location of HRP labelled neurons in the basal telencephalon at the coronal planes indicated at the top left. Reproduced with permission from Barstad and Bear.

ing possibility that the cortically-projecting cholinergic BF cells actually consist of a series of subsystems that become active under different behavioral conditions. In any case, the scattered distribution of neurons with projections to somatosensory cortex presents a technical challenge for producing complete lesions of the cortical cholinergic inputs. Even large lesions, which include a significant fraction of the substantia innominata, globus pallidus, putamen and adjacent structures, rarely deplete the cortex of all AChE-positive axons. Nonetheless, it is likely that the degree of depletion attained after these lesions is sufficient to help elucidate cholinergic contributions to cortical function. For example, excitotoxic lesions of the cat basal telencephalon have been found to reduce the metabolic activity evoked in somatosensory cortex by repetitive tactile stimulation (Juliano et al., 1988), an effect that is also mimicked by topical application of atropine. And as we discuss below, BF lesions can also disrupt experience-dependent synaptic modification in the sensory neocortex.

THE ELECTROPHYSIOLOGY OF ACETYLCHOLINE IN SENSORY CORTEX

The classic effects of ACh in cerebral cortex were described many years ago by Krnjević and Phillis (1963a,b) and others (Stone, 1972). Krnjević (1988) has recently reviewed this literature. In these early studies the direct effects of ACh iontophoresis in cortex were apparent only in about 15% of the cells. In the "cholinoceptive" neurons, ACh caused a slow depolarization, thought to be due to a reduction in potassium permeability.

Twenty years later Sillito and Kemp (1983) showed in visual cortex that when ACh was administered iontophoretically while neurons were stimulated with optimally oriented visual stimuli, 92% of the cells dis-

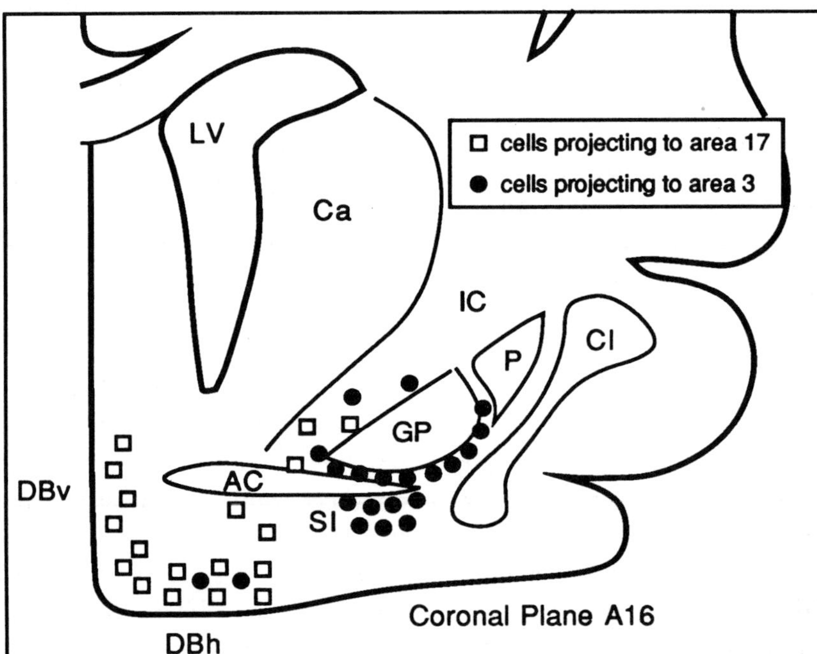

Figure 3. Cartoon of a coronal section through the cat basal forebrain, approximately 16 mm anterior to the interaural line. Schematically illustrated is the location of BF neurons with projections to visual or somatic sensory cortices.

played altered responsiveness to the stimuli in the presence of ACh: 61% showed an enhancement of the response magnitude without reducing receptive field selectivity to visual stimuli and without an increase in the level of spontaneous activity, while 31% showed a decrease in their firing rates and of their evoked responses. Cells depressed by ACh were found in laminae III and IV while those facilitated were found in all cortical laminae. In this study it was not clear whether nicotinic or muscarinic receptors were involved.

Sato et al. (1987a) reported a facilitatory effect in 74% of the 137 cells tested in cat visual cortex and a suppression in 16%. These effects could be blocked by atropine (muscarinic antagonist) but not hexamethonium (nicotinic antagonist) in 93% of the 56 cells tested, indicating that the ACh effects were mediated through muscarinic receptors. Sato et al. (1987a) suggested the existence of endogenously released ACh, presumably by terminals of cholinergic fibers of the BF, since iontophoretic administration of atropine in absence of ACh suppressed visual responses of 60% of the cells facilitated by ACh.

They (Sato et al., 1987b) tested this hypothesis by depleting the cat visual cortex of its extrinsic cholinergic inputs with unilateral chemical lesions in the BF. In the depleted cortex, the proportion of cells facilitated by administration of ACh was significantly larger than it was in the contralateral cortex. This was attributed to a supersensitivity of presumable muscarinic receptors and/or a reduction in rate of catabolism of ACh. Twenty percent of the cells had either no detectable or very weak visual responses in the depleted cortex, an unexpectedly high value in comparison to the normal visual cortex. During the administration of ACh, the responsiveness of many of these cells was greatly improved and they became clearly responsive. Atropine administration no longer affected responsiveness suggesting that the origin of the tonically released ACh in normal cortex had been from the BF.

In the primary somatosensory cortex of the rat, Donoghue and Carroll (1987) observed an increase in discharges elicited by whisker stimulation during ACh administration and the appearance of responses in previously unresponsive cells. Although the enhancement of sensory-evoked discharges was observed in all cortical layers, inhibitory responses to ACh were seen mostly in the granular layer IV, a location similar to that found for inhibitory effects of ACh in visual cortex (Sillito and Kemp, 1983). In the somatosensory cortex of the cat, Metherate el al. (1988a) found that changes in response to somatic stimuli during ACh administration tended to be facilitatory. Sixteen percent of the 203 cells tested were overtly excited by ACh administration while 5% were inhibited; the responsiveness to somatic stimuli of 29% were modulated and 7% were both modulated and driven. Responses to somatic stimuli during ACh administration were often increased by as much as 200%. These data demonstrate an important role for ACh in sensory cortex and suggest that it must have a marked ameliorative effect on function when it is released by BF activity during periods of arousal and motivated behavior (Richardson and Delong, 1986). That BF activity might lead to long term changes in neuronal excitability is less obvious, however, there are several lines of evidence that suggest it must do so.

ACETYLCHOLINE AND LONG-TERM NEOCORTICAL PLASTICITY

Modulation of Ocular Dominance Plasticity in the Kitten Striate Cortex

Perhaps the best model of experience-dependent synaptic plasticity in the neocortex is the kitten striate cortex (area 17). The classic example of experience-dependent modification of functional circuitry in the striate cortex is the change induced by the temporary closure of one eye (monocular deprivation, MD). Normally, most neurons in area 17 are binocularly activated, and this binocularity can be measured with the physiological assay of ocular dominance (OD) introduced by Hubel and Wiesel (1962). After brief periods of MD, the OD of cortical neurons is shifted dramatically to the eye that remained open — that is, most neurons lose their ability to respond to stimuli presented through the deprived eye and are activated solely by stimulation through the open eye (Wiesel and Hubel,1963).

This ocular dominance shift appears to require more than simply an imbalance of afferent activity from the two eyes. Stimulus conditions that are sufficient to activate the sensory (lateral geniculate) afferents but do not activate cortical neurons (diffuse light, for example) will not shift OD (Singer et al., 1977). This has led to the idea that postsynaptic activation of cortical neurons is a necessary condition for synaptic modification. However, there is evidence that OD plasticity will not always occur even under conditions in which striate cortical neurons are activated robustly by visual stimulation. For example, no OD shift occurs with MD in anesthetized or paralyzed kittens (Freeman and Bonds, 1979; Singer and Rauschecker, 1982). This has led to the concept of an extra-retinal gating signal that depends on the state of the animal and is required for synaptic modifications to occur. Over the past decade, several attempts have been made to determine the neural substrate of this hypothetical gate. Among the candidates examined so far are the projections to striate cortex that arise from the noradrenergic locus coeruleus (Kasamatsu and Pettigrew, 1979), the thalamic intralaminar nuclei (Singer, 1982; Bear et al., 1988) and the cholinergic basal forebrain (Bear and Singer, 1986).

The pioneering work of Kasamatsu and Pettigrew (1976, 1979) first directly tested the idea that the extrathalamic inputs to the neocortex were important for the modification of circuitry by use. They initially focused their attention on the noradrenergic input that arises from the locus coeruleus in the pons. Their strategy was to destroy this projection and then test for a deficit in the OD shift that normally results from brief periods of monocular deprivation. They reported that cortical depletion of norepinephrine (NE) prevented OD plasticity (Kasamatsu and Pettigrew, 1976, 1979). Based on these results, they formulated the "catecholamine hypothesis of visual cortical plasticity, " which states that the noradrenergic projection is essential for synapse modification to occur in the striate cortex.

The methods that Kasamatsu and Pettigrew used to deplete NE involved either repeated intraventricular or continuous intracortical administration of the neurotoxin 6-hydroxydopamine (6-OHDA). While these methods have the advantage of restricting the NE depletion to cortex, they both involve the continuous exposure of cortex to 6-OHDA during the period of monocular experience. Bear and Daniels (1983) used another method of catecholamine depletion that had proved effective in rodents, the systemic administration of 6-OHDA to neonates. High pressure liquid chromatography confirmed that the two injections of 6-OHDA given shortly after birth would indeed cause a drastic and long lasting depletion of NE in kitten striate cortex; however, subsequent neurophysiological recording revealed that this method of NE depletion had no detectable effect on the cortical response to MD. Paradiso et al. (1983), in the same laboratory, were able to repeat Kasamatsu and Pettigrew's original experiment (1976) by directly infusing the 6-OHDA from an osmotic minipump into visual cortex as the animal was monocularly deprived. Under these conditions, a 50-80% depletion of NE was accompanied by a loss of ocular dominance plasticity (Bear et al., 1983; Paradiso et al., 1983).

There are at least two possible explanations for these conflicting results (cf. Gordon et al., 1988). On the one hand, it is possible that mechanisms exist to compensate for the early destruction of the NE system. On the other hand, 6-OHDA might directly disrupt plasticity in a way that is independent of the NE depletion. Evidence in favor of the latter explanation has come from the work of Daw et al. (1984) and Adrien et al. (1985). Both groups report that methods ranging from locus coeruleus lesions (Adrien et al., 1985) to interruption of the dorsal noradrenergic bundle (DNAB) (Daw et al., 1984) leave visual cortical plasticity intact despite a significant depletion of cortical NE (60-90%). However, this explanation fails to account for the finding that infusion of exogenous NE into the visual cortex apparently will restore susceptibility to lid closure in adult cats (Kasamatsu et al., 1979). Nonetheless, it seems likely that other factors besides NE contribute importantly to critical period plasticity.

The cholinergic projection seemed like another good candidate for the hypothetical gating mechanism for three main reasons. First, there is biochemical evidence that the striate cortex is heavily innervated by cholinergic fibers during the critical period (Potempska et al., 1979; Shaw et al., 1984). Second, the facilitatory action of ACh on excitatory transmission in striate cortex (Sillito and Kemp, 1983) increases the probability of postsynaptic activation, a condition thought to be required for OD plasticity. Third, the cholinergic projection is thought to be an important component of the ascending reticular activating system, and reticular activation of striate cortex appears to be necessary for OD plasticity (reviewed by Singer, 1982).

The first step in this inquiry was the characterization of the anatomical organization and development of the cholinergic projection to striate cortex (Bear et al., 1985a,b). This work confirmed that striate cortex is heavily innervated by cholinergic fibers during the critical period, and that these fibers arise largely from cells in the BF. The next step, was to destroy these cholinergic neurons with the excitotoxin N-methyl aspartate, and then to test for a deficit in the ocular dominance shift that normally results from MD. Bear and Singer (1986) found that a substantial depletion of cortical ACh had no effect on OD plasticity. However, when the NE and ACh projections were both destroyed in the same animal, the normal OD shift was reliably prevented. In these experiments, the NE projection was destroyed with injections of 6-OHDA into the DNAB which normally have no effect on OD plasticity (Daw et al., 1984). Thus, while BF and DNAB lesions are ineffective alone, the combined destruction of these structures results in a significant loss of OD plasticity in striate cortex (Fig. 4).

A second way to deplete both ACh and NE in the striate cortex is to transect the cingulum bundle at the level of the genu of the corpus callosum. Bear and Singer (1986) found that this procedure also prevented the normal OD shift after MD. This effect was recently replicated by Gordon et al. (1989).

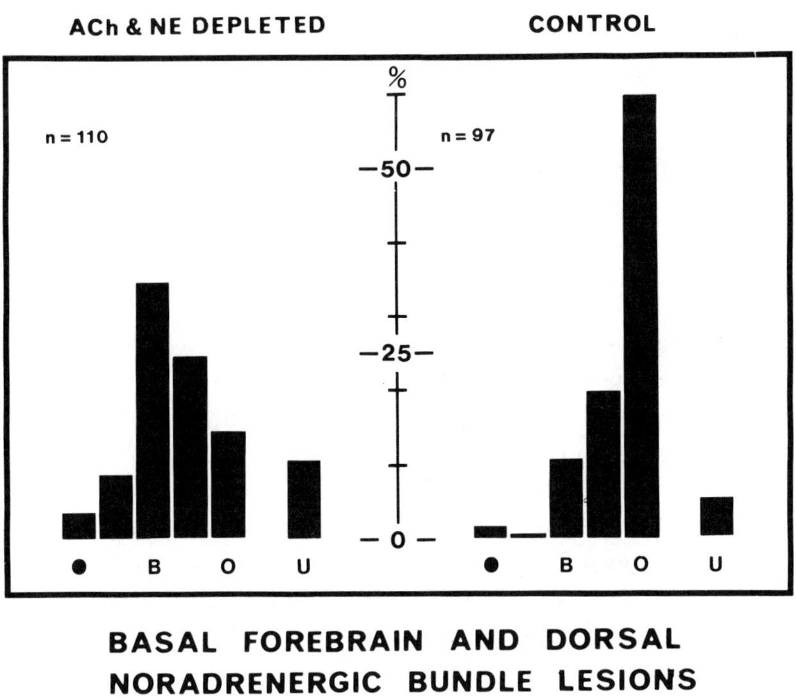

Figure 4. Pooled ocular dominance histograms from hemispheres ipsilateral (left; ACh and NE depleted) and contralateral (right; control) to a combined basal forebrain and dorsal noradrenergic bundle lesion. The animals had been monocularly deprived for 10 days prior to recording. Neurons in the ocular dominace (OD) category marked with a B were equally responsive to stimulation of the two eyes; those in the OD category marked with an open circle were responsive only to the non-deprived eye; and those in the category marked with a filled circle were responsive exclusively to the deprived eye.

Bear and Singer (1986) also described iontophoretic experiments in the visual cortex which indicated that directly applied 6-OHDA can interfere with cholinergic transmission. Thus, three different methods that prevent OD plasticity—combined lesions of the BF and DNAB, transection of the cingulum bundle, and intracortical infusion of 6-OHDA—all apparently disrupt both cholinergic and noradrenergic neurotransmission in the striate cortex. These data suggest that NE and ACh can substitute for one another in the modulation of cortical plasticity, and raise the possibility that they facilitate synaptic modifications via a common molecular mechanism. This interpretation, if correct, resolves the controversy surrounding the "catecholamine hypothesis" of Kasamatsu and Pettigrew (cf. Trombley et al., 1986).

In summary, although the cholinergic innervation of striate cortex does not appear to be essential for visual cortical plasticity in young animals, (the loss of cortical ACh evidently can be compensated for by the noradrenergic system), the evidence clearly indicates that ACh released by fibers from the BF promotes the synaptic modifications which underlie the OD shift in kittens.

Modulation of "Map Plasticity" in Adult Sensory Cortex

The modification of binocular connections in the visual cortex following brief MD only occurs in the first few months after birth. However, in the other sensory systems neuronal plasticity has been demonstrated to occur in adults. Kalaska and Pomeranz (1979) were the first to suggest that somatosensory cortical neurons acquire new receptive fields following transection of the nerves to the cat forepaw. In owl monkeys, Merzenich et al. (1983a, b) showed that soon after median nerve transection neurons, located in the region of the somatosensory cortex originally serving the skin surfaces innervated by the median nerve, could be driven by inputs from adjacent skin surfaces. Although these changes began within hours after a median nerve transection, changes continued during the following weeks until new inputs gradually began to excite the cells in patterns that formed a new somatotopically ordered map. More recently, experiments in which portions of the cochlear membrane are destroyed in the adult have shown that a similar kind of reorganization and rebuilding of a cochleotopic map will occur in primary auditory cortex (Robertson and Irvine, 1989).

Thus, rather dramatic reorganizational processes can occur in adult sensory regions following radical alterations of the sensory receptor sheet. Post-hoc reasoning suggests that these processes may be a reflection of the extremes of a dynamic process which is constantly active in cortex and which serves to maintain an up-to-date correspondence between the sensory representation and the sensory receptors which that representation serves (Clark et al., 1988). Further, one can imagine that changes in these cortical sensory representations might be modified by use or by activity in a process related to certain kinds of learning and memory (cf. Olton et al., this volume).

The hypothesis being explored here is whether or not this cortical map plasticity could be dependent upon extrathalamic inputs in general, and the cholinergic input in particular. Support for such a role for ACh in somatosensory cortex comes from the work of Metherate el al. (1988b) who showed that pairing neuronal excitation by glutamate with ACh administration led to long-lasting changes in the responsiveness of those neurons to glutamate. If the ACh was administered while atropine was present to block its effect on muscarinic receptors, the long-lasting change in neuronal excitability did not occur. Metherate et al. (1988b) demonstrated that this phenomenon could play a role in reorganization of somatosensory cortex by showing that stimulation of the cutaneous receptive field of a somatosensory cortical neuron in the presence of iontophoretically administered ACh could lead to enhanced responses from the cutaneous receptive field for periods of time measured in 10s of minutes or as long as the cell was studied (up to 1.5 hrs.) In addition, when somatosensory cortical neurons lacking overt receptive fields were treated with ACh while the skin was stimulated, overt receptive fields appeared in many of the cases and these uncovered afferent inputs often lasted for as long as the cells were studied (Dykes et al., 1988; Metherate el al., 1988b).

These observations are consistent with the hypothesis that somatosensory cortical neurons depolarized in the presence of ACh undergo a long-term enhancement of neuronal excitability by a mechanism similar to that described by Woody et al. (1978) and Woody and Gruen (1988) in the motor cortex of the cat. Such a mechanism is capable of changing the pattern of afferent inputs which excite somatosensory cortical neurons in adult animals and may be the process whereby the excitability of cortical neurons is changed following deafferentation. Further, such a mechanism might be involved in the changes in excitability seen in somatosensory cortex following extensive but selective use of particular surfaces (Clark et al., 1988, Jenkins et al., 1990).

If such a mechanism is to play a role in somatosensory cortex, ACh must be released by some physiological process in quantities sufficient to produce the same alterations in neuronal excitability that occur following the pharmacological administration of ACh using iontophoresis. Recently, Tremblay et al. (1990a,b) have tested the hypothesis that the ACh released in the cortex by activity in the cholinergic BF neurons is sufficient to produce neuronal plasticity similar to that observed in the somatosensory cerebral cortex during iontophoretic administration of ACh. Stimulating electrodes were implanted in the BF of cats anesthetized with halothane and single neurons were isolated by recording in primary somatosensory cortex with multibarrel iontophoretic pipettes using an experimental paradigm similar to that employed by Metherate et al. (1988a). Tremblay et al (1990a,b) tested the excitability of cells before and after the ACh was liberated in cortex by stimulating electrodes placed in the BF. When the BF stimulus was paired with neuronal excitation by glutamate that neuron showed an enhancement of responsiveness for an extended period of time. This phenomenon did not occur in the presence of atropine, and when excitation by glutamate was replaced by excitation from the cutaneous receptive field of a cortical neuron, pairing the BF stimulus with stimulation of the receptive field produced an enhancement in excitability lasting at least for 10s of minutes.

These data suggest that a mechanism exists whereby the endogenous release of ACh during the excitation of a somatosensory cortical neuron leads to a long-term enhancement of that neuron's responsiveness. It is apparent that this mechanism might play a role in learning or memory or the enhanced performance that follows repeated practice. The evidence is also consistent with the hypothesis that ACh contributes to the neuronal plasticity which follows deafferentation.

Further evidence in favor of this hypothesis has recently been presented by Juliano et al. (1989). In adult cat somatic sensory cortex, using the method of 2-deoxyglucose (2-DG) autoradiography, these workers studied the expansion of the digit 3 representation following amputation of the adjacent digit 2. They found that the total cortical surface area of 2-DG uptake evoked by digit 3 stimulation was doubled several weeks after digit 2 removal. However, if the cortical cholinergic input was depleted with a BF lesion, the expansion failed to occur. These exciting

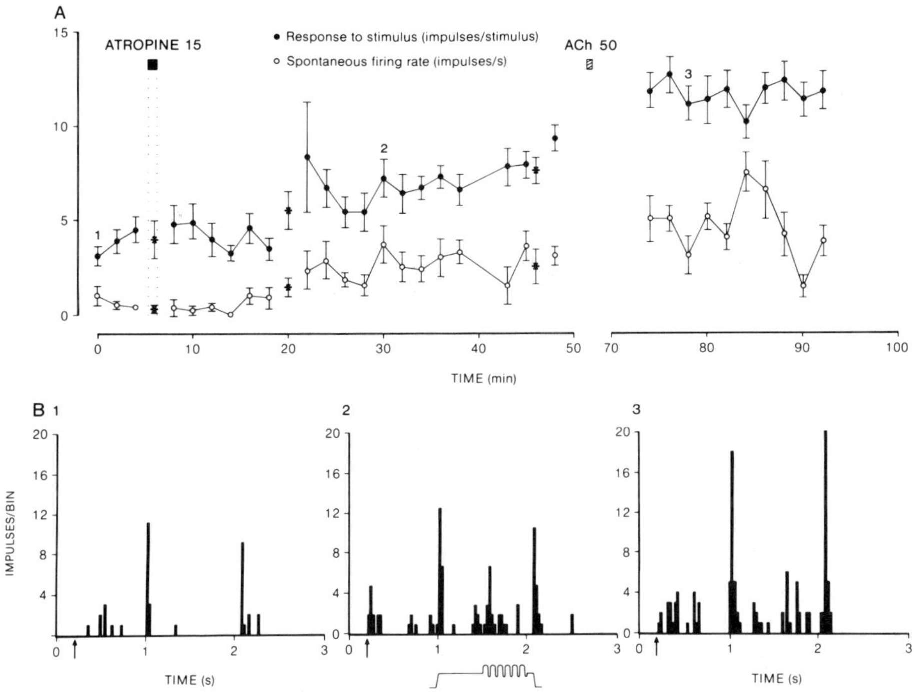

Figure 5. The effect of stimulation of the basal forebrain (BF) on the responsiveness of a neuron in cat somatosensory cortex. (A) filled circles show the mean response (impulses/stimulus) to a brief vibratory stimulus to the cutaneous receptive field of a single cortical neuron. The open circles show the ongoing spontaneous rate (imp/s). Six min after data collection began, the BF was stimulated while atropine was administered to the cell. At filled triangle on time axis there was no change for the next 12 min until the BF was stimulated while the skin was stimulated and atropine was not administered. At open triangle on time axis the mean response increased to approximately twice the value before BF stimulation. Twenty-five min later the BF was stimulated again and 50 nA of acetylcholine was administered to the cell whose receptive field was being stimulated. At filled circle on time axis the responsiveness increased further and was still enhanced when the cell was abandoned 1.5 hours after data collection began. (B) Three time histograms illustrate the response to 10 vibratory stimuli before (B1) the BF stimulus, following the BF stimulus (B2) and following the BF stimulus and acetylcholine treatments (B3) at the times numbered in (A). Modified with permission from Tremblay et al. (1990a,b): Cortex of the cat (II) cortical neurons excited by somatic stimuli. *J. Neurophysiol.* (in press).

data support the idea that ACh facilitates the modification of cortical maps by sensory experience.

SUMMARY AND CONCLUSIONS

We have reviewed evidence suggesting that in the cat, (1) sensory cortex is richly innervated by cholinergic fibers arising from the BF, (2) ACh released from BF fibers usually leads to a facilitation of the responses evoked by sensory stimulation, (3) the enhancement of cortical responses by ACh can be long-lasting, and (4) destruction of the BF projection can interfere with both OD plasticity in kitten visual cortex and with map plasticity in adult somatic sensory cortex. We propose that cortically released ACh facilitates synaptic modification and that the mechanisms of cortical plasticity are fundamentally similar in all areas of sensory neocortex at all postnatal ages.

Completely unknown at present is the mechanism by which ACh exerts its effects on synaptic plasticity, although it seems clear that muscarinic receptors are involved. Muscarinic receptor activation leads to the hydrolysis of membrane phosphoinositides, resulting in the generation of two second messengers, inositol triphosphate (IP_3) and diacyl glycerol (DG). IP_3 liberates intracellular stores of Ca^{2+} and subsequently activates Ca-dependent enzymes such as calcium-calmodulin dependent protein kinase II; DG activates protein kinase C. It is not surprising that this rich biochemistry can play a role in synapse modification. One of the possible consequences of this biochemical cascade may be decreases in the potassium conductances mediated by muscarinic receptors (McCormick and Prince, 1988; Nicoll et al., 1990).

How might an increase in membrane excitability enhance lasting synaptic modifications in the neocortex? Recent evidence indicates that long-term synaptic potentiation in the hippocampus and cortex requires the activation of N-methyl-D-aspartate (NMDA) receptors (Collingridge et al., 1983; Artola and Singer, 1987). NMDA receptors normally become effective only upon sufficient postsynaptic membrane depolarization (Dingledine, 1983). Thus BF inputs (as well as other modulatory inputs such as NE) could facilitate cortical modifications by raising neuronal excitability enough for NMDA receptors to become active. Indeed, recent evidence suggests that NMDA receptor activation is a necessary condition for OD plasticity (Kleinschmidt et al., 1987; Bear et al., 1990).

It will be of considerable interest to examine the possible involvement of NMDA receptors in somatosensory map plasticity, and to investigate more generally the interactions of ACh with cortical NMDA receptor mechanisms.

REFERENCES

Adrien, J., Blanc, G., Buisseret, P., Frégnac, Y., Gary-Bobo, E., Imbert, M., Tassin, J.P. and Trotter, Y. (1985): Noradrenaline and functional plasticity in kitten visual cortex: a reexamination. *J. Physiol.* (Lond.) 367:73-98

Artola, A. and Singer, W. (1987): Long-term potentiation and NMDA receptors in rat visual cortex. *Nature* 330:649-652

Barstad, K.E. and Bear, M.F. (1990): Basal forebrain projections to somatic sensory cortex in the cat. *J Neurophysiol.*, in press

Bear, M.F., Carnes, K.M. and Ebner, F.F. (1985a): An investigation of cholinergic circuitry in cat striate cortex using acetylcholinesterase histochemistry. *J. Comp. Neurol.* 234:411- 430

Bear, M.F., Carnes, K.M. and Ebner, F.F. (1985b): Postnatal changes in the distribution of acetylcholinesterase in kitten striate cortex. *J. Comp. Neurol.* 237:519-534

Bear, M.F., Gu, Q., Kleinschmidt, A. and Singer, W. (1990): Disruption of experience-dependent synaptic modifications in the striate cortex by infusion of an NMDA receptor antagonist. *J. Neurosci.*, in press

Bear, M.F., Kleinschmidt, A. and Singer, W. (1988): Experience-dependent modifications of kitten striate cortex are not prevented by thalamic lesions that include the intralaminar nuclei. *Exp. Brain Res.* 70:627-631

Bear, M.F., Paradiso, M.A., Schwartz, M., Nelson, S.B., Carnes, K.M. and Daniels, J.D. (1983): Two methods of catecholamine depletion in kitten visual cortex yield different effects on plasticity. *Nature* 302:245-247

Bear, M.F. and Daniels, J.D. (1983): The plastic response to monocular deprivation persists in kitten striate cortex after chronic depletion of norepinephrine. *J. Neurosci.* 3:407-416

Bear, M.F. and Singer, W. (1986): Modulation of visual cortical plasticity by acetylcholine and noradrenaline. *Nature* 320:172-176

Butcher, L.L. (1977): Nature and mechanisms of cholinergic-monoaminergic interactions in the brain. *Life Sci.* 21:1207-1226

Clark, S.A., Allard, T., Jenkins, W.M. and Menzenich, M.M. (1988): Receptive fields in the body surface map in adult cortex defined by temporally correlated inputs. *Nature* 332:444-445

Cole, A.E., Nicoll, R.A. (1983): Acetylcholine mediates a slow synaptic potential in hippocampal pyramidal cells. *Science* 221:1299-1301

Collingridge, G.L., Kehl, S.L. and McLennan, H. (1983): Excitatory amino acids in synaptic transmission in the Schaffer collateral-commisural pathway of the rat hippocampus. *J. Physiol.* (Lond.) 334:33-46

Daw, N.W., Robertson, T.W., Rader, R.K., Videen, T.O. and Coscia, C.J. (1984): Substantial reduction of cortical noradrenaline by lesions of adrenergic pathways does not prevent effects of monocular deprivation. *J. Neurosci.* 4:1354-1360

DeLima, A.D. and Singer, W. (1986): Cholinergic innervation of cat striate cortex: a choline acetyltransferase immunocytochemical analysis. *J. Comp. Neurol.* 250:324-338

Dingledine, R. (1983): N-methylaspartate activates voltage-dependent calcium conductance in rat hippocampal pyramidal cells. *J. Physiol.* 343:385-405

Donoghue, J.P. and Carroll, K.K. (1987): Cholinergic modulation of sensory responses in rat primary somatic sensory cortex. *Brain Res.* 408:367-371

Dykes, R.W., Metherate, R. and Tremblay, N. (1988): Cholinergic modulation of neuronal excitability in cat somatosensory cortex. Chapter In: *Neurotransmitters and Function: From Molecules to Mind.* Avoli, M., Reader, T., Dykes, R. and Gloor, P., eds. New York: Plenum Press

Fibiger, H.C. (1982): The organization and some projections of cholinergic neurons of the mammalian forebrain. *Brain Res.* 257:327-388

Freeman, R.D. and Bonds, A.B. (1979): Cortical plasticity in monocularly deprived immobilized kittens depends on eye movement. *Science* 206:1093-1095

Gordon, B., Allen, E.E. and Tromblay, P.Q. (1988): The role of norepinephrine in plasticity of visual cortex. *Prog. Neurobiol.* 30:171-199

Gordon, B., Mitchell, B., Mohtadi, K., Roth, E., Tseng, Y. and Turk, F. (1989): Effect of norepinephrine and acetylcholine depletion on plasticity in kitten visual cortex. *Neurosci. Abst.* 15:796

Houser, C.R., Crawford, G.D., Salvaterra, P.M. and Vaughn, J.E. (1985): Immunocytochemical localization of choline acetyltransferase in rat cerebral cortes: a study of cholinergic neurons and synapses. *J. Comp. Neurol.* 234:17-34

Hubel, D.H. and Wiesel, T.N. (1962): Receptive fields, binocular interactions and functional architecture in the cat's visual cortex. *J. Physiol.* (Lond.) 160:106-154

Hubel, D.H. and Wiesel, T.N. (1970): The period of susceptibility to the physiological effects of unilateral eye closure in kittens. *J. Physiol.* (Lond.) 206:419-436

Jenkins, W.M., Merzenich, M.M., Ochs, M.T. Allard, T. and Guic-Robles, E. (1990): Functional reorganization of primary somatosensory cortex in adult owl monkeys after behaviorally controlled tactile stimulation. *J. Neurophysiol.*, in press

Johnston, M.V., McKinney, M. and Coyle, J.T. (1981): Neocortical cholinergic innervation: a description of extrinsic and intrinsic components in the rat. *Exp. Brain Res.* 43:159-172

Juliano, S.L., Ma, W., Bear, M.F. and Eslin, D. (1988): Manipulation of cortical cholinergic innervation alters stimulus-evoked metabolic activity in cat somatosensory cortex. *Soc. Neurosci. Abstr.* 14:8448

Juliano, S.L., Eslin, D and Ma, W. (1989): Lesions disrupting cortical cholinergic innervation prevent plasticity of somatosensory maps in cat somatosensory cortex. *Soc. Neurosci. Abstr.* 15:19

Kalaska, J.F. and Pomeranz, B. (1979): Chronic paw denervation causes an age-dependent appearance of novel responses from forearm in "paw cortex" of kittens and adults rats. *J. Neurophysiol.* 42:618-633

Kasamatsu, T., and Pettigrew, J.D. (1976): Depletion of brain catecholamines: failure of ocular dominance shift after monocular occlusion in kittens. *Science* 194:206-209

Kasamatsu, T. and Pettigrew, J.D. (1979): Preservation of binocularity after monocular deprivation in the striate cortex of kittens treated with 6-hydroxydopamine. *J. Comp. Neurol.* 185:139-162

Kasamatsu, T., Pettigrew, J.D. and Ary, M. (1979): Restoration of visual cortical plasticity by local microperfusion of norepinephrine. *J. Comp. Neurol.* 185:163-182

Kleinschmidt, A., Bear, M.F. and Singer, W. (1987): Blockade of "NMDA" receptors disrupts experience-dependent modifications of kitten striate cortex. *Science* 238:355-358

Krnjević, K. (1988): Acetylcholine as transmitter in the cerebral cortex. Chapter In: *Neurotransmitters and Function: From Molecules to Mind.* Avoli, M., Reader, T., Dykes, R. and Gloor, P., eds. New York: Plenum Press

Krnjević, K. and Phillis, J.W. (1963a): Acetylcholine-sensitive cells in the cerebral cortex. *J. Physiol.* (Lond.) 166:296-327

Krnjević, K. and Phillis, J.W. (1963b): Pharmacological properties of acetylcholine sensitive cells in the cerebral cortex. *J. Physiol. (Lond.)* 166:328-350

Lindvall, O. and A. Björklund (1974): The organization of the ascending catecholamine neuron systems in the rat brain. *Acta. Physiol. Scand. (Suppl.)* 412:1-45

Ma, W., Hohmann, C.F., Coyle, J.T. and Juliano, S.L. (1989): Lesions of the basal forebrain alter stimulus-evoked metabolic activity in mouse somatosensory cortex. *J. Comp. Neurol.* 288:414-427

McCormick, D.A. and Prince, D.A. (1985): Two types of muscarinic response to acetylcholine in mammalian cortical neurons. *Proc. Natl. Acad. Sci. USA* 82:6344-6348

McCormick, D.A. and Prince, D.A. (1988): Noradrenergic modulation of firing pattern in guinea pig and cat thalamic neurons, *in vitro*. *J. Neurophysiol.* 59:978-996

Merzenich, M.M., Kaas, J.H. Wall, J.T., Nelson, R.J., Sur, M. and Felleman, D.J. (1983a): Topographic reorganization of somatosensory cortical areas 3b and 1 in adult monkeys following restricted deafferentation. *Neurosci.* 8:33-55

Merzenich, M.M., Kaas, J.H., Wall, J.T., Nelson, R.J. and Felleman, D.J. (1983b): Progression of change following median nerve section in the cortical representation of the hand in areas 3b and 1 in adult owl and squirrel monkeys. *Neurosci.* 10:639-665

Metherate, R., Tremblay, N. and Dykes, R.W. (1988a): The effects of acetylcholine on response properties of cat somatosensory cortical neurons. *J. Neurophysiol.* 59:1231-1252

Metherate, R., Tremblay, N. and Dykes, R.W. (1988b): Transient and prolonged effects of acetylcholine on responsiveness of cat somatosensory cortical neurons. *J. Neurophysiol.* 59:1253-1276

Morrison, R.S. and Dempsey, E.W. (1942): A study of thalamo-cortical relations. *Amer. J. Physiol.* 135:281-292

Moruzzi, G. and Magoun, H.W. (1949): Brainstem reticular formation and activation of the EEG. *EEG Clin. Neurophysiol.* 1:155-473

Nicoll, R.A., Malenka, R.C. and Kauer, J.A. (1990): Functional comparison of neurotransmitter receptor subtypes in mammalian central nervous system. *Physiol. Rev.* 70:513-565

Paradiso, M.A., Bear, M.F. and Daniels, J.D. (1983): Effects of intracortical infusion of 6-hydroxydopamine on the response of kitten visual cortex to monocular deprivation. *Exp. Brain Res.* 51:413-422

Potempska, A., Skangiel-Kramska, J. and Kossut, M. (1979): Development of cholinergic enzymes and adenosinetriphosphatase activity of optic system of cats in normal and restricted visual input conditions. *Dev. Neurosci.* 2:38-45

Rauschecker, J.P. and Singer, W. (1979): Changes in the circuitry of the kitten's visual cortex are gated by postsynaptic activity. *Nature* 280:58-60

Richardson, R.T. and Delong, M.R. (1986): Nucleus basalis of Meynert neuronal activity during a delayed response task in monkey. *Brain Res.* 399:364-368

Robertson, D. and Irvine, D.R.F. (1989): Plasticity of frequency organization in auditory cortex of guinea pigs with partial unilateral deafness. *J. Comp. Neurol.* 282:456-471

Sato, H., Hata, Y., Masui, H. and Tsumoto, T. (1987a): A functional role of cholinergic innervation to neurons in cat visual cortex. *J. Neurophysiol.* 58:765-794

Sato, H., Hata, Y., Hagihava, K. and Tsumoto, T. (1987b): Effects of cholinergic depletion on neuron activities in the cat visual cortex. *J. Neurophysiol.* 58:781-794

Shaw, C., Needler, M.C. and Cynader, M. (1984): Ontogenesis of muscarinic acetylcholine binding sites in cat visual cortex: reversal of specific laminar distribution during the critical period. *Dev. Brain Res.* 14:295-299

Shute, C.C.D. and Lewis, P.R. (1967): The ascending cholinergic reticular system: neocortical, olfactory and subcortical projections. *Brain* 90:497-521

Sillito, A.M. and Kemp, J.A. (1983): Cholinergic modulation of the functional organization of the cat visual cortex. *Brain Res.* 289:143-155

Singer, W. (1979): Central core control of visual cortex functions. In: *The Neurosciences: Fourth Study Program.* Schmitt, F.O. and Worden, F.G., eds. Cambridge, MA: MIT Press. pp 1093-1109

Singer, W. (1982): Central core control of developmental plasticity in the kitten visual cortex: I. Diencephalic lesions. *Exp. Brain Res.* 47:209-222

Singer, W., and Rauschecker, J. (1982): Central core control of developmental plasticity in the kitten visual cortex: II. Electrical activation of mesencephalic and diencephalic projections. *Exp. Brain Res.* 47:223-233

Singer, W., Rauschecker, J. and Werth, R. (1977): The effect of monocular exposure to temporal contrasts on ocular dominance in kittens. *Brain Res.* 134:568-572

Stichel, C.C. and Singer, W. (1987): Quantitative analysis of the choline acetyltransferase-immunoreactive axonal network in the cat primary visual cortex: I. Adult cats. *J. Comp. Neurol.* 258:91-98

Stone, T.W. (1972): cholinergic mechanisms in the rat somatosensory cerebral cortex. *J. Physiol* (Lond.) 225:485-499

Szerb, J.C. (1967): Cortical ACh release and EEG arousal. *J. Physiol.* (Lond.) 192:329-343

Tremblay, N., Warren, R.A. and Dykes, R.W. (1990a): Electrophysiological studies of acetylcholine and the role of the basal forebrain in the somatosensory cortex of the cat. (I) Cortical neurons excited by glutamate. *J. Neurophysiol.*, in press

Tremblay, N., Warren, R.A. and Dykes, R.W. (1990b): Electrophysiological studies of acetylcholine and the role of the basal forebrain in the somatosensory cortex of the cat (II) cortical neurons excited by somatic stimuli. *J. Neurophysiol.* in press

Trombley, P., Allen, E.E., Soyke, J., Blaha, C.D., Lane, F.F. and Gordon, B. (1986): Doses of 6-hydroxydopamine sufficient to deplete norepinephrine are not sufficient to decrease plasticity in the visual cortex. *J. Neurosci.* 6:266-273

Wiesel, T.N. and Hubel, D.H. (1963): Single cell responses in striate cortex of kittens deprived of vision in one eye. *J. Neurophysiol.* 28:1029-1040

Woody, C.D. and Gruen, E. (1988): Evidence that acetylcholine acts *in vivo* in layer V pyramidal cells of cats via GMP and a GMP-dependent protein kinase to produce a decrease in an outward current. In: *Neurotransmitters and Cortical Function: From Molecules to Mind.* Avoli, M., Reader, T., Dykes, R.W. and Gloor, P., eds. New York: Plenum Press

Woody, C.D., Swartz, B.E. and Gruen, E. (1978): Effects of acetylcholine and cyclic GMP on input resistance of cortical neurons in awake cats. *Brain Res.* 158:373-395

The Cholinergic Basal Forebrain as a Cognitive Machine

Nancy J. Woolf and Larry L. Butcher

INTRODUCTION

The processing of information is the primary function of the central nervous system, the organ of behavior. Determination of how the brain and spinal cord receive, store, access, transform, and transmit information has been a major quest of cognitive neuroscience. Valid brain mechanisms of cognition have remained elusive, however, not only because of the intricacies of the neural systems designed to perform those functions but also because of the inherent complexity of cognitive processes in general. The very nature of cognition, for example, implies in most instances relationships among different information domains (e.g., perceiving, knowing) rather than seemingly less labyrinthine events as might be encountered in the study of sensations at first-order levels.

In this treatise, we present a model of brain function based on the proposition that a large number of cognitive operations in the brain can be performed by a relatively small number of neurons, including those comprising the cholinergic basal nuclear complex (for nomenclature, see Butcher and Semba, 1989), that project widely to the cerebral mantle and maintain their capacity for structurofunctional plasticity throughout the lifespan (Butcher and Woolf, 1989). These neurons will be called "network" neurons to emphasize their potential for connectional multiplicity, both among themselves and with other cellular elements and configurations. By contrast, the vast majority of neurons in the brain, designated "hierarchical" neurons in our schema, are proposed to be essentially "hard-wired," to comprise systems having generally more restricted projections and interconnections, and to be organized in modular chunks of information representing specific microfeatures (e.g., lines, tones) of the external and internal environment. It is proposed that the interactions between network neurons and those comprising hierarchical systems, particularly those involving cholinergic neurons of the basal nuclear complex and their pyramidal cell targets in the hippocampus and cortex, form an important substrate for cognitive function.

THE BASALO-PYRAMIDAL CELL CIRCUIT AS A COGNITIVE PROCESSING UNIT

Although relatively complex behavioral responses can occur at comparatively "primitive" levels (e.g., spinal cord) of the nervous system (Shurrager and Culler, 1940), it is generally believed that the telencephalon, especially as it has been elaborated in the human brain, is the locus of the most complex manipulations of information relevant to cognition. Although such a contention is likely to be valid, the disproportionate attention given to the hippocampus and cerebral cortex in this regard and the lesser role(s) attributed to the basal nuclear complex which projects to those brain regions represents, in our opinion, a major shortcoming of current theorizing. We will argue that the cholinergic basal forebrain, by virtue of its unique anatomy and physiology, is particularly well-suited to perform complex cognitive operations, even though the component neurons are relatively few in number. As will be considered in greater detail later in this treatise, the key to understanding how a relatively small number of cells can be involved in a seemingly vast number of cognitive tasks may lie in parallel distributed processing of information (Rumelhart and McClelland, 1986), which permits the same units to participate in different operations at different times, and which views the activity of the system as a whole to be more important than the properties of individual neurons themselves. We maintain further that analyses of the cognitive functions of the telencephalon must consider specifically interactions between the most highly evolved component of the embryologic sensory or alar plate (i.e., the cerebral cortices) and the most highly evolved part of the motor or basal plate (i.e., the basal forebrain and basal ganglia), as well as the functions of the various telencephalic subunits alone.

Although the cerebral cortex contains considerably more neurons than the basal forebrain and is seemingly more elegant cytoarchitecturally, this beauty may only be skin deep. With respect to strategies of information processing (i.e., computational styles), the cerebral cortex may be less sophisticated than the basal forebrain. Specifically, the neurons in the cerebral cortex appear to be well-suited for gathering information quickly, as well as for clearing the record of that information rapidly. For example, many cortical neurons use fast-acting small amino acid transmitters like glutamate (Fagg and Foster, 1983; Conti et al., 1988) and can maintain high frequency spike trains (Eccles, 1966). The comparative rapidity with which such events transpire is consonant with observations that visual sensory information is processed very quickly and that much of this information escapes encoding in memory (Sperling et al., 1971; Reeves and Sperling, 1986). This computational style is ideally suited to transmit ever-changing sensory events continually impinging on the various receptive fields. Other modes of operation need to be considered in relation to cognitive function, however, since we know that the telencephalon is capable of much more than just providing a continually updated view of the external and internal worlds, of outer as well as inner space.

The cholinergic neurons of the basal forebrain, like cholinergic and monoaminergic neurons of brainstem reticular networks, appear to exhibit a fundamentally different computational style than do cortical neurons. The former neurons – network neurons – fire more slowly, have longer refractory periods, and, perhaps most importantly, produce regular spontaneous patterns of action potentials even when isolated from other neural tissue (Griffith and Matthews, 1986). This capacity for generating endogenous pacemaker-like activity, which is lacking in isolated cortical tissue (Burns, 1958), could provide each network cell with its own unique profile of patterned activity upon which incoming patterns of activation could be superimposed, compared, and analyzed. Moreover, the fact that activation patterns can be transmitted throughout the basal nuclear complex from one neuron to its neighbors (Petsche et al., 1965) gives the network at large enormous computational ability to generate and compare the vast number of relationships needed to account for the complexity of higher cognitive processes.

It is known that rich interconnections exist between the neurons of the cholinergic basal forebrain and those of the cerebral mantle. Cholinergic basal forebrain cells project to every region of the cerebral cortex, including the hippocampus and olfactory bulb, as well as to the amygdala (Bigl et al., 1982; Butcher and Woolf, 1986). It is not inconsequential

(a) that the slab of cortex innervated by a single cholinergic neuron in the basal nuclear complex, approximately 1-2 mm^2 (Bigl et al., 1982; Price and Stern, 1983), is of the same dimensions as a cortical module, and (b) that basal forebrain cells projecting to totally different regions of the cerebral mantle can lie in close proximity (Bigl et al., 1982).

Particularly dense inputs to pyramidal cells are provided by basal forebrain neurons (Luiten et al., 1989). Pyramidal cells from deep layers of many cortical regions also reciprocally innervate the cholinergic basal forebrain, and afferents from a number of cortical areas have been suggested to terminate directly on those neurons (Lemann and Saper, 1985; Haring and Wang, 1986; Irle and Markowitz, 1986). Although evidence is currently most compelling for direct reciprocal innervation between basal forebrain neurons and their targets in the limbic telencephalon, information conveyed from other cortical regions could influence basal nuclear cells in a reciprocating fashion as well, even if by non-synaptic mechanisms. Many cholinergic basal forebrain neurons and/or their processes are embedded in or traverse the corticofugal fiber tracts from the cortical region to which they project (see data in Saper, 1984). Neurons projecting to the visual cortex, for example, lie in the path of the occipitogeniculate projections (see Saper, 1984). As illustrated in Fig. 1, cholinergic neurons of the basal forebrain possess dense plexuses of dendrites extending into fiber tracts such as the diagonal band, which contains corticofugal fibers arising from the limbic cortex (Fig. 1A), and the posterior internal capsule, which contains corticofugal fibers deriving from the visual and parietal cortices (Fig. 1B). The existence of cholinergic dendrites highly interdigitated with fiber bundles deriving from the cortex provides seemingly ample opportunities for cortically derived axons to communicate with basal forebrain neurons. Even in the absence of synaptic linkages, transneuronal field effects, which do not require specialized junctions (Korn and Faber, 1979), could mediate the transfer of information from the cerebral cortex to the basal forebrain.

A large number of studies further indicate that within the telencephalon, the pyramidal cells of the cerebral cortex and hippocampus and the cholinergic basal forebrain cells are critical to cognitive function (see Table 1). All of these findings, coupled with data contained in the foregoing discourse, provide reasonable indication that the transfer of information from the hierarchical processing units of the cerebral cortex to the cholinergic network, and the possible reverberation of that

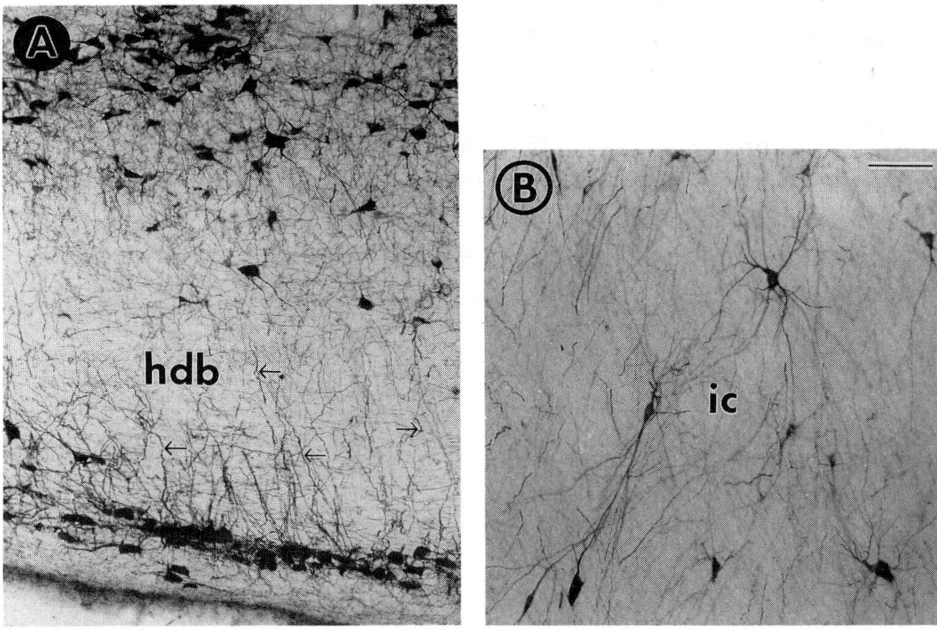

Figure 1. Neurons demonstrating choline acetyltransferase-like immunoreactivity and associated with the horizontal limb of the diagonal band (hdb, frame A) and the nucleus basalis (frame B) of the cat. Immunohistochemical procedures were performed as described in Woolf et al., 1984. In A, individual cholinergic neurons possess dendritic processes (arrows) that traverse almost perpendicularly the fibers of the diagonal band. In B, cholinergic somata and their processes are embedded within the myelinated fibers of the posterior limb of the internal capsule (ic). Scale bar in B equals 100 μm and applies to both frames.

information within reciprocal circuits, comprise an integral component of cognition.

ROLE OF THE TROPHIC FACTORS IN COGNITION

A conceivably important feature of any cognitive processing unit is its ability to be modified as a function of experience. In other words, cognitive processing units must somehow be able to learn. Among the various alterations that might occur, morphologic restructuring of neurons has been repeatedly suggested as a potential neural mechanism for various aspects of the learning process (e.g., Hebb, 1949; see also Butcher and Woolf, 1989). The biochemical mechanisms underlying alterations in neuronal architecture, however, remain to be established. Nonetheless, endogenous compounds such as "trophic factors" (i.e., those that enable and maintain the differentiated state of cells) are known to affect neurite outgrowth, in addition to influencing cell survival (e.g., see Purves, 1988). It is not surprising, therefore, that speculations have been advanced that one role of these agents is to mediate neuronal plasticity associated with the acquisition and storage of information (Purves, 1988).

A number of endogenous substances which could be considered to have trophic-like properties (e.g., nerve growth factor, thyroid hormone,

Table 1. Evidence that the basalo-pyramidal cell circuit is a primary cognitive processing unit of the telencephalon.

Damage to the basalo-pyramidal cell circuit is a prominent lesion in Alzheimer's dementia.	Butcher & Woolf, 1989 Woolf & Butcher, 1990
In the hippocampus, pyramidal cells are the predominant cell type to express changes during conditioning.	Berger & Thompson, 1978
Changes in cortical pyramidal cell excitability exhibited during conditioning can be mimicked by the application of acetylcholine.	Woody et al., 1970 Woody et al., 1978
Changes in cortical pyramidal cell responses exhibited during conditioning can be blocked by cholinergic agonists or by lesion of the nucleus basalis.	Rigdon & Pirch, 1986
Neurons throughout the entire extent of the cholinergic basal forebrain exhibit changes in activity during conditioning before such changes are observed in the cerebral cortex.	Linseman & Olds, 1974

estrogen) have been shown to have effects on the structure of pyramidal cells of the cerebral cortex and hippocampus (Ruiz-Marcos et al.,1982; Woolf et al., 1989a,b) and the cholinergic cells of the basal forebrain (Hefti et al., 1985; Luine, 1985; Butcher and Woolf, 1987; Gould and Butcher, 1989). Nerve growth factor and thyroid hormone, in fact, appear to have preferential effects on cholinergic neurons of the basal nuclear complex (Seiler and Schwab, 1984; Patel et al., 1988; Gould and Butcher, 1989). Furthermore, their molecular actions have been studied extensively. Evidence exists, for example, that the synthesis of a number of proteins important in determining neuronal architecture can be regulated or modified by nerve growth factor and thyroid hormone (Table 2), not only during development but also in the mature organism (Isaacson et al., 1989; Mathes et al., 1989). In particular, cytoskeletal proteins associated with cholinergic basal forebrain cells and their pyramidal cell targets, to the extent that they have been examined, appear to be regulated by these agents (Fig. 2; see also Woolf et al., 1989b)

Other proteins important for cell growth, the maintenance of cell-to-cell contacts, and synapse formation appear to be regulated by relatively long-acting molecules, such as nerve growth factor and thyroid hormone (Table 2). The apparent sensitivity of adult cholinergic neurons to such compounds (Isaacson et al., 1989; Mathes et al., 1989) raises the possibility that the structurofunctional organization of responsive cells is dynamically controlled by substances possessing trophic-like actions in the mature organism (see also Butcher and Woolf, 1987). Complex neurotrophic control, finely tuned by the activity of individual basal forebrain cells (see Kalil, 1989), could mediate connectional variability, resulting in either the strengthening or weakening of connections between cholinergic cells and their neighbors or between cholinergic cells and their pyramidal cell targets (Fig. 3).

There is evidence for at least two kinds of structurofunctional changes which could result in modified connectivity between cholinergic basal forebrain cells with other basal forebrain cells and cortical pyramidal cells as illustrated in Fig. 3. These include changes in fiber diameter and redistribution of synapses, conditions which in either case could profoundly alter the computation parameters of the basalo-cortical loop and the flow of information through the cholinergic network (Fig. 3).

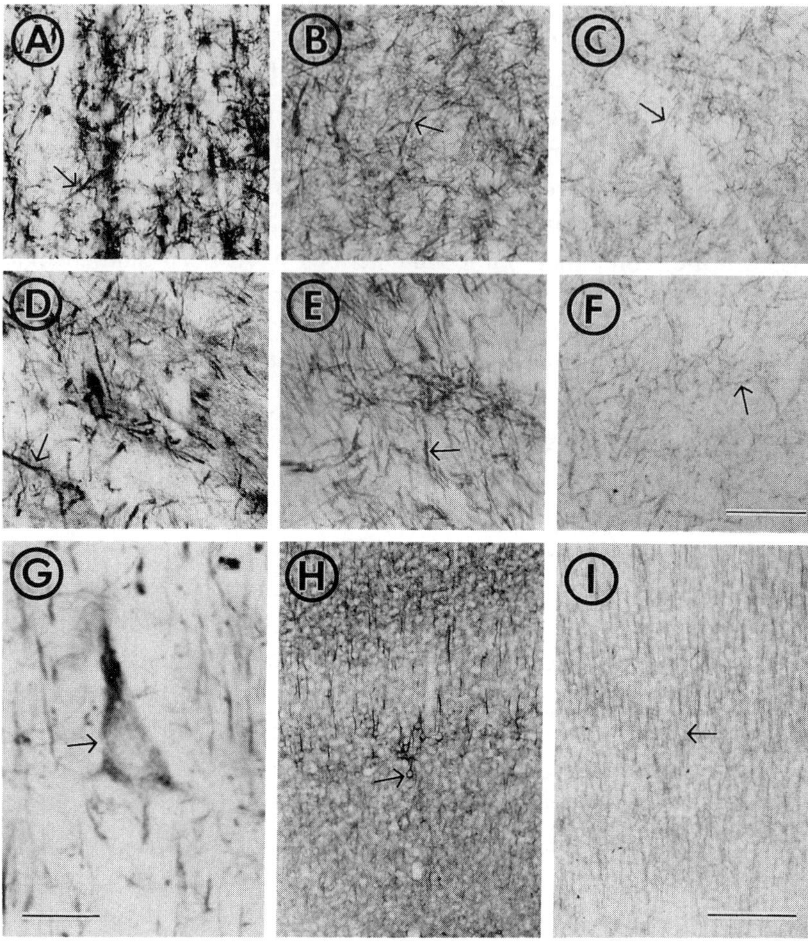

Figure 2. Microtubule associated protein-1 (MAP1) immunoreactivity associated with processes of neurons in the vertical limb of the diagonal band (A-C, examples indicated by arrows) and nucleus basalis (D-F, examples indicated by arrows) and with pyramidal cells of the parietal cerebral cortex (G-I, examples indicated by arrows) of developing rats sacrificed 1-3 weeks after birth. Compared to controls (B, E) from all three regions, drug treatment producing hyperthyroidism enhanced and accelerated the development of MAP1 expression (A,D,H), whereas drug manipulation inducing hypothyroidism decreased and delayed the expression of that cytoskeletal protein (C,F,I). Normal immunoreactivity for a cortical pyramidal cell is shown at higher power in G. Thyroid manipulations on developing rat pups were performed as described in Gould and Butcher (1989). Scale bar in F is 50 mm and applies also to frames A-F. Scale bar in G equals 20 μm. Scale bar in I is 200 μm and applies also to H.

Table 2. Endogenous factors regulate the expression of proteins that determine cellular features which could be dynamically modified during cognitive processing.

MOLECULAR CHARACTERISTIC	CELLULAR FEATURE	FUNCTIONAL PROPERTY RELEVANT TO COGNITION
Proteins regulated by nerve growth factor or thyroid hormone	*Dynamic control over*	
cytoskeletal proteins	cell shape	connectional variability
neurofilaments[1]	axonal growth	
microtubules[2]	axonal transport	
MAPs[3]	synapses	
tubulin[4]		
membrane proteins	cell-cell contact	connectional variability
N-CAM[5]	axonal growth	
GAP-43[6]	synapses	
receptors[7]		
ion channels	excitability	multiple physiologic states
Na +[8]		
Ca+ +[9]		

[1] Dickson et al., 1986; Lindenbaum et al., 1988; Plioplys et al., 1986

[2] Marc and Rabie, 1985

[3] MAPs = microtubule-associated proteins; Drubin et al., 1985; Hargreaves et al., 1988

[4] Fernyhough and Ishii, 1987

[5] N-CAM = neural cell adhesion molecule; Prentice et al., 1987; Seilheimer and Schachner, 1987

[6] GAP-43 = growth-associated protein-43; Federoff et al., 1988

[7] Milbrandt, 1988; Viana et al., 1988

[8] Rudy et al., 1987

[9] Takahashi et al., 1985

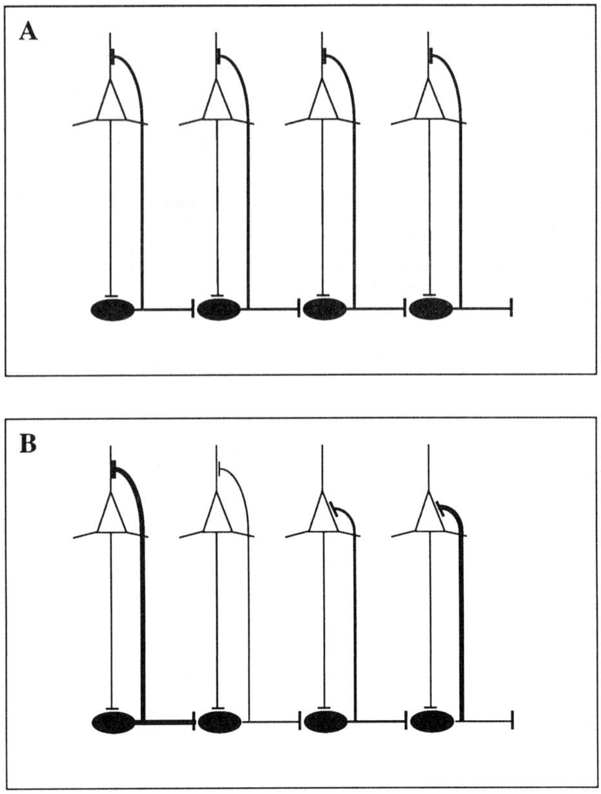

Figure 3. Schematic representation of possible remodeling strategies exhibited by basalo-pyramidal cell circuits during periods of heightened plasticity such as might occur during maturation and/or as a function of learning. For purposes of figure construction, a four-neuron ensemble is portrayed. The initial state of the ensemble is diagrammed in A, and the end stage deriving from the operation of processes determining morphological plasticity is indicated in B. Filled ovals represent cholinergic basal forebrain neurons that project onto cortical pyramidal cells (open triangles) and have interconnections with other basal forebrain cells. The following types of structural changes could occur in cholinergic axons (left to right in B, compare with A): (a) increased caliber of different axonal branches, (b) decreased diameters of different axonal branches, (c) altered topography of inputs to target cells, or, perhaps more likely, (d) combinations of increased and decreased calibers of different axonal branches accompanied by altered organization of afferents to target cells. No morphologic remodeling is indicated for putative pyramidal cell projections directly onto cholinergic basal forebrain neurons or those comprising descending fiber bundles traversed by dendrites of basal nuclear cells (see Fig. 1). The reason for this latter stipulation is that pyramidal axons have been shown to be relatively non-plastic in the adult (Tolbert and Der, 1987).

During maturation cholinergic basal forebrain axons develop increasingly variable axon calibers. In the adult animal, thick, as well as thin, cholinergic fibers can be traced to the cerebral cortex (e.g., Figure 4; see also de Lima and Singer, 1986). Since fiber diameter is generally correlated with conduction velocity, these observations are compatible with reports indicating a wide range of variable conduction velocities in basal forebrain cells projecting to the neocortex (e.g., Aston-Jones et al., 1984).

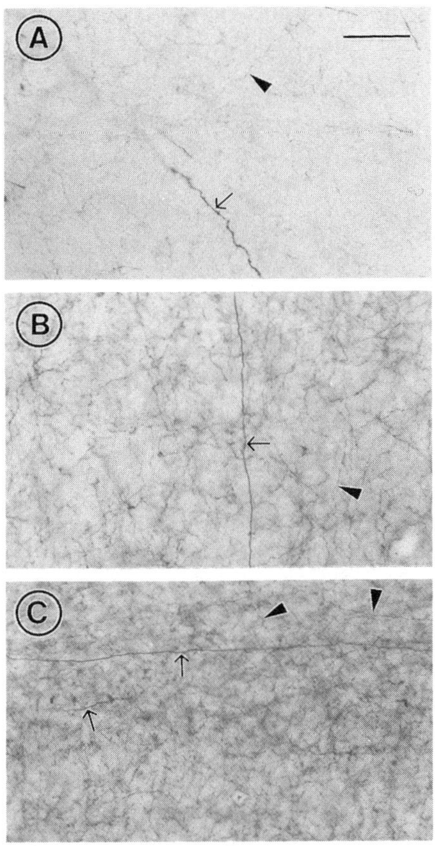

Figure 4. Axon segments of cholinergic neurons in various cortical layers and regions of the cat. Observe the range of fiber diameters, which appears to be correlated positively with intensity of choline acetyltransferase immunoreactivity. Arrows in each frame point to fibers having larger calibers, whereas arrowheads indicate axons with thinner diameters. Fibers in A are from layer 6 and those in B are from layer 2 of the midectosylvian gyrus. Axon segments in C are from layer 2 of the cingulate cortex. Scale bar in A equals 50 μm and applies to all frames.

The axon calibers of cholinergic basal forebrain neurons may be influenced in turn by the electrical activity patterns of those cells. Neurofilament proteins have been implicated in the determination of axon caliber (Hoffman et al., 1985). Furthermore, these proteins are sensitive to nerve growth factor (Dickson et al., 1986; Lindenbaum et al., 1988) and appear to participate in the restructuring of cholinergic basal forebrain axons following injury (Woolf and Butcher, 1990). It is conceivable that the structure-activity relationships that exist for cholinergic motor neurons (Ribchester and Taxt, 1983) also exist for cholinergic basal forebrain neurons and that nerve growth factor may be one of the agents that modulates such behavior.

The topography of cholinergic innervation patterns also can be modified by nerve growth factor and the putative growth factor release inhibitory factor, somatostatin (Butcher and Woolf, 1987), giving rise to the conjecture that within certain structural limits these kinds of modifications could occur normally. Given that most structures of the adult brain are relatively hard-wired (Cajal, 1928), even structurally plastic systems will be confined by a relatively rigid matrix. Thus, in the adult brain, endogenous trophic factors could likely have limited effects upon individual axonal fiber branches rather than having massive effects on the total axonal arbor (Fig. 3B). There is evidence that nerve growth factor, for example, can specifically affect only those neurites it directly contacts, leaving other neurites of the same cell unaltered (Campenot, 1977).

Changes in the distribution of cholinergic fibers, as assessed by acetylcholinesterase, have been demonstrated in response to damage to a competing set of afferents (Lynch et al., 1972), in association with dementia (Geddes et al., 1985), in response to enriched environment (Rosenzweig et al., 1972), and as a function of maturation in humans (Mesulam and Geula, 1988). In the latter case, acetylcholinesterase staining was shown to increase in pyramidal cells as a function of increasing age (Mesulam and Geula, 1988). To the extent that acetylcholinesterase staining in pyramidal cells is concentrated at postsynaptic sites of cholinergic inputs, as it is at the neuromuscular junction (Donoso et al., 1987), this finding can be interpreted as evidence that over time cholinergic synapses in the human cerebral cortex are redistributed to evince a greater concentration in the proximal regions of the pyramidal cell (Fig. 3B).

MULTIPLE PHYSIOLOGICAL STATES

Although verification of the structurofunctional plasticity of the basalo-pyramidal loop is important for its role as a major cognitive processing unit, of perhaps even greater significance is how such units function in the first place. The necessity of addressing this issue becomes increasingly clear when one attempts to speculate how the weakening or strengthening of particular network connections will impact upon the functioning of the system. To what end does neuronal plasticity exist?

Recent connectionist models provide some indications as to how the strengthening and weakening of inputs within a highly interconnected network could result in various activation states for units of that network (e.g., Rumelhart and McClelland, 1986). Cholinergic basal forebrain neurons appear to be highly interconnected with each other (see Bigl et al., 1982). These neurons possess axon collaterals terminating in the immediate vicinity of their own parent cell bodies and dendritic arbors (Semba et al., 1987), and choline acetyltransferase-positive nerve terminals on other cholinergic basal forebrain neurons have been identified electron microscopically (Bialowas and Frotscher, 1987; Meeker et al, 1988). In addition, the confluence of cholinergic dendrites in the basal forebrain could provide another locus of interaction (Bigl et al, 1982). Although cholinergic-cholinergic synapses appear to be sparse in the basal forebrain, a number of studies indicate that cholinergic neurons nonetheless have significant physiological effects on adjacent cholinergic neurons. Neighboring basal forebrain neurons that discharge in synchronous bursts are frequently found (Petsche et al., 1965). Cholinomimetics applied to regions of the basal forebrain can induce alterations of basic firing patterns of the neurons found there and can even precipitate changes in sleep-wakefulness state (Hernandez-Peon and Chavez-Ibarra, 1963; Petsche et al., 1965; Lamour et al., 1984;1986). Moreover, cholinergic stimulation of cholinergic cells can result in either increased or decreased firing rates (Petsche et al., 1965; Lamour et al., 1984, 1986), providing a possible basis for units in connectionist networks which can at some times excite and at other times inhibit other units (for alternate point of view, see Crick and Asanuma, 1986).

Based upon the aforementioned considerations, the cholinergic basal forebrain can be envisioned as a highly interconnected network of neurons which, by means of interactions with adjacent cells, has the capacity to affect the activity of other neurons in the network through a cascade of connections. It is further proposed that these individual cholinergic neurons operate by computing the weights of all their inputs and, based upon that information, assume a particular state of activation, much in the manner proposed in connectionist models. A critical question to be answered, however, is whether or not cholinergic basal forebrain neurons exhibit multiple activation states, and, if so, what are their bases?

Physiological studies suggest that cholinergic basal forebrain neurons exhibit a range of regular firing rates that can be equated with several relatively stable levels of activation. Rhythmic bursting activity ranging 12-18 Hz, with an average of 4 burst cycles per second, has been noted for cholinergic basal forebrain cells (Petsche et al., 1965; Lamour et al., 1984; Lamour et al., 1986; Detaríet al., 1987; Szymusiak and McGinty, 1989). The periods of the burst cycles, moreover, appear to be determined by the cortical inputs back onto the basal forebrain (Lamour et al., 1984). Additionally, regular firing at intermediate rates (1-8 Hz), as well as at very low rates of firing (<1 Hz), have been recorded from cells in these regions (Petsche et al., 1965; Lamour et al., 1984; Lamour et al.,1986; Szymusiak and McGinty, 1989). That these cells demonstrate intermediate firing rates (1-7 Hz) during synchronized sleep, in contrast to the heterogeneous pattern of firing during wakefulness and desynchronized sleep (Szymuziak and McGinty, 1989), suggests that the firing rate of approximately 1 spike per burst cycle may represent a basal activation state for those neurons. Multiple spikes per burst cycle or missed bursts on cycles could represent more positive and more negative levels of activation. Although these basic firing patterns appear to be relatively stable, basal forebrain cells can be induced to change their burst frequencies in response to sensory stimulation, reticular stimulation, and the application of cholinergic drugs (Petsche et al., 1965; Lamour et al., 1984, 1986), indicating that those neurons are highly responsive to afferent information.

With respect to the molecular basis of multiple physiological states exhibited by cholinergic basal forebrain neurons, the proteins that are regulated by trophic-like factors may again serve as a starting point in unraveling this complex question. In addition to a number of proteins with clear roles in maintaining the integrity of the cytoskeleton, nerve growth factor has additionally been shown to effect the expression of certain ion channels (Table 2). Thus, it can be hypothesized that the regulation of these ion channels are also under dynamic control in cholinergic basal forebrain cells and that their concentrations and patterns of synthesis bear conceivably complex relationships to ongoing activity patterns. Such an arrangement can be modeled to account for multiple states of activation, as well as for the apparent self-organization of activity that individual units of the network evince as may occur in relation to the sleep-wakefulness cycle. On the sole basis of minor variations in the conductance to Ca^{2+} ion, for example, pancreatic β-cells modify their endogenous firing rates to achieve a number of stable regular firing rates as well as a number of transitional "unstable" states (Chay and Rinzel, 1985). These firing patterns resemble those exhibited by cholinergic basal forebrain cells. It is conceivable, therefore, that cholinergic basal forebrain cells utilize a similar mechanism to autoregulate seemingly complex trains of patterned activity by making relatively small modifications in the availability of certain ion channels, possibly in a self-activating, trophic factor-dependent manner.

THE MICROSTRUCTURE OF COGNITION

The conjecture that cholinergic basal forebrain neurons possess the ability to generate unique sequential trains of patterned activity in response to particular inputs is consistent with a number of empirical results and, furthermore, enables the modeling of a very basic neural computational mode with potential relevance to higher cognition. It seems reasonable to suppose, for example, that during quiet waking the neurons of the cholinergic basal forebrain exhibit various pseudostable states of activation with occasional spontaneous deviations to unstable states. Since many of these units are presumed to be interlinked (e.g., see Bigl et al., 1982), spontaneous fluctuations in activity would be expected to affect neighboring cells. The extent of spreading activation (or deactivation) would presumably be determined by factors such as the intensity of the initial source of activation and the states of the recipient cells. Since sequences of unstable transitional states appear to be expressed in a deterministically chaotic manner (for definition and discussion of chaos, see Chay and Rinzel, 1985), networks of cholinergic cells exhibiting these transitional unstable states would be expected to produce a kind of chaotic background activity in the cortical targets that they innervate, which could serve to poise the basalo-cortical loops for rapid activation. Chaotic background activity has been measured from EEG recordings taken from the surface of the olfactory bulbs (Freeman and Viana Di Presco, 1986). Since this activity is not present in isolated olfactory bulbs (Skarda and Freeman, 1987), and since cholinergic mechanisms play a major role in determining the cortical EEG pattern (Stewart et al., 1984), this kind of chaotic background activity could very well be produced by cholinergic basal forebrain afferents to the olfactory bulb.

Given that cholinergic basal forebrain neurons are in a position to be influenced by cortical pyramidal cells and are capable of transitions in activational state, such cells could detect relationships that occur among low level sensory cues such as those relayed to primary sensory cortices. In this sense, cholinergic basal forebrain neurons could function as minihypothesis makers. Minihypotheses are defined here as discrete changes in neuronal activation state which signify that a putative relationship between several low level sensory cues may have occurred. That a line of a particular orientation has been presented to the visual field, for example, could be a minihypothesis. The simultaneous excitation of several pyramidal cells from various cortical modules, which all are selectively sensitive to that orientation, could provide the information upon which such a minihypothesis could be drawn. A critical feature of the minihypothesis, however, is its susceptibility to further revision. If additional information is presented which contradicts the preliminary minihypothesis, then that hypothesis is abandoned. For example, if more visual information becomes available such that a putative line appears to be part of a large circle, the minihypothesis that a straight line is detected is discarded and the neuron(s) encoding it revert back to baseline state(s) of activation.

In order to illustrate this point, a simple model of visual recognition is illustrated (Fig. 5). Recognition in this case is taken to mean the simplest form possible, such as would be encountered by a naive person who had no previous experience with the stimulus. It is not meant to imply recognition in the sense that any associations to the stimulus are elicited. A model incorporating these latter constraints would require a richly developed network. Over time, however, repeated events of the type indicated here could serve to encode not only for the simple relationships discussed in this example, but additionally to relate these sensations or perceptions to other previously experienced relationships.

Cholinergic basal forebrain neurons are anatomically arranged to receive multifarious combinations of sensory information. The large dendritic arbors of cholinergic basal forebrain neurons and the preferential localization of afferents on their distal dendrites (see Fig. 1; Lemann and Saper, 1985; Semba et al., 1987) invariably result in considerable spacing between inputs onto the different dendrites of these neurons. Given that the distalmost aspects of cholinergic dendritic arbors sample diverse portions of topographically organized corticofugal fibers tracts, each basal forebrain neuron should be influenced by a number of pyramidal cells from different scattered cortical modules. This anatomic arrangement could in many instances provide a steady flow of unrelated inputs onto the basal forebrain units which could enable, in part, the maintenance of their baseline firing rates. Similar to the proposal of Segundo et al. (1968), unrelated constellations of inputs, as well as conceivable patterns of inputs which are familiar or which are deemed irrelevant, could function to energize or drive the regular baseline firing pattern in recipient basal forebrain cells but do not cause a transition in activation state. Conversely, patterns of inputs that are novel or are of particular relevance to some motivational state could produce specific perturbations in the recipient cholinergic cells causing a change in activation state. For example, when a novel pattern of visual stimuli is projected onto a small part of the visual field, those basal forebrain neurons that receive a relatively large proportion of their cortical afferents from those excited pyramidal cells will be perturbed (Fig. 5). A minihypothesis is postulated to have been formulated when the affected neurons settle upon a new stable state of activation. As depicted in Fig. 5, complex stimuli presented to a small enough part of the receptive field would presumably result in the perturbation of very few or even single basal forebrain units. In the case where an isolated basal forebrain neuron or set of neurons detects a relationship, the lack of competing hypotheses is predicted to result in a rapid resolution of the hypothesis — a rapid transition to another stable state of activation.

Three such cholinergic neurons are schematically drawn on the left side of Fig. 5 intended to represent three separate minihypotheses that (a) an ascending oblique, (b) a horizontal, and (c) a descending oblique line were detected over a very small region of the visual field. The ability of these particular cholinergic neurons to derive these particular hypotheses is wholly based upon the particular sets of pyramidal cells which provide afferent information to these basal forebrain neurons. It is further assumed that each basal forebrain unit would be capable of detecting relationships between more than one set of inputs, given the multiplicity of those inputs. Conceivably, one of the many multiple activation states (e.g., 2, 3, or 4 spikes per burst cycle or 1, 2, or 3 skipped cycles between spikes) could be utilized for each separate minihypothesis.

These kinds of minihypotheses which deal directly with low level sensory cues would be expected to be formed most extensively during the earliest stages of cognitive development. Therefore, minihypotheses should be most prevalent in basal forebrain cells reciprocally connected

---

Figure 5. Schematic representation of cholinergic basal forebrain neurons (filled ovals) and their interactions with cortical modules (cylinders, pyramidal cells represented by triangles) in primary visual cortex (left column) and secondary visual cortex (right column). Suppose that a small triangle is presented to the visual field. Cholinergic basal forebrain cells reciprocally linked to primary visual cortex would presumably be able to make guesses or minihypotheses about the nature of the visual stimulus, albeit low-level sensory features, on the basis of information from cortical columns signaling line orientation. In our example, pyramidal-cell axons (thin lines) approximate dendrites (thick lines connected to ovals) of relevant cholinergic cells in the basal forebrain. The testing of a minihypothesis is modeled as a perturbation in the endogenous patterns of basal nuclear cell firings as a function of cortical input. One possibility is that a shift occurs from a particular type of firing schema (e.g., regular beating exemplified by one spike per burst cycle) to another pattern (e.g., regular bursting exemplified by multiple spikes per burst cycle), followed by a shift back to the original state when the stimulus is removed or ignored. When minihypotheses are presented to basal forebrain cells, such as the three illustrated on the left that three orientation specific lines had been detected, the activity associated with those lines may be transmitted to other cholinergic basal forebrain cells, some of which presumably are reciprocally linked to secondary visual cortex. These second echelon cholinergic cells could formulate slightly larger hypotheses (e.g., that the three lines formed a triangle or that two of them formed acute angles as indicated on the right), although it is likely that more information than that illustrated would be required (e.g., whether or not the corners were connected). Determination of the most likely of these hypothesis would depend on the degree of activation of the recipient neurons, which in the example shown would be greatest in the middle cell. These slightly larger hypotheses (e.g., that a triangle existed rather than a line of a particular orientation) might be expected to take longer times to test, as competing hypotheses would be available and, in the settling process, the relevant neurons would be expected to exhibit unstable transitional firing states such as chaotic beating and chaotic bursting. For further explanation, see text.

See Figure 5 on next page

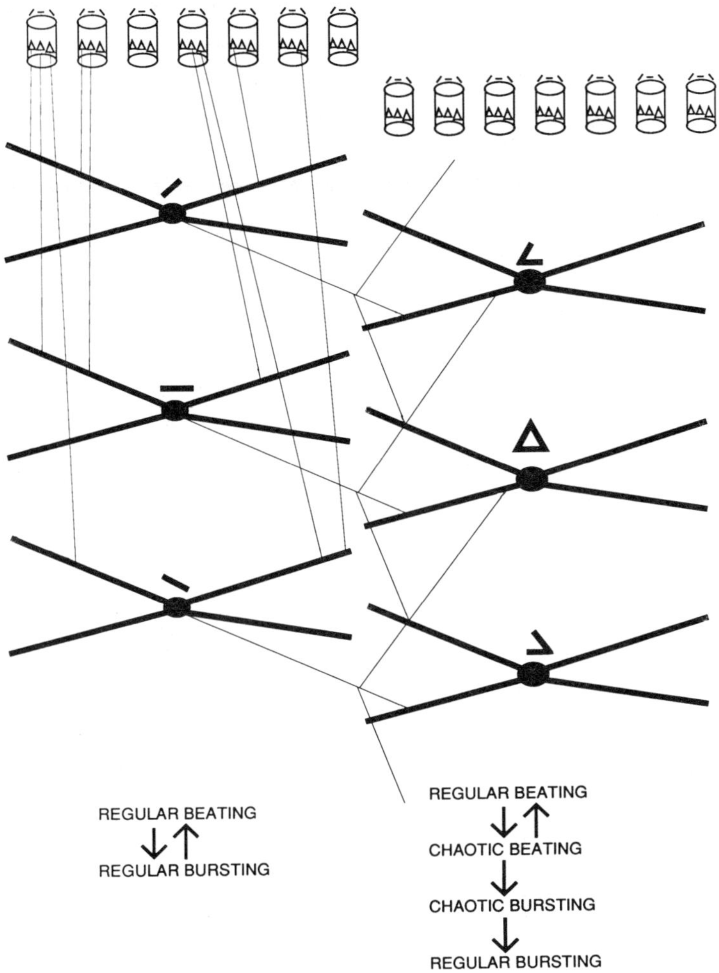

Figure 5.

to first order sensory areas of the cerebral cortex, such as primary visual cortex, in order to be consistent with the trend for primary areas to begin to develop earlier than secondary areas (Zilles et al., 1986). Presumably, basal forebrain neurons connecting to secondary sensory areas would also be capable of generating minihypotheses regarding relationships between low level sensory cues since these cortical areas also process low level sensory information (DeYoe and Van Essen, 1988). However, since secondary visual areas begin to develop a few weeks later than primary visual areas (Zilles et al., 1986), it is conceivable that basal forebrain neurons linked to these regions participate to a greater extent in the generation of larger hypotheses built upon a number of minihypotheses. In other words, cholinergic neurons linked to secondary cortical areas would additionally assess relationships between information relayed to them from cholinergic neurons linked to primary cortical regions. This notion is supported by the fact that complete bilateral removal of primate secondary visual cortex, while sparing fundamental visual abilities, severely disrupts the acquisition of pattern discrimination tasks (Zeki, 1969). Clearly, pattern discrimination tasks, which are disrupted following lesions to secondary visual areas, involve the determination of seemingly more complex relationships between visual inputs than could be accounted for by the minihypotheses described in this paper. Given that the cholinergic cells which are reciprocally linked to secondary visual cortex would invariably be disrupted when this cortical mass was removed, the learning deficits could very well reflect diminished computational capacities for these cholinergic cells to make the kinds of larger hypotheses regarding relationships between minihypotheses as mentioned above.

On the right side of Fig. 5, three basal forebrain neurons connecting to secondary visual cortices, are presumed to receive inputs from the cholinergic basal forebrain neurons on the left, and on the basis of these inputs make the following three competing hypotheses: (a) a two-sided (right side open) figure, (b) a three-sided closed figure, or (c) a two-sided (left side open) figure is detected in a small part of the visual field. Since three hypotheses are cogenerated in this example, a resolution will involve the settling upon the best hypothesis, and therefore it is likely that reaching a new state of activation will take longer and will involve more transitional steps during which activity will be recirculated between the adjacent hypothesizing neurons and their neighbors. Eventually, however, one would predict that the symmetry of activity surrounding the three-sided figure hypothesis would strengthen that hypothesis by increasing the relatedness of its inputs, whereas the lack of symmetry surrounding the two-sided hypotheses would weaken those hypotheses by decreasing relatedness of inputs — resulting in a new activation state for the three-sided hypothesis neurons and a return to the previous activation state for the two-sided hypotheses. Presumably, over time the repeated expression of these hypotheses would increase the efficiency of the transition to the final activation state, so that eventually even very elaborate hypotheses could be settled very rapidly.

The notion that at least initially, hypotheses take longer to resolve in basal forebrain neurons connected to secondary as opposed to primary sensory areas is perhaps compatible with the finding of more instances of long-term potentiation in pyramidal cells of secondary as compared to primary sensory cortices, and in fact, association areas of neocortex and hippocampus exhibit the phenomenon most robustly (Teyler and Discenna, 1984). That these kinds of prolonged pyramidal cell response are related to basal forebrain input is supported by evidence that long term potentiation is suppressed by drugs that block cholinergic action (Hirotsu et al., 1989; Tanaka et al., 1989) and can be enhanced or inhibited by drugs that increase cholinergic activation (Williams and Johnston, 1988; Tanaka et al., 1989). Additionally, the optimal pattern of stimuli which will induce long-term potentiation in hippocampal cells is similar to the theta rhythm (Larson and Lynch, 1986), a pattern of activity produced by cholinergic afferents from the medial septal region (Bland, 1986).

BUILDING THE MACROSTRUCTURE

According to the present model, the kinds of hypotheses individual basal forebrain neurons make will be entirely dependent upon the inputs that those cells receive. In addition to information received from the cerebral cortices, information relayed from other basal forebrain neurons should affect information processing in each recipient cell, and the direction that activity flows through the basal forebrain network is likely to be of critical importance. Although no data are available that directly address this topic, it seems reasonable to assume that since the cholinergic basal forebrain is intimately connected with the cerebral cortices, the flow of information through the cholinergic network should more or less mirror the flow of information through the hierarchically organized structures with which they are reciprocally linked. Details regarding the flow of information through the major cortical pathways are certainly available. In general, feedforward projections usually consist of primary sensory areas projecting to secondary sensory areas, which in turn project to tertiary, and quaternary sensory areas, eventually relaying to association areas. In the visual system, for example, streams of visual information are hierarchically relayed through several levels of visual cortex, finally reaching temporal and parietal association cortices (DeYoe and Van Essen, 1988). Feedback projections also exist which can be distinguished from feedforward projections on the basis of the cortical layers within which they terminate, and in many cases, are weaker and reciprocal to feedforward connections (Pandya and Yeterian, 1985).

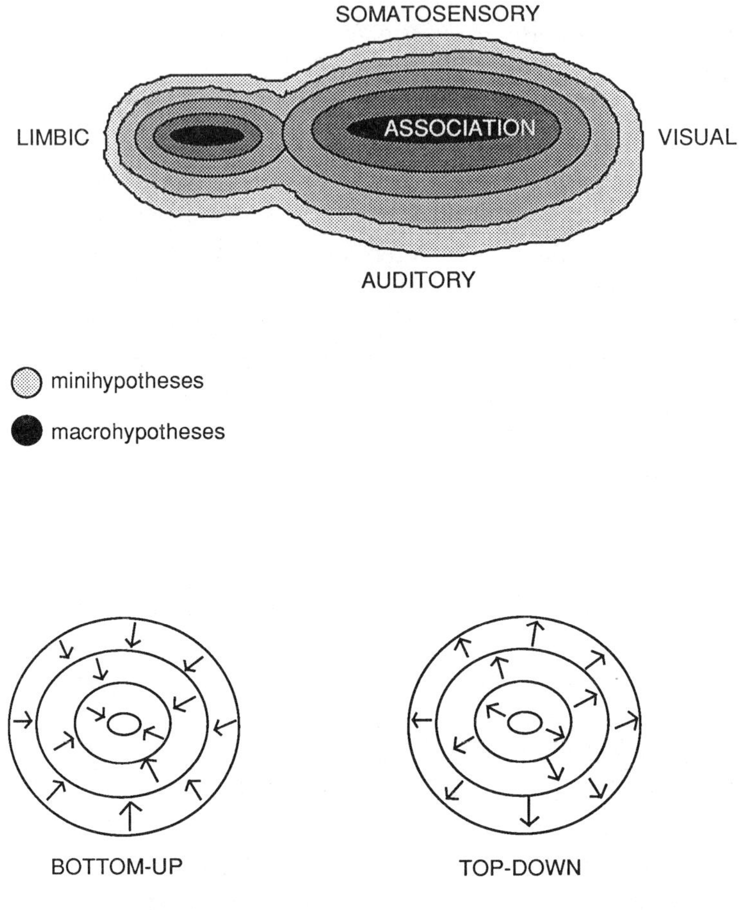

Figure 6. Concentric flow of information within the network of cholinergic basal forebrain neurons. Information relayed from primary sensory areas of the cerebral cortex or primary regions of limbic cortex is proposed to be transmitted to the schematically represented "outer layers" of the network (e.g., basal nuclear cells receiving input from primary sensory cortex) where minihypotheses are formed. The concentric levels of processing derive from the corresponding hierarchical levels of reciprocally linked cortical regions. As information flows inward, minihypotheses grow exponentially in complexity to become macrohypotheses. Feedforward flow of information within the concentric organizational scheme is analogous to bottom-up processing and feedback flow of information is analogous to top-down processing. For further explanation, see text.

As schematically illustrated in Fig. 6, a reflected version of the flow of information through hierarchical pathways superimposed upon the reciprocally linked cholinergic basal forebrain would presumably result in parallel streams of information flowing from basal forebrain cells linked to primary sensory areas to cells linked to secondary, tertiary, and quaternary sensory regions, and finally converging in basal forebrain cells linked to association cortices. The reflected version of feedforward projections through the basal forebrain would produce a predominant trend of bottom-up flow of information (i.e., minihypotheses to macrohypotheses). A reflected version of feedback projections would be expected to follow with a weaker flow in the opposite or top-down direction (Fig. 6). It is proposed that cholinergic basal forebrain neurons reciprocally linked to increasingly higher hierarchical levels of cerebral cortex make increasingly more sophisticated hypotheses based upon a layering of hypotheses upon hypotheses. Consider, for example, that cholinergic basal forebrain units reciprocally linked with primary receiving cortex make minihypotheses regarding putative relationships between 2 to 5 low level sensory cues. Cholinergic basal forebrain neurons linked to secondary regions could make hypotheses regarding relationships between 2 to 5 minihypothesis. Each layer of hypothesizing within the cholinergic network exponentially increases the number of relationships that can be detected between low level sensory cues. The number of functional computational layers within the cholinergic basal forebrain network will be equivalent to the number of hierarchical processing levels for each sensory domain. Although the precise number of hierarchical levels for human cerebral cortex is not known, non-human primates are known to relay sensory information of various sensory domains in a stepwise fashion through several modality specific association regions, on to several multimodal association areas and to prefrontal and paralimbic cortices (Pandya and Yeterian, 1985). Given that one can conservatively estimate at least 10 hierarchical cortical layers process sensory information in each sensory domain, cholinergic basal forebrain neurons connected to the highest hierarchical levels, such as association, prefrontal, and paralimbic cortices, should be able generate hypotheses for specific relationships existing between tens of thousands of low level sensory cues.

Thus, the enormous increase in cognitive ability attendant with the addition of ascending hierarchical cortical areas may be directly attributable to the fact that these regions contribute exponentially to the computation ability of reciprocally linked basal forebrain neurons. This is an attractive conjecture for a number of reasons. First of all, this premise seems to offer a rational explanation for why units in relatively high levels of cerebral cortex (i.e., association cortex) still show sensitivity to relatively low level sensory cues (DeYoe and Van Essen, 1988). In many respects, neural processing in higher cortical regions appears to be redundant reorganization of information within a given sensory domain. While the stepwise reorganization of sensory information may additively contribute to the richness of the sensory experience, these gains may be less consequential than the explosion in the number of low level cues between which relationships can be detected in reciprocally linked basal forebrain neurons. The fact that higher level cortical neurons can also be selectively responsive to more complex stimuli such as faces (Perrett et al., 1982; Yamane et al., 1988) does not contradict the current model, since it would be expected that cortical cell activity would reflect, to some extent, computations done by cholinergic basal forebrain neurons. One would expect, however, that these responses would be infrequently encountered in the cerebral cortex, as does appear to be the case.

Second, having relationships between stimuli of different sensory modalities being encoded in reciprocally linked basal forebrain neurons rather than in the cerebral cortical units overcomes the necessity for

Figure 7. Clustering of cholinergic neurons in the basal nuclear complex of the rat (A), cat (B), and monkey (C). The nucleus basalis is shown in each frame, visualized by use of choline acetyltransferase immunohistochemistry (Woolf et al., 1984). Clusters of cholinergic neurons in the basal forebrain were described first by Bigl et al. (1982), wherein it was noted that the dendrites of many individual cholinergic basal forebrain neurons were confluent, indicating the possibility of functional linkages and giving rise to the speculation that the cells of a given cluster could operate as a unit within the basal nuclear complex. The presence and size of such cellular aggregates appears to be species related. First, the tendency for cholinergic cells of the nucleus basalis to aggregate in soma clusters of three or more neurons is much less common in the rat and cat than in the monkey, and, second, the number of cells (>15) comprising a single cluster in thc non-human primate is greater than in the rat or cat, both latter species demonstrating maximum cluster sizes of 3-5 neurons. Scale bar in A equals 50 μm and applies to all frames. *See Figure 7 on next page*

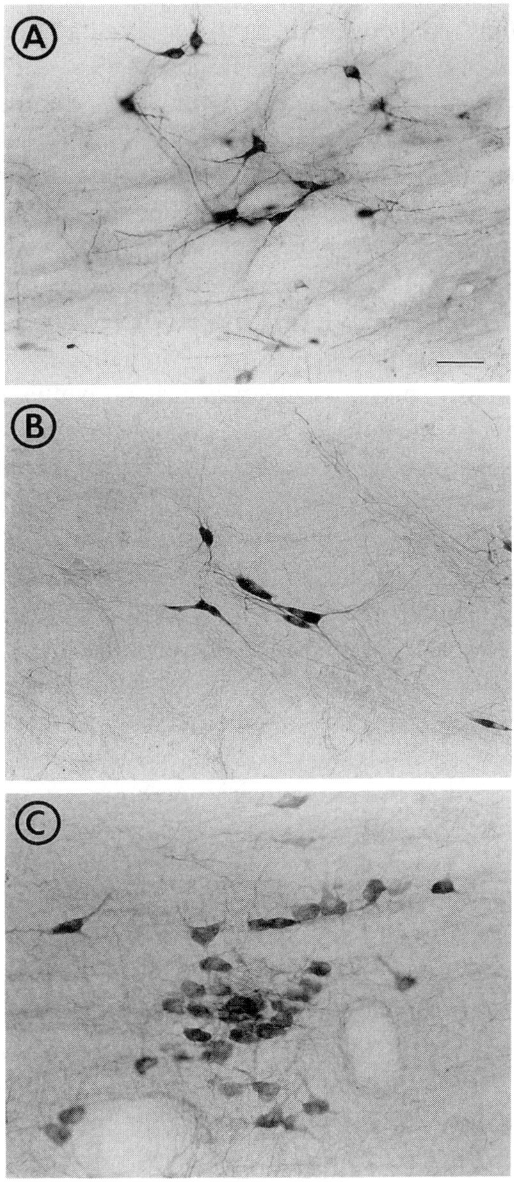

Figure 7

sensory convergence in a particular part of the cortex, a caveat that has posed some difficulties in reconciling certain experimental data. Various experimental paradigms, for example, have revealed that the prefrontal cortex exhibits highly integrative functions which appears in many cases to involve relationships between information from a number of sensory domains (Bignall and Imbert, 1969; Fuster, 1989). An anatomic substrate for integration between sensory modalities appears to exist for prefrontal cortex insofar as a large number of sensory association areas do project to that area. However, modality-specific information is discretely relayed to individual subregions of that brain area and there is little convergence of multimodal information onto most individual regions of the prefrontal cortex (Goldman-Rakic, 1988). Convergence could occur in reciprocally linked cholinergic basal forebrain neurons, however, especially since these neurons are known to only roughly reproduce topographic relationships in hierarchical structures. Individual basal forebrain neurons projecting to one cortical regions may be located next to another basal forebrain cell projecting to a cortical region several millimeters away from the first cortical region (Bigl et al., 1982; Woolf et al., 1984). In the rat, several millimeters between cortical regions is tantamount to a completely different cortical zone. In humans and non-human primates several millimeters would generally separate different subregions of a particular cortical zone. Thus, it is very possible for reciprocally linked basal forebrain neurons to encode for relationships between different modalities even if this information never converges in the cerebral cortex.

The conjecture that cholinergic basal forebrain neurons are likely to generate increasingly lengthy patterns of unstable transitional states as increasingly elaborate hypotheses are constructed, additionally enables the modeling of temporal relationships. One can envision a particular stimulus triggering an individual basal forebrain unit to produce a sequence of patterned activity which in turn triggers another sequence in another unit, and this pattern cascading to encode for particular temporal relationships between complex stimuli. Neurons which maintain various firing outputs during the delay period of delayed discrimination tasks have been found in prefrontal cortex (Fuster, 1989). Since the prefrontal cortex is at the highest end of the hierarchical tier, reciprocally linked basal forebrain cells would be expected to be generating macrohypotheses that would presumably have some of the longest transitional unstable periods.

The capability of cholinergic basal forebrain neurons to modify their architecture in response to activity raises the possibility that the connections determining the flow of activity through the network and through the loops with the cerebral cortex could be continually strengthened and weakened to produce the desired spatial and temporal patterns of activity. One morphologic feature of cholinergic basal forebrain neurons found increasingly in non-human primates as compared to cats and rodents is the increased tendency for those neurons to form clusters (Fig. 7). Such clustering of some cholinergic neurons closely together along with the isolation of that group from the other cholinergic basal forebrain neurons could conceivably result from morphologic restructuring over time, and could conceivably function to group together similar hypotheses derived from similar sets of inputs.

CONCLUSION

A highly speculative model has been presented addressing the basic neural computation style that cholinergic basal forebrain cells could use in order to perform cognitive operations upon incoming information gathered by the hierarchically-organized neurons which comprise the vast majority of neurons in the mammalian telencephalon. One of the strengths of the model is that it can be applied to any sensory domain and any cortical region. Basalo-pyramidal loops presumably exist for hippocampus, limbic cortex, primary sensory cortices, and association cortex. The general computational devices could be applied in modified form to similar interactions between hierarchical and network neurons in the lower brain stem and spinal cord to develop models of more primitive cognitive operations. Additionally, a variation of the present model could be extrapolated to account for the programming of voluntary motor output by the basal ganglionic structures. Although the computational mechanisms proposed in this treatise are consistent with what is currently known about the physiologic behavior of cholinergic basal forebrain cells, much more information is needed. Perhaps the greatest strength of the mechanisms presently proposed is that they are amenable to empirical verification, and experiments testing these notions could very well lead to the discovery of additional or fundamentally different computation mechanisms. The approach of identifying the basic computational mechanisms that are generally applicable to a large number of neuronal interactions is likely to be a topic of continued interest.

REFERENCES

Aston-Jones, G., Shaver, R. and Dinan, T. (1984): Cortically projecting nucleus basalis neurons in rat are physiologically heterogeneous. *Neurosci. Lett.* 46: 19-24

Berger, T.W. and Thompson, R.F. (1978): Identification of pyramidal cells as the critical elements in hippocampal neuronal plasticity during learning. *Proc. Nat. Acad. Sci.* 75:1572-1576

Bialowas, J. and Frotscher, M. (1987): Choline acetyltransferase-immunoreactive neurons and terminals in the rat septal complex: a combined light and electron microscopic study. *J. Comp. Neurol.* 259:298-307

Bigl, V., Woolf, N.J. and Butcher, L.L. (1982): Cholinergic projections from the basal forebrain to frontal, parietal, temporal, occipital, and cingulate cortices: a combined fluorescent tracer and acetylcholinesterase analysis. *Brain Res. Bull.* 8:727-749

Bignall, K.E. and Imbert, M. (1969): Polysensory and cortico-cortical projections to frontal lobe of squirrel and rhesus monkeys. *EEG Clin. Neurophysiol.* 26: 206-215

Bland, B.H. (1986): The physiology and pharmacology of hippocampal formation theta rhythms. *Prog. Neurobiol.* 26:1-54

Burns, B.D. (1958): *The Mammalian Cerebral Cortex.* London: Edward Arnold

Butcher, L.L. and Semba, K. (1989): Reassessing the cholinergic basal forebrain: nomenclature schemata and concepts. *Trends Neurosci.* 12:483-485

Butcher, L.L. and Woolf, N.J. (1986): Central cholinergic systems: synopsis of anatomy and overview of physiology and pathology. In: *The Biological Substrates of Alzheimer's Disease*, Scheibel, A.B., Wechsler, A.F., eds. New York: Academic Press

Butcher, L.L. and Woolf, N.J. (1987): Cholinergic neuronal regeneration can be modified by growth factors. In *Cellular and Molecular Basis for Cholinergic Function.* Dowdall, M.J., Hawthorne, J.N., eds. Chichester, U.K.: Ellis Horwood.

Butcher, L.L. and Woolf, N.J. (1989): Neurotrophic agents exacerbate the pathologic cascade of Alzheimer's disease. *Neurobiol. Aging* 10:557-570

Cajal, S.R. (1928): *Degeneration and Regeneration of the Nervous System.* London: Oxford University Press

Campenot, R.B. (1977): Local control of neurite development by nerve growth factor. *Proc. Nat. Acad. Sci.* 74:4516-4519

Chay, T.R. and Rinzel, J. (1985): Bursting, beating, and chaos in an excitable membrane model. *Biophys. J.* 47:357-366

Conti, F., Fabri, M. and Manzoni, T. (1988): Immunocytochemical evidence for glutamatergic cortico-cortical connections in monkeys. *Brain Res.* 462:148-153

Crick, F. and Asanuma, C. (1986): Certain aspects of the anatomy and physiology of the cerebral cortex. In: *Parallel Distributed Processing, Vol. 2:*

Psychological and Biological Models. McClelland, J.L., Rumelhart, D.E., eds. Cambridge, MA: MIT Press

de Lima, A.D. and Singer, W. (1986): Cholinergic innervation of the cat striate cortex: a choline acetyltransferase immunocytochemical analysis. *J. Comp. Neurol.* 250:324-338

Detarí, L., Juhasz, G. and Kukorelli, T. (1987): Neuronal firing in the pallidal region: firing patterns during sleep-wakefulness cycle in cats. *EEG Clin. Neurophysiol.* 67:159-166

DeYoe, E.A. and Van Essen, D.C. (1988): Concurrent processing streams in monkey visual cortex. *Trends Neurosci.* 11:219-226

Dickson, G., Prentice, H., Julien, J.-P., Ferrari, G., Leon, A. and Walsh, F.S. (1986): Nerve growth factor activates Thy-1 and neurofilament gene transcription in rat PC12 cells. *EMBO J.* 5:3449-3453

Donoso, J.A., Stiles, J.R. and Fernandez, H.L. (1987): Intracellular acetylcholinesterase of adult rat myofibers is more concentrated in endplate than non-endplate regions. *J. Neurosci. Res.* 17:146-153

Drubin, D.G., Feinstein, S.C., Shooter, E.M. and Kirschner, M.W. (1985): Nerve growth factor-induced neurite outgrowth in PC12 cells involves the coordinate induction of microtubule assembly and assembly-promoting factors. *J. Cell Biol.* 101:1799-1807

Eccles, J.C. (1966): Cerebral synaptic mechanisms. In: *Brain and Conscious Experience*, Eccles, J.C., ed. Berlin: Springer-Verlag

Fagg, G.E. and Foster, A.C. (1983): Amino acid neurotransmitters and their pathways in the mammalian central nervous system. *Neurosci.* 9:701-719

Federoff, H.J., Grabczyk, E. and Fishman, M.C. (1988): Dual regulation of GAP-43 gene expression by nerve growth factor and glucocorticoids. *J. Biol. Chem.* 263:19290-19295

Fernyhough, P. and Ishii, D.N. (1987): Nerve growth factor modulates tubulin transcript levels in pheochromocytoma PC12 cells. *Neurochem. Res.* 12:891-899

Freeman, W. and Viana Di Prisco, G. (1986): EEG spatial pattern differences with discriminated odors manifest chaotic and limit cycle attractors in olfactory bulb of rabbits. In: *Brain Theory*. Palm, G., Aertsen, A., eds. Berlin: Springer-Verlag

Fuster, J.M. (1989): *The Prefrontal Cortex: Anatomy, Physiology and Neuropsychology of the Frontal Lobe*. New York: Raven Press

Geddes, J.W., Monaghan, D.T., Cotman, C.W., Lott, I.T., Kim, R.C. and Chui, H.C. (1985): Plasticity of hippocampal circuitry in Alzheimer's disease. *Science* 230:1179-1181

Goldman-Rakic, P.S. (1988): Topography of cognition: parallel distributed networks in primate association cortex. *Ann. Rev. Neurosci.* 11:137-156

Gould, E. and Butcher, L.L. (1989): Developing cholinergic basal forebrain neurons are sensitive to thyroid hormone. *J. Neurosci.* 9:3347-3358

Griffith, W.H. and Matthews, R.T. (1986): Electrophysiology of AChE-positive neurons in basal forebrain slices. *Neurosci. Lett.* 71:169-174

Hargreaves, A., Yusta, B., Aranda, A., Avila, J. and Pascual, A. (1988): Triiodothyronine (T3): induces neurite formation and increases synthesis of a protein related to MAP 1B in cultured cells of neuronal origin. *Dev. Brain Res.* 38:141-148

Haring, J.H. and Wang, R.Y. (1986): The identification of some sources of afferent input to the rat nucleus basalis magnocellularis by retrograde transport of horseradish peroxidase. *Brain Res.* 366:152-158

Hebb, D.O. (1949): *Organization of Behavior: A Neuropsychological Theory.* New York: Wiley and Sons, Inc.

Hefti, F., Hartikka, J., Eckenstein, F., Gnahn, H., Heumann, R. and Schwab, M. (1985): Nerve growth factor increases choline acetyltransferase but not survival or fiber outgrowth of cultured fetal septal cholinergic neurons. *Neurosci.* 14:55-68

Hernandez-Peon, R. and Chavez-Ibarra, G. (1963): Sleep induced by electrical or chemical stimulation of the forebrain. *EEG Clin. Neurophysiol.* Suppl. 24: 188-198

Hirotsu, I., Hori N., Katsuda N. and Ishihara T. (1989): Effect of anticholinergic drug on long-term potentiation in rat hippocampal slices. *Brain Res.* 482:194-197

Hoffman, P.N., Griffin, J.W. and Price, D.L. (1985): The role of neurofilaments in the control of axonal caliber In: *Intermediate Filaments: Annals of the New York Academy of Sciences* 455, Wang, E., Fischman, D., Liem, R.K.H., Sun T.-T, eds. pp 785-786

Irle, E. and Markowitsch, H.J. (1986): Afferent connections of the substantia innominata/basal nucleus of Meynert in carnivores and primates. *J. Hirnforsch.* 27:343-367

Isaacson, L.G., Saffran, B.N. and Crutcher, K.A. (1989): NGF-induced sprouting of mature, uninjured neurons. *Soc. Neurosci. Abstr.* 15:91

Kalil, R.E. (1989): Synapse formation in the developing brain. *Sci. Amer.* 261:76-85

Korn, H. and Faber, D.S. (1979): Electrical interactions between vertebrate neurons: field effects and electrotonic coupling. In: *The Neurosciences Fourth Study Program.* Schmitt, F.O., Worden, F.G., eds. Cambridge, MA: MIT Press

Lamour, Y., Dutar, P. and Jobert, A. (1984): Septo-hippocampal and other medial septum-diagonal band neurons: electrophysiological and pharmacological properties. *Brain Res.* 309:227-239

Lamour, Y., Dutar, P., Rascol, O. and Jobert, A. (1986): Basal forebrain neurons projecting to the rat frontoparietal cortex: electrophysiological and pharmacological properties. *Brain Res.* 362:122-131

Larson, J. and Lynch, G. (1986): Induction of synaptic potentiation in hippocampus by patterned stimulation involves two events. *Science* 232:985-988

Lemann, W. and Saper, C.B. (1985): Evidence for a cortical projection to the magnocellular basal nucleus in the rat: an electron microscopic study. *Brain Res.* 334:339-343

Lindenbaum, M.H., Carbonetto, S., Grosveld, F., Flavell, D. and Mushynski, W.E. (1988): Transcriptional and post-transcriptional effects of nerve growth factor on expression of the three neurofilament subunits in PC-12 cells. *J. Biol. Chem.* 263:5662-5667

Linseman, M.A. and Olds, J. (1973): Activity changes in rat hypothalamus, preoptic area, and striatum associated with Pavlovian conditioning. *J. Neurophysiol.* 36:1038-1050

Luine, V.N. (1985): Estradiol increases choline acetyltransferase activity in specific basal forebrain nuclei and projection areas of female rats. *Exp. Neurol.* 89:484-490

Luiten, P.G.M., Gaal, G., Gaykema, R.P.A., Strosberg, A.D. and Schroeder, H. (1989): Immunohistochemical demonstration of muscarinic acetylcholine receptor proteins in rat and human neocortex. Interactions with cortical projections from the magnocellular basal nucleus. *Soc. Neurosci. Abstr.* 15:811

Lynch, G., Matthews, D.A., Mosko, S., Parks, T. and Cotman, C. (1972): Induced acetylcholinesterase-rich layer in rat dentate gyrus following entorhinal lesions. *Brain Res.* 42:311-318

Marc, C. and Rabie, A. (1985): Microtubules and neurofilaments in the sciatic nerve fibres of the developing rat: effects of thyroid deficiency. *Int. J. Devel. Neurosci.* 3:353-358

Mathes, C.W., Woolf, N.J., Lee, C. and Butcher, L. L. (1989): Thyroid hormone alters cholinergic expression in adult basal forebrain. *Soc. Neurosci. Abstr.* 15:782

Meeker, R.B., Swanson, D.J. and Hayward, J.N. (1988): Local synaptic organization of cholinergic neurons in the basolateral hypothalamus. *J. Comp. Neurol.* 276:157-168

Mesulam, M.-M. and Geula, C. (1988): Acetylcholinesterase-rich pyramidal neurons in the human neocortex and hippocampus: absence at birth development during the life span and dissolution in Alzheimer's disease. *Ann. Neurol.* 24:765-773

Milbrandt, J. (1988): Nerve growth factor induces a gene homologous to the glucocorticoid receptor gene. *Neuron* 1:183-188

Pandya, D.N .and Yeterian, E.H. (1985): Architecture and connections of cortical association areas. In: *Cerebral Cortex, Vol 4: Association and Auditory Cortices*. Peter, A., Jones, E.G., eds. New York: Plenum Press

Patel, A.J., Hayashi, M. and Hunt, A. (1988): Role of thyroid hormone and nerve growth factor in the development of choline acetyltransferase and other cell-specific marker enzymes in the basal forebrain of the rat. *J. Neurochem.* 50:803-811

Perrett, D.I., Rolls, E.T. and Caan, W. (1982): Visual neurons responsive to faces

Petsche, H., Gogolak, G. and van Zwieten, P.A. (1965): Rhythmicity of septal cell discharges at various levels of reticular excitation. *EEG Clin. Neurophysiol.* 19:25-33

Plioplys, A.V., Gravel, C. and Hawkes, R. (1986): Selective suppression of neurofilament antigen expression in the hypothyroid rat cerebral cortex. *J. Neurol. Sci.* 75:53-68

Prentice, H.M., Moore, S.E., Dickson, J.G., Doherty, P. and Walsh, F.S. (1987): Nerve growth factor-induced changes in neural cell adhesion molecule (N-CAM) in PC12 cells. *EMBO J.* 6:1859-1863

Price, J.L. and Stern, R. (1983): Individual cells in the nucleus basalis-diagonal band complex have restricted axonal projections to the cerebral cortex in the rat. *Brain Res.* 269:352-356

Purves, D. (1988): Body and Brain: A Trophic Theory of Neural Connections. Cambridge, MA: Harvard University Press

Reeves, A. and Sperling, G. (1986): Attention gating in short-term visual memory. *Psychol. Rev.* 93:180-206

Ribchester, R.R. and Taxt, T. (1983): Motor unit size and synaptic competition in rat lumbrical muscles reinnervated by active and inactive motor axons. *J. Physiol.* 344:89-111

Rigdon, G.C. and Pirch, J.H. (1986): Nucleus basalis involvement in conditioned neuronal responses in the rat frontal cortex. *J. Neurosci.* 6:2535-2542

Rosenzweig, M.R., Bennett, E.L. and Diamond, M.C. (1972): Brain changes in response to experience. *Sci. Amer.* 226:22-29

Rudy, B., Kirschenbaum, B., Rukenstein, A. and Greene, L.A. (1987): Nerve growth factor increases the number of functional Na channels and induces TTX-resistant Na channels in PC12 pheochromocytoma cells. *J. Neurosci.* 7:1613-1625

Ruiz-Marcos, A., Sanchez-Toscano, F., Obregon, M.J., Del Rey, F.E. and de Escobar, G.M. (1982): Thyroxine treatment and recovery of hypothyroidism-induced pyramidal cell damage. *Brain Res.* 239:559-574

Rumelhart, D.E. and McClelland, J.L. (1986): *Parallel Distributed Processing. Vol. 1 Foundations*. Cambridge, MA: MIT Press

Saper, C.B. (1984): Organization of cerebral cortical afferent systems in the rat. I. Magnocellular basal nucleus. *J. Comp. Neurol.* 222:313-342

Segundo, J.P., Perkel, D.H., Wyman, H., Hegstad, H. and Moore, G.P. (1968): Input-output relations in computer-simulated nerve cells: influence of the statistical properties, strength number and inter-dependence of excitatory presynaptic terminals. *Kybernetik* 5:157-171

Seiler, M. and Schwab, M.E. (1984): Specific retrograde transport of nerve growth factor (NGF): from neocortex to nucleus basalis in the rat. *Brain Res.* 300:33-39

Seilheimer, B. and Schachner, M. (1987): Regulation of neural cell adhesion molecule expression on cultured mouse Schwann cells by nerve growth factor. *EMBO J.* 6:1611-1616

Semba, K., Reiner, P.B., McGeer, E.G. and Fibiger, H.C. (1987): Morphology of cortically projecting basal forebrain neurons in the rat as revealed by intracellular iontophoresis of horseradish peroxidase. *Neurosci.* 20:637-651

Shurrager, P.S. and Culler, E. (1940): Conditioning in the spinal dog. *J. Exp. Psychol.* 26:133-159

Skarda, C.A. and Freeman, W.J. (1987): How brains make chaos in order to make sense of the world. *Behav. Brain. Sci.* 10:161-195

Sperling, G., Budiansky, J., Spivak, J.G. and Johnson, M.C. (1971): Extremely rapid visual search: the maximum rate of scanning letters for the presence of a numeral. *Science* 174:307-311

Stewart, D.J., MacFabe, D.F. and Vanderwolf, C.H. (1984): Cholinergic activaiton of the electrocorticogram: role of the substantia innominata and effects of atropine and quinuclidinyl benzilate. *Brain Res.* 322:219-232

Szymusiak, R. and McGinty, D. (1989): Sleep-waking discharge of basal forebrain projection neurons in cats. *Brain Res. Bull.* 22:423-430

Takahashi, M., Tsukui, H. and Hatanaka, H. (1985): Neuronal differentiation of Ca^{2+} channel by nerve growth factor. *Brain Res.* 341:381-384

Tanaka, Y., Sakurai, M. and Hayashi, S. (1989): Effect of scopolamine and HP 029, a cholinesterase inhibitor, on long-term potentiation in hippocampal slices of the guinea pig. *Neurosci. Lett.* 98:179-183

Teyler, T.J. and Discenna, P. (1984): Long-term potentiation as a candidate mnemonic device. *Brain Res. Rev* 7:15-28

Tolbert, D.L. and Der, T. (1987): Redirected growth of pyramidal tract axons following neonatal pyramidectomy in cats. *J. Comp. Neurol.* 260:299-311

Viana, G.B., Davis, L.H. and Kauffman, F.C. (1988): Effects of organophosphates and nerve growth factor on muscarinic receptor binding number in rat pheochromocytoma PC12 cells. *Toxicol. Appl. Pharmacol.* 93:257-266

Williams, S. and Johnston, D. (1988): Muscarinic depression of long-term potentiation in CA3 hippocampal neurons. *Science* 242:84-87

Woody, C.D., Swartz, B.E. and Gruen, E. (1978): Effects of acetylcholine and cyclic GMP on input resistance of cortical neurons in awake cats. *Brain Res.* 158:373-395

Woody, C.D., Vassilevsky, N.N. and Engel, J. (1970): Conditioned eye blink: unit activity at coronal precruciate cortex of the cat. *J. Neurophysiol.* 33:851-864

Woolf, N.J. and Butcher, L.L. (1990): Dysdifferentiation of structurally plastic neurons initiates the pathologic cascade of Alzheimer's disease: toward a unifying hypothesis In: *Brain Cholinergic Systems*. Steriade, M., Biesold, D., eds. New York: Oxford University Press

Woolf, N.J., Eckenstein, F. and Butcher, L.L. (1984): Cholinergic systems in the rat brain: I Projections to the limbic telencephalon. *Brain Res. Bull.* 13:751-784

Woolf, N.J., Gould, E. and Butcher, L.L. (1989a): Nerve growth factor receptor is associated with cholinergic neurons of the basal forebrain but not the pontomesencephalon. *Neurosci.* 30:143-152

Woolf, N.J., Oh, J.D. and Butcher, L.L. (1989b): Thyroid hormones alter the postnatal development of the 68kD neurofilament protein in the cerebral cortex: an immunocytochemical analysis. *Soc. Neurosci. Abstr.* 15:1017

Yamane, S., Kaji, S. and Kawano, K. (1988): What facial features activate face neurons in the inferotemporal cortex of the monkey? *Exp. Brain Res.* 73:209-214

Zeki, S.M. (1969): The secondary visual areas of the monkey. *Brain Res.* 13:197-226

Zilles, K., Werners, R., Büsching, U. and Schleicher, A. (1986): Ontogenesis of the laminar structure in areas 17 and 18 of the human visual cortex. *Anat. Embryol.* 174:339-353

Subject Index